## WITH THE PRITIKIN PROGRAM
## THE "IMPOSSIBLE" IS POSSIBLE:

- The 81-year-old woman who has congestive heart failure, angina and hypertension. Today, at 90, she is a gold medal Senior Olympics winner.

- The 58-year-old airline pilot who, because of hypertension and diabetes, was suspended. After only one month with the Pritikin Program, he was able to resume flying.

- Nathan Pritikin, founder of the Pritikin Program, who twenty years ago reversed a serious heart condition with a diet and exercise regimen that achieved almost miraculous results.

## PEOPLE OF *ALL* AGES
## ARE DISCOVERING LONGER LIFE.

Thousands of Americans—young and old alike—have paid more than $3,000 to enroll in the Pritikin Program, now detailed for the first time in this book. It has been called the most exciting breakthrough in the age-old quest for vigorous longevity, and probably the most feasible method yet discovered for adding twenty to thirty years to your lifespan.

The Pritikin Program is a program you can live with. Not just for two weeks, but for the rest of your long, healthy, active life!

# The PRITIKIN PROGRAM
## for DIET & EXERCISE

by
### Nathan Pritikin
with Patrick M. McGrady, Jr.

BANTAM BOOKS
TORONTO · NEW YORK · LONDON

THE PRITIKIN PROGRAM FOR DIET AND EXERCISE

*A Bantam Book / published by arrangement with
Grosset & Dunlap, Inc*

*PRINTING HISTORY*

*Grosset & Dunlap edition published May 1979
Ten printings through January 1980
Literary Guild edition November 1979
Macmillan Book Club edition February 1980
Excerpts appeared in Family Circle, November 1978;
Cosmopolitan, November 1979;
Book Digest between September 1979 and December 1979
Serialized in The New York Post between April 30 and May 4,
1979
and the United Features Syndicate
between July and December 1979.
Bantam edition / June 1980*

ISBN 0-553-13026-9

*Published simultaneously in the United States and Canada*

PRINTED IN THE UNITED STATES OF AMERICA

0 9 8 7 6 5 4 3 2 1

## Caution

This book is meant primarily for those who consider themselves healthy or who have minor problems, such as a little high blood pressure, borderline diabetes, morning stiffness, a touch of tennis elbow, or the like.

We warn those who are on prescription drugs for angina, hypertension, diabetes, claudication, or generalized atherosclerosis (narrowing or closure of the arteries) against trying to doctor themselves.

If you wish to try the therapeutic approach outlined in this book for such serious conditions, we advise you to find a physician familiar with the Pritikin Program who can supervise you and modify your drug requirements.

There is a serious risk for sick people to attempt to solve medical problems without trained medical supervision. We caution the reader against it.

## ACKNOWLEDGMENTS

The authors express their deepest appreciation to the following people: members of the Longevity Center staff, especially Janet Leon who helped with many phases of the preparation of the book, and Merisa Smith and Esther Taylor who helped with the food selections; Paul Glenn who was instrumental in bringing the authors together; and to other members of the Pritikin Research Foundation Advisory Board who gave valuable suggestions; Judith Gray and Ilya, Vanessa, and Ian McGrady.

*To my wife, Ilene,*
*whose faith, guidance, and dedication*
*made my nutritional career possible.*

# Contents

## ONE
### The First Mode: Dieting

## TWO
### The Second Mode: Walking

## THREE
## Getting Down to Cases

## FOUR
## The Maximum Weight Loss Diet

## FIVE
## The Pritikin Kitchen

## SIX
## Selected Pritikin Program Recipes

# Appendix:

# Foreword
## by
# C. Richard Harper, M.D.

I first became acquainted with the Pritikin Program in November 1975, when Nathan Pritikin presented the results of his Long Beach Study in Atlanta, Georgia, to the American Congress of Rehabilitation Medicine and the American Academy of Physical Medicine and Rehabilitation. At that time, I was Medical Director and President of the Aviation Insurance Agency in Atlanta.

While in Atlanta, Nathan Pritikin came to see me to tell me about his data and philosophy on the effect of diet in degenerative diseases in his Long Beach Study. His results, frankly, seemed too good to be true. I was very skeptical that such results could be achieved by medical therapy of any kind and least of all by a diet-exercise regimen alone.

After discussing the Pritikin Program with other physicians, I became even more convinced that the claims had to be exaggerated. If some *were* factual, I was sure they were not reproducible.

My employer was the agent for an insurance policy held by thousands of airline pilots against their being permanently "grounded" for medical reasons. The stringent health requirements of the Federal Aviation Administration (FAA) prevent a pilot from flying for a variety of medical conditions, including hypertension, diabetes, etc. Pritikin suggested that such grounded pilots be sent to the rehabilitation center he was inaugurating.

I expressed interest in his work but admitted I was skeptical of his claims.

Although Pritikin's claims of success sounded exaggerated, he was extremely well versed in human physiology and disease states. I nevertheless visited his newly opened rehabilitation center in Santa Barbara, California, in February, 1976, and I returned to Atlanta feeling very op-

timistic. However, I still did not *really* believe what I had
seen and heard at the Center. I made another visit the following month, again reviewing the medical records and
interviewing patients with angina, diabetes and other degenerative diseases. Again, I was amazed by the results
and decided to "experiment" by sending one of our dis-
abled pilot claimants to the Center.

Our first pilot, J. H., was thirty-five years old. He had
been treated with the best conventional care available.
Despite anti-hypertensive medication, his blood pressure
was 160/110. The FAA had suspended his certificate.

During the first month on the program, his blood
pressure dropped from 160/110 to 130/80. His medication had been discontinued by the final week. His blood
lipid levels also responded quickly to therapy. His cholesterol fell from 293 to 165, and triglycerides from 230 to
105. He lost twenty-three pounds.

When he returned home, it was thought the "spa effect" of Santa Barbara had been responsible for his improvement and that in a week or two, his blood pressure
would rise. We watched him for two months before we
were convinced that the return to normal blood pressure
was real. He was re-certified for flying sixty days after returning from the Center.

Flying again, J. H. stays fit by jogging regularly and
faithfully following the diet. When traveling, he admits to
some difficulty with the diet, depending on what food is
available to him. He enjoys the full cooperation of his
family on the diet program.

Since that first success, I have not only sent many pilots
to the Longevity Center, but have the approach in
my own practice of aviation medicine. The results have
been excellent.

Another success was W. C., a thirty-seven-year-old airline pilot who had recently been diagnosed as an insulin
dependent juvenile diabetic. He had attained his ideal
weight on the usual diabetic diet and had stabilized on
twenty-five units of insulin. At the end of his thirty-day
trial on the diet-exercise regime, he no longer required insulin and demonstrated blood sugars acceptable to the
FAA. He returned to flying sixty days later and is still fly-

ing today—a person whose career and health had been salvaged.

Needless to say, the return of many pilots to flying saved my company hundreds of thousands of dollars. Equally important, it established that in motivated people, a nutritional therapy could be more effective than the best conventional care available in dealing with many degenerative diseases.

Although I am no longer associated with the Aviation Insurance Agency, I continue to utilize the Pritikin concept in my current position as Vice President, Medical Services for one of the world's largest airlines.

Based on my observations, my convictions became so firm that I have sent personal friends and members of my own family to the Pritikin Center.

Although Pritikin's results are still viewed skeptically by many in the medical world, I feel his nutritional methods are the very foundation of sound management of various degenerative diseases.

C. Richard Harper, M.D.

# Foreword
# by
# Denis P. Burkitt, M.D.

In January, 1977 I first visited Nathan Pritikin and examined his work. This visit and follow-up visits in January, 1978 and 1979, convinced me that good results were being achieved in the cardiovascular diseases and some other diseases that were being specifically investigated.

My colleague, Dr. Hugh Trowell, and I were impressed by the similarities between the dietary and exercise regime being recommended by him and his staff and the style of life practiced in communities in the third world who have minimal prevalences of many diseases that are characteristic of modern Western culture.

Nathan Pritikin has put maximum emphasis on reduction of fat and cholesterol intake, but almost inevitably his low fat diet of unrefined foods is high in fibre-rich carbohydrates. There is almost invariably a reciprocal relationship between the amount of fat and fibre consumed. There is now good epidemiological, clinical, and in some cases experimental, evidence indicating a relationship between fibre-depleted diets and prevalences of such common diseases as large bowel cancer, gallstones, varicose veins, hemorrhoids, diverticular disease of the colon, appendicitis and hiatus hernia.

It might be best in our present state of knowledge to consider fibre as potentially protective against these diseases. This does not rule out the possibility of several causes. All of these diseases have been shown to have their maximum prevalences in communities in which, as a direct result of an inadequate fibre intake, intestinal content is small in volume and firm in consistency and slow in its transit through the bowel. Hypotheses that are consistent with epidemiological and other evidence have been formulated to explain the relationship between fibre-depleted diets and these diseases. Although there is no way where by they can be proved short of studies lasting over several decades, the evidence is certainly strong enough to warrant advising an increase in fibre intake. Cigarette smoking is, for example, rightly condemned on strong circumstantial evidence short of absolute proof.

Although the effect of Mr. Pritikin's low-fat and high-fibre diets on these diseases (large bowel cancer, gallstones, varicose veins, hemorrhoids, diverticular disease of the colon, appendicitis, and hiatus hernia) has not yet been evaluated, I believe its protective effect against some, if not all of these diseases, could be as great as it is with regard to diseases that have been evaluated, such as ischemic heart disease and diabetes.

Denis P. Burkitt,
M.D., C.M.G., F.R.S.

# Preface

The diets of faddists and ordinary American share common features. Both are high in fats, cholesterol, and protein, and their followers are unlikely to live long, healthy lives.

Did your ancestors live to a ripe old age? This factor is probably in your favor, but it's not enough to protect your health.

What about the many dieters who exercise regularly? Unfortunately, even *optimal* exercise is not enough to remove them from jeopardy.

If you take the time to check your cholesterol, triglycerides, total lipids, blood pressure, and stress-treadmill heartbeat, you might be unpleasantly surprised. Those readings can give you a fair idea of what your life-style has done to your body, particularly to your arteries and heart.

If you are an average American, you have a fifty-fifty chance of dying of stroke or heart disease before your time. Your risk of getting arthritis and diabetes and cancer rises dramatically as you grow older. Your hearing acuity almost certainly is diminishing. Your eyesight may be failing. Your ability to taste and smell differences in food declines with age. Your touch perceptions also diminish. In sum, you are slowing down. This diet can do something about that.

You might be interested in the Pritikin Program if you'd like to go swimming with your great-grandchildren when your peers are either in the grave or playing checkers in a nursing home. You might want to keep a job you like when your colleagues have all retired. In other words, when others your age have grown old and tired of existence, you may be able to find pleasure in living, loving, working, and playing.

For convenience I call the diet by my name, but its principles are as old as man. For centuries the hardiest, most long-lived peoples in the world have thrived on these foods.

It is also a diet the poorest can afford. You find its fundamental foods among history's *descamisados,* the havenots, humble peasants: people who simply cannot afford the sauces, viands, desserts, liquors, salty appetizers, and elegant and inelegant nonfoods that foster heart attacks, strokes, gout, diabetes, and arthritis. Traditionally, it has been the diet of societies that have remained largely immune to aging-related, degenerative pathologies.

On the Pritikin Program you will feel years younger— and look it, too. Your new eating patterns will enhance the acuity of all your senses, give you boundless new energy, take away that tired feeling, and may even reduce your daily sleep requirement. Some symptoms of aging even disappear in the time that it normally takes to shake a cold. Others, of course, take longer.

Within the limits of our present scientific knowledge and our ability to test nutritional results, the Pritikin Diet comes closest to the optimal diet. To a huge extent, it frees even far-gone victims from further ravages of cardiovascular diseases and other nutrition-related conditions. At the Longevity Center, we have found at least twenty major ailments that respond to this program. It can also spare symptom-free dieters from developing these diseases at all.

At first, the success of the program was mainly spread by word-of-mouth, emanating from the therapeutic successes achieved at the Longevity Center in Santa Barbara. Since then, there has been an unending spate of national press, magazine, television, and radio publicity. (The rudiments of the diet were spelled out in the bestselling book *Live Longer Now.*)

The Longevity Center treats patients* with a four-week regimen of nutrition and a walking program as strenuous as it is safe—nothing else. Drugs are reduced or dropped to correspond with the body's lessened need for them. Most patients leave dramatically improved in their physical and mental functioning, with symptoms reduced, better blood profiles, lower blood pressure, emancipation

---

* The term "patient" used throughout the book indicates a participant in the Longevity Center program who was at the same time under the care of the resident physician staff associated with the Center.

from medication, a happier outlook, and loads of extras such as improved sleeping, better digestive and bowel habits, and regained sexual potency and interest.

A word of caution here. If you are on drugs, you qualify as a patient requiring a physician's monitoring. Or, you may be interested in the Longevity Center's medically supervised twenty-six-day crash program. If you are not on drugs, you should have no problem in following the Pritikin Program using this book as a guide. You may, however, find it helpful to be part of one of the community-based Pritikin Better Health Programs. For information on either program, write to the Longevity Center, P.O. Box 5335, Santa Barbara, California 93108.

At the Longevity Center, during each day of the program, each patient has a blood pressure check taken once or more, walks to his or her comfortable capacity, has the mileage computed, eats eight meals, and listens to lectures on the whys of the program.

When patients return home, they are highly motivated to continue the program for two reasons. The first is an almost unbelievable positive change in their health and feelings that seems eminently worth preserving. The second is a comprehensive understanding of why they feel so good and why it's important to stick to the program. Most, overwhelmingly, do just that.

The Pritikin Diet is no run-of-the-mill, starvation weight-loss diet. Patients at the center eat eight low-calorie meals a day without any quantity restrictions. Nor do they experience any loss of energy or appetite pangs. They lose, in their four-week stay, an average of 13.3 pounds. A special program for those interested in rapid weight reduction is described in Part Four of this book.

The blood tests are the most easily quantifiable, and there the results have been most impressive. The complete data on the first 900 Center patients appear in "For the Health Professional" in the appendix. We may note the following:

• A significant drop in *serum cholesterol* levels. The patients' cholesterol levels averaged 235 mg./percent at the start of the program and dropped to 175 mg./percent by month's end. Many patients had levels exceed-

ing 300 mg./percent, and from an average group-level
of 344 mg./percent, they fell to 227 mg./percent.

- The lowering of *serum triglyceride* levels was equally
  impressive. The group began with an average level of
  174 mg./percent and finished the four weeks with 130
  mg./percent. In the 300 mg./percent range and over,
  the average level was 553 mg./percent at the start of
  the program and 194 mg./percent at the end.
- Blood pressure and uric acid levels also fell consistently.

Aside from its healthfulness, gustatorily the diet can be
superb. By withholding greasy, sweet, and salty taste-kill-
ers from pot and plate, you will start to enjoy the inherent savoriness of foods you've been polluting all your life.

The diet revives old food friends unjustly scorned by
fad diets: breads, cereals, pastas, fruits, vegetables, soups,
rice, potatoes.

Thanks to a foremost cook, June Roth, we have discovered that with some ingenuity you can produce gourmet delights in every meal category with the permissible
foods. Her recipes appear in Part Six.

It is also the finest, safest weight-loss diet there is.
Used either as a weight-loss or weight-maintenance diet, it
is a natural, high-fiber nutritional program that can make
well people look and feel better than they have in years
and can give sick people a new lease on life.

This is not an easy diet. It requires a reversal of lifelong bad habits and nutritional fallacies.

For example, people who feel protected by eating so-
called wholesome foods will be startled to learn that many
of those foods are just as damaging to the body as "junk"
foods. Harmful foods include such hallowed items as fer-
tile eggs, raw milk, cheeses, most soy bean products,
cold-pressed oils, and granola.

Individuals who diet may be equally astonished to learn
that honey, molasses, and various shades of brown sugar
are no improvement over refined white sugar. The seeds-
'n'-nuts snacking habit of many misguided dieters can be
harmful because of the high fat levels of these foods.

This diet amounts to a declaration of war against the

American diet's dependence on processed foods, fats, sugars, proteins, salt, caffeine, alcohol, and nonfoods. Dietary bad habits are the thorniest to overcome. But this book will give you good reasons and valuable techniques for overcoming them.

If this diet was once the province of people too poor to afford the rich American diet, such is no longer the case. Today the Pritikin Program is being followed by men and women whose education and self-esteem prompt them to want the best for their bodies.

You see these knowledgeable people everywhere: toting vegetable-and-fruit setups to what once would have been a three-martini business lunch; jogging at the crack of dawn on highway shoulders, down country lanes, and over asphalt city streets; asserting a firm "Yes, I *do* mind" to the smoker; sipping water with a lemon wedge at cocktail parties; pressuring PTAs to replace school candy-vending machines with fruit or juice machines; bicycling into town instead of driving; playing tennis instead of watching the football games on TV; banishing sodas, whole milk, and other harmful foods from the refrigerator and replacing them with fresh fruit, whole-grain breads and pita, skim-milk products, and salad fixings for snacks.

These are a few of the many signs of a revolution in self-preservation and life-enrichment. This revolution has had a special impact in the realm of sports. For a considerable time now, long-distance runners have used diets resembling the Pritikin diet for endurance and stamina. Recently the rest of the sports world has taken a cue from them.

The old and highly mythical "fortifiers"—steaks, chops, ice cream—have largely gone by the board. "In" foods are basically complex carbohydrates, which give an athlete a much better crack at charging the Miami Dolphins' front line, or lofting a baseball into the Yankee Stadium bleachers, or lasting fifteen rounds with Muhammad Ali.

In a comment made before the Olympic Games in Montreal to a *New York Times* reporter, Walter H. Gregg, chairman of health and physical education at Northwestern University, noted:

Athletes are forever looking for more energy. But they are leaning toward carbohydrates to be sure of an energy supply. . . . You'll see more [glycogen-loading*]. . . . Most athletes are off the vitamin kick, because their doctors are convincing them it doesn't work as well. . . . But things like steak aren't really as effective as people think. What athletes need are carbohydrates.

The switch from fats and proteins to carbohydrates comes with enlightenment. And the list of people who have found out what can be gained from low-fat, low-protein, high-carbohydrate diets is long. It includes actors Peter Sellers, Gloria Swanson, Twiggy, Dennis Weaver, David Carradine, Marty Feldman, Candice Bergen, and Marisa Berenson; musicians George Harrison, Ravi Shankar, and Yehudi Menuhin; authors Laura Huxley and Isaac Bashevis Singer; basketball player Bill Walton, long-distance runner Lasse Viren, and labor organizer Cesar Chavez.

The poet Lord Byron kept his boyish figure on such a diet, supping on cold potatoes, rice, fish, and vegetables sprinkled with vinegar and snacking on biscuits and sparkling water. The venerable physician-educator Sir William Osler noted as far back as 1896 that coronary artery disease was rare among the poor, not only because of the absence of stressful ambition, but because of their carbohydrate diets.

President Thomas Jefferson, who lived to be eighty-three, believed his longevity was because of his vegetarian menus. "I have lived temperately, eating little animal food, and not as an aliment, so much as a condiment for the vegetables which constitute my principal diet," he wrote.

When I first proposed my views on diet about ten years ago, it appeared that acceptance on this diet concept would take a hundred years. Now I'm convinced that in

---

* Glycogen is often called "animal starch." It is a carbohydrate form stored in the muscles and liver and is made of units of glucose synthesized from blood sugar. As energy demands require, it is then broken down again into blood sugar.

five years large segments of our country will have changed to this kind of diet.

True, cooperation from those agencies most concerned with Americans' dietary habits has not been as whole-hearted as one would have wished. But the new research in nutrition almost daily confirms one or another aspect of our basic hypotheses, which we have seen borne out in our own clinical programs in Santa Barbara and else-where. These confirmatory studies have obliged many nu-tritionists to reexamine their nutritional beliefs.

The McGovern Senate Select Committee on Nutrition and Human Needs issued a report on nutrition that jibes very closely with the Pritikin Diet, but does not go quite as far in its fat- and cholesterol-cutting recommendation. *It is, nonetheless, a big step forward.* It proposes that Americans reduce *all* fat intake from 42 percent to 30 percent and specifies that this reduction be in *both animal and vegetable fats* (i.e., saturated and unsaturated fats). This is an important step forward because most official bodies (such as the American Heart Association) recom-mend replacement of animal with vegetable fats. You will learn later on in this book why both kinds are equally hazardous to your health.

The committee report also stresses the urgency of cut-ting cholesterol levels by half and of using more fish and fowl and less meat, more vegetables and fruits and grains, and far less sugar and salt.

The purpose of these changes, as the report states, is to reduce the risk of heart disease, hypertension, gall bladder disease, liver disease, and cancers of the breast and colon. Words were not minced. Our eating habits, the report as-serted, "may be as profoundly damaging to the nation's health as the widespread contagious diseases of the early part of the century."

This book will steer you around the shoals, guide you through supermarkets and restaurants, show you how to plan your menus, prepare meals, eat out, travel, and—once you've got your new, healthy life-style under your belt—extend those benefits to family and friends.

This is not idle talk. The co-author, who has spent twelve years researching, writing, and lecturing on the ag-ing process, believes that the Pritikin Diet is the single most impressive rejuvenation treatment among the hundreds he has investigated. Biochemist Johan Bjorksten, author of the molecular cross-linkage aging theory and a foremost gerontologist, has stated that the Pritikin Diet is probably the most feasible method of attaining an extra twenty to thirty years of vigorous life!*

Clearly, this is the most significant breakthrough in man's age-old quest for rejuvenation. Nothing comes near it. There is no pill, no injection, no drug, no powder, no yoga, no potion, no other process that produces the revitalizing effects achieved by the Pritikin Program of diet and exercise.

In Part One, you will learn exactly *why* this is the world's healthiest diet.

* Positive proof of this claim would require controlled human longevity computations over a period of generations. However, experimental animal evidence and the available, if imperfect, clinical data permit reasonable speculation that this program gives humans their best chance to make the most of their genetic potential.

# ONE

# The First Mode: Dieting

# 1

## What the Pritikin Diet Is

The Pritikin Diet is the nutritional mode of the Pritikin Program. It represents a significant departure from other diets and nondiets in a manner calculated to enable you to live longer and better.

The Pritikin Diet is *low* in fats, cholesterol, protein, and highly refined carbohydrates, such as sugars. It is *high* in starches, as part of complex, mostly unrefined carbohydrates, and is basically "food as grown," eaten raw or cooked.

There is a second mode of the Pritikin Program, and that is exercise. The main exercise we recommend (in fact, you don't have to do anything else) is regular, sustained walking. All sustained isotonic exercises that work your long muscles, particularly your legs, so as to pump the blood back up to your heart are acceptable. We shall talk more about exercise in Part Two.

Not only is the Pritikin Diet safe and healthy, but it maintains your ideal weight—without *any* restrictions on food quantity. You can eat as much as you like of many of the permissible foods. All day long, if you wish.

For accelerated, maximum weight loss, we offer a variation on the regular diet. It is described later in Part Four.*

* The Maximum Weight Loss plan is your safest, most effective way to shed excess pounds and achieve an attractive figure. It is superior by far to any fast. A total fast, for instance, would produce only 6 more pounds of weight reduction in one month than this plan, as well as unpleasant and worrisome side effects, which the Maximum Weight Loss plan does not have. Strictly monitored testing at the Pritikin Center shows that patients on this version of the optimal diet can lose up to 31 pounds in the four-week period

3

If you are an average American, your diet is probably the polar opposite of the Pritikin Diet. It is almost surely dangerously high in fats, cholesterol, protein, and sugars, and low in complex carbohydrate foods with their starch, fiber, and natural vitamins and minerals.

There is also an excellent probability that many readers of this book smoke too much, drink too much, and lead a sedentary life.

The Pritikin Diet is not easy to begin because its menus are so different from what you're used to. Once you've tried it and understand it, however, the chances are high that you will stick with it. Only a foolish or unmotivated person would voluntarily abandon its enormous rewards.

This is not a faddist diet. It is a most basic regimen that revives the types of food available when our physiology evolved to its present complexity. It is a diet in harmony with the digestive and metabolic machinery we've had these several hundreds of thousands of years.

The convenience-food diet most Americans live by, on the other hand, *is* faddist and reckless. Our systems are plainly uncomfortable with the chemical hocus-pocus that parades as, or invades, our food supply. In one way or another, some 3,500 new chemicals have found their way into our food—and common sense tells us that our bodies simply aren't ready for them.

## CARBOHYDRATES—THE BEST FOOD YOU CAN EAT

The Pritikin Diet is not vegetarian, but meat and fish intake is restricted to under ¼ pound daily. If you can do with animal protein only three times a week, so much the better. Ideally, meat and fish become *condiments* to flavor other dishes, rather than main courses. This means your diet will be very high in carbohydrates.

Surprised? In all probability you thought that carbohydrates were a big no-no. After all, most of the popular di-

---

—and still eat up to 4 pounds of food every day. The average monthly weight loss of these patients is 13.3 pounds.

ets of the past few years have pilloried carbohydrates—and praised protein and fat.

Well, some carbohydrates are banned by this diet, too. Those are the highly refined sugars of all kinds, honey, molasses, and syrups. They are basically monosaccharides and disaccharides—and are bad for you. We eliminate them altogether.

Foods high in complex carbohydrates, however—grains, vegetables, and fruits—are the best foods you can eat. They are most valuable when minimally processed or refined. Not the least of the virtues of these foods is that they do no harm—while still providing us with an ample supply of the necessary vitamins, minerals, dietary fiber, and energy.

If this is a diet rich in complex carbohydrates, that makes it a high-starch diet, too.

I'm sure that you, like me, have memories of some authority figure—be it a parent, a doctor, a sweetheart, or someone else ardently trying to cajole you into trimming your paunch—waggling a finger at you and warning you to avoid those horrible "starchy" foods.

Starch foods are most valuable when closest to their natural form, such as brown rice (cultivated rice with only the woody husk removed), or grains that haven't been milled to death and therefore deprived of their vitamins, minerals, and fiber. Whole-wheat flour is therefore superior to white flour. White flour that has been bleached has had insult added to injury because of the dangerous chemicals used in the bleaching process. It should never be used.

Is this *the* optimal diet for man? No. There isn't enough known about nutrition to make such a claim. But it is as close as I've been able to come to it during thirty years of intensive nutritional research and my experience at the Pritikin Center.

Nonetheless, the Pritikin Diet can spare mankind much of the scourge of degenerative "aging pathologies." *We are saying that the Pritikin Diet is the most important step taken by nutritional science in that direction.*

After analyzing the available information on which food constituents and nutrients enable the body to work most efficiently and continuously over many decades, we

## TABLE OF FOODS TO USE AND TO AVOID

| CATEGORY | FOODS TO USE | QUANTITY PERMITTED | FOODS TO AVOID |
|---|---|---|---|
| FATS, OILS | None. | | All fats and oils, including butter, margarine, shortening, lard, meat fat, all oils, lecithin (as in vegetable spray). |
| SUGARS | None. | | All extracted sugars, including syrups, molasses, fructose, dextrose, sucrose, and honey. |
| POULTRY, FISH, SHELLFISH AND MEAT | Chicken, turkey, Cornish hen, game birds (white meat preferred; remove skin before cooking). | Limit acceptable poultry, fish, and meat to a total of 1-½ lbs./week or 3-½ oz./day. | Fatty poultry:[1] duck, goose, etc. |
| | Lean fish and shellfish.[2] | Lobster: 3-½ oz./day (replaces entire daily allotment of poultry, fish or meat)<br>Shrimp, oysters, crab, clams or scallops: 1-¾ oz./day (replaces entire daily allotment of poultry, fish or meat) | Fatty fish:[1] sardines, fish canned in oil, mackerel etc.<br>Fatty meats:[1] marbled steaks, fatty hamburger and other fatty ground meat, bacon, spareribs, sausage, frankfurters, luncheon meat, etc.<br>Organ meats: liver, kidneys, hearts, sweetbreads.<br>Smoked, charbroiled or barbecued foods. |
| | Lean meat. | | |
| EGGS | Egg whites. | 7/week max. (raw: 2/week max.). | Egg yolks.<br>Fish eggs: caviar, shad roe, etc. |
| DAIRY FOODS | Nonfat (skim milk, nonfat buttermilk (up to 1% fat by weight), or nonfat yogurt.<br>Nonfat (skim) powdered milk. | 8 oz./day. | Cream, half-and-half, whole milk and lowfat milk or products containing or made from them, such as sour cream, lowfat yogurt.<br>Non-dairy substitutes: creamers, whipped toppings, etc. |
| | Evaporated skim milk. | 5 level tbsp./day (replaces entire allotment of fluid skim milk or equivalents). | |
| | 100% skim milk cheeses, primarily uncreamed cottage cheese such as hoop cheese or dry curd cottage cheese, or cheeses up to 1% fat by weight. Sap Sago (Green) cheese. | 4 oz./day (occasional) use) only; replaces entire allotment of fluid skim milk or equivalents).<br>2 oz./day.[3] | Cheeses containing over 1% fat by weight. |
| | | 1-2 oz./week max. | |
| BEANS, PEAS | All beans and peas (except soybeans). | Limit to 1-1½ lbs. (cooked)/week max. In addition, may substitute 8 oz. serving for each 3-½ oz. serving of acceptable, poultry, fish, shellfish or meat. | Soybeans unless substituted:<br>1 oz. soybeans = 1 oz. poultry, fish, shellfish or meat allotment. |
| | Tofu (bean curd). | Limit to 2 oz. serving twice/week substituted for day's cheese allotment or equivalent. | |

| CATEGORY | FOODS TO USE | QUANTITY PERMITTED | FOODS TO AVOID |
|---|---|---|---|
| NUTS, SEEDS | Chestnuts. | Not limited. | All nuts (except chestnuts). All seeds (except in small quantities for seasoning as with spices). |
| VEGETABLES | All vegetables except avocados and olives. | Limit vegetables high in oxalic acid, such as spinach, beet leaves, rhubarb, and swiss chard. | Avocados. Olives. |
| FRUITS[4] | All fresh fruits. Unsweetened cooked, canned, pureed or frozen fruit. Dried fruit: Unsweetened fruit juices. Frozen concentrates, undiluted. | 5 servings/day max. 24 oz./week max. 1 oz./day max. (28 oz./week). 4 oz./day max. (28 oz./week). 1 oz./day max. (7 oz./week). | Cooked, canned or frozen fruit with added sugars. Jams, jellies, fruit butters, fruit syrups with added sugars. Fruit juices with added sugars. |
| GRAINS | All whole or lightly milled grains: rice, barley, buckwheat, millet, etc. Breads, cereals, crackers, pasta, tortillas, baked goods and other grain products without added fats, oils, sugars or egg yolks. | Unlimited. Limit refined grains and grain products (i.e., with bran and germ removed) such as white flour, white rice, white pasta, etc. | Extracted wheat germ. Grain products made with added fats, oils, sugars or egg yolks. Bleached white flour, soy flour. |
| SALT | Salt[5] | Limit salt intake to 3-4 g./day by eliminating use of high salt or sodium (Na) foods such as soy sauce, pickles, most condiments, prepared sauces, dressings, canned vegetables and MSG (monosodium glutamate). | Salt from all sources in excess of permitted amount. |
| CONDIMENTS, SALAD, DRESSINGS, SAUCES, GRAVIES AND SPREADS | Wines for cooking. Natural flavoring extracts. Products without fats, oils, sugars or egg yolks. | Dry white wine preferable. Moderate use. | Products containing fats, oils, sugars or egg yolks such as: mayonnaise, prepared sandwich spreads, prepared gravies and sauces and most seasoning mixes, salad dressings, catsups, pickle relish, chutney, etc. |
| DESSERTS OR SNACKS | Dessert and snack items without fats, oils, sugars or egg yolks. | Plain gelatin (unflavored); 1 oz./week max. | Desserts and snack items containing fats, oils, sugars or egg yolks such as: most bakery goods, package gelatin desserts and puddings, candy, chocolate and gum. |

| CATEGORY | FOODS TO USE | QUANTITY PERMITTED | FOODS TO AVOID |
|---|---|---|---|
| BEVERAGES[6] | Mineral water, carbonated water.<br>Nonfat (skim) milk or nonfat buttermilk.<br>Unsweetened fruit juices.<br>Vegetable juices.<br>Linden or Red Bush tea. | Limit variation with added sodium.<br><br>See restrictions under *Dairy Foods* above.<br><br>See restrictions under *Fruit* above.<br>Carrot juice: 2 glasses/week max. | Alcoholic beverages.<br><br>Beverages with caffeine: coffee, tea, cola drinks, etc.<br><br>Beverages with added sweeteners such as soft drinks.<br>Diet and other soft drinks with artificial sweetener. |

[1]See Caloric Ratios of Common Foods, pages 213-222.

[2]Our revised recommendations are based on a conservative interpretation of the newest data concerning cholesterol and other possibly atherogenic sterols in shellfish.

[3]Cheese and nonfat milk allotments may be exchanged: 2 oz. cheese = 8 oz. nonfat milk or equivalents

[4]If triglycerides are above 125 mg.%, eat only fresh fruit in the permitted amount.

[5]Normal salt (sodium) needs are provided by food in their natural state and additional intake should be kept to a minimum.

[6]Recommendations on herb tea (other than the two given), decaffeinated coffee and coffee substitutes are under study.

## FOLLOWING THE PRITIKIN DIET SUGGESTIONS:

Adhere carefully to the Do's and Dont's of the *Table of Foods to Use and to Avoid* and to the following rules:

1. Eat two or more kinds of whole grain daily (wheat, oats, brown rice, barley, buckwheat, etc.) in the form of cereals side dishes, pasta, bread, etc.
2. Eat two or more servings of raw vegetable salad and two or more servings of raw or cooked green or yellow vegetables daily. Potatoes may be eaten every day.
3. Eat one piece of citrus fruit and up to three or four fresh fruit servings daily.
4. Do not use sugar or honey of any kind. When sweeteners are necessary, use pureed fresh fruit or fruit juices.
5. Eat beans or peas one to three times weekly, as you wish.
6. Limit protein intake from animal sources as follows:
   Up to 24 ounces per week of low fat, low cholesterol meat, fish, shellfish or fowl.
   Up to 8 ounces (1 glass) skim milk and 2 ounces of uncreamed cottage cheese per day or equivalent in skim milk products.
7. If you have constipation problems, add some unprocessed wheat bran flakes, (starting with 1 tablespoon daily) to your cereal, soup, or other foods.
8. Eat three full meals daily. Don't go hungry between meals; snacks are encouraged. For snacks, eat fruit (not exceeding daily fruit allotment), vegetables and raw salad, or whole-grain bread or crackers that are free of oil, fat, added wheat germ or sweeteners.
9. Flavor with herbs and spices, instead of salt. Keep salt intake minimal.
10. If you need to lose weight, increase vegetables and decrease grains. If you need to gain weight, decrease vegetables and increase grains.

*Vegetarians eating no animal protein at all may require a supplement of Vitamin B12 once every several weeks.

are convinced that the Pritikin Diet is your best opportunity to help yourself live a long life at your mental and physical peak.

The average American diet runs to about 40 or 45 percent of total calories in fat, 15 to 20 percent in protein, and 40 to 45 percent in (mostly refined) carbohydrates. The Pritikin Diet's fat level, on the other hand, runs from 5 to 10 percent, the protein from 10 to 15 percent, and the carbohydrates (mostly complex and unrefined) to 80 percent.

## A TYPICAL DAY'S FARE

Here is what the co-author of this book might eat on any given day:

*Breakfast*

Half grapefruit
Bowl of cooked whole-wheat grain cereal with sliced banana, skim milk, cinnamon, and bran

*Lunch*

Bowl of lentil soup
Whole-wheat pita bread (warmed or toasted) stuffed with raw salad greens, pickled vegetables (pepper, pimento, onions, cauliflower, celery, etc.) and sprinkled with vinegar or lemon juice and bran
Glass of water with lemon wedge

*Dinner*

Oxtail soup (defatted)
Steamed broccoli and yellow squash
Long-grain brown rice
String bean salad
Sourdough or whole-grain rye bread
Applesauce mixed with skim-milk yogurt

*Snacks* (at any time)

Scandinavian flatbreads
A few pieces of fresh raw fruit (apples, pears, grapes, peaches, or plums)
Whole-wheat pita bread stuffed with salad material as per lunch menu
The table on pages 6-8 will give you some idea of the foods the Pritikin Diet approves of, restricts in quantities, or disapproves of. The chapters that follow take up each diet component—and noncomponent—in turn.

# 2

## What Fats Do

The Pritikin Diet is low in fat for the very simple reason that high fat levels damage the body. Of the calories that we Americans consume, about 40 or 45 percent come in the form of fats. Many health authorities recommend cutting this down to about 30 percent. We feel that fats are so bad for you that you should eat no more than 5 to 10 percent fat.

### THE DAMAGE FATS CAUSE

Essentially, fats do three kinds of damage. First of all, they suffocate your tissues by depriving them of oxygen. Second, they raise the level of cholesterol and uric acid in your tissues, contributing to atherosclerosis and gout. Third, they impede carbohydrate metabolism and foster diabetes.

If the suffocation factor sounds a bit far out, it isn't. In fact, it's easily demonstrated. In one clinical experiment, fourteen heart patients suffering from angina pectoris drank a glass of heavy cream after an overnight fast. Within five hours, their blood became six times cloudier than normal and, though they had been at rest during this entire procedure, most of them suffered a severe angina attack within minutes of each other. Normally, angina strikes only under the stress of strenuous physical activity. But the fats had deprived the heart of enough oxygen—just as exertion might have.

When this test was repeated with a *fat-free* drink containing the same calories and volume, *no* angina attacks or abnormalities occurred!

11

# WHY ALL EXCESS FATS ARE BAD FOR YOU

All fats—animal and vegetable, saturated and unsaturated—have a common effect. They form a fatty film around the formed elements in the blood—particularly red blood cells and platelets—and cause them to stick together. When they stick together, they cannot function properly. With this clumping, small blood vessels and capillaries become plugged and shut down. That means that from 5 to 20 percent of your blood circulation is also shut down.

By the way, if you smoke in addition to eating a meal heavy in fats, your oxygen tie-up is *colossal!* (You can actually knock yourself out with a combination of heavy fats and carbon monoxide from smoke in the blood.) The brain cannot sustain that kind of poisoning. This is why many people fall asleep after a heavy dinner.

## WHAT WE MEAN BY FATS

Generically, *fat* comprises both fats (solid at room temperature) and oils (liquid at room temperature). Fat constitutes almost half of the total caloric intake of most Americans. It comes in obvious forms as butter, margarine, shortening, and cooking and salad oils. It also comes in less obvious forms as an important constituent of certain foods, such as peanuts, dairy products, eggs, meats, nuts, and seeds. There are about 9 calories in each gram of fat—and about half that number in carbohydrates.

Both animal fats and vegetable fats are made of fatty acids. Animal fats, however, are made largely of *saturated* fatty acids. This means that each carbon atom in the chain has a hydrogen atom stuck onto it. Cholesterol blood levels are raised by animal saturated fatty acids.

Vegetable fats are made mostly of *unsaturated* fatty acids. There are two notable exceptions to the rule: cocoa oil and coconut oil, which are *nearly* saturated. (Nondairy creamers are made of coconut oil and are a *big* no-no.)

In unsaturated fatty acids, at least two of the carbon

atoms have no hydrogen atoms attached. You find unsaturated fatty acids in corn, safflower, cottonseed, and soybean oils. Fish tend to have more unsaturated than saturated fatty acids.

While it is true that unsaturated fats lower cholesterol levels in the blood, they create havoc by raising triglyceride levels and creating metabolic suffocation by the resultant sludge in the blood.

## KETOSIS

A dietary trick that has become popular in recent years employs a high-fat, low-carbohydrate regimen to achieve rapid weight loss. It can be a very risky trick, as many dieters have found to their dismay.

Since the diet is largely fat, the free glucose (sugar) in the blood is rapidly burned off, forcing the body to depend on its fat reserves for energy.

The fatty acids derived from the fat reserve burn rather inefficiently, producing acid metabolites called ketones. This abnormal increase of ketones is called ketosis.

But ketosis isn't a good way to lose weight for a number of reasons. The brain is at least partially starved by the absence of glucose, which is its *only* source of food. Ketones are acid metabolites that may actually change your blood's pH. If the blood becomes acid enough, you can go into ketosis shock—which is sometimes fatal.

Moreover, a highly acid blood makes it hard for the body and the brian to function properly. Fatty acids liberated from fat reserves are extremely mischievous. They circulate in the bloodstream, sometimes cause irregular heartbeats, and can invade the liver and cause problems. This can be quite serious, by the way, since you need a healthy liver in order to ward off disease, neutralize toxins, and maintain high energy reserves and optimal health.

Finally, the high amounts of cholesterol accompanying fats on diets such as the Atkins or Stillman diets create an environment conducive to the growth of plaque—deposits of fatlike matter—in the arteries. As plaque deposits proliferate, there is less and less space for the blood to flow. We'll say more about cholesterol in the next chapter.

## QUESTIONS AND ANSWERS

*How much is bad? Suppose I just have a teaspoon of olive oil on my salad. Will that hurt me?*

Any added oil or fat is unnecessary and potentially damaging. Even a teaspoonful of olive oil will boost your serum triglyceride level within an hour and a half. How harmful it will be depends on the fat backlog in your system. If you're relatively fat free, it won't harm you much. The blood fat levels will rise and then fall quickly. If there's a lot of fat, the blood levels will stay higher longer—and do much more damage.

*The American Heart Association recommends substituting unsaturated fats for saturated fats—e.g., margarine made of corn oil for butter. Do you?*

We do not. In several respects, unsaturated fats may be worse for you than saturated fats. Human experiments show that when certain people drink either heavy cream (saturated fat) or safflower oil (unsaturated fat), their blood tends to sludge and undergo capillary blockage. Both kinds of fats raise the triglyceride levels in the blood, but with safflower oil, they stay higher much longer. Polyunsaturates also deplete the body's vitamin E, are implicated in gallstone formation, and may well stimulate tumor growth.

*If I don't eat any fats, don't I run the risk of a fat deficiency?*

No. All foods have *some* fat. On a diet of grains, vegetables, and fruits (which excludes nuts and seeds, processed fats such as oils, margarine, butter, cheese, other dairy products, and most animal fat), you will still be taking in 5 to 10 percent of your total calories in fat.

Your body can manufacture all the fats it needs from other foods. The only one it cannot make is linoleic acid, of which we need no more than one 1/10 ounce to correct a deficiency. An ounce of oatmeal contains more than enough linoleic acid for your daily requirement.

*I'm pregnant. Shouldn't·I be drinking whole milk instead of the nonfat milk you recommend?*

No. Nonfat milk is still your best bet. You need nonfat milk's calcium so that your baby doesn't take the calcium it needs from your bones and teeth. Neither you nor your baby needs the fat part of whole milk.

*Will this diet help to keep me safe from cancer?*

We can't promise that. But it is safe to say that the diet you're probably on now is highly carcinogenic. World Health Organization statistics show a persuasively high correlation between dietary fat and colon cancer. High-fat diets produce up to ten times the normal amount of bile acids and large quantities of anerobic bacteria. Anerobic bacteria convert bile acids into carcinogens. There is also a correlation between fat levels and breast cancer, which is the Number One killer of women in their late thirties, forties, and early fifties.

*You said that fats are a factor in diabetes. Isn't it sugar instead?*

Just because there is a lot of sugar in a diabetic's urine doesn't mean that there is a sugar intolerance. That's false. The reason for the sugar in the urine is that fats in the blood keep the body from making use of the sugar—from metabolizing it. Since the sugar goes unmetabolized, the body must call upon fat reserves for energy. When free fatty acids flow into the blood, you are working on fat alone. The by-product of fat metabolism is ketones, which may produce ketosis shock, as we've just mentioned.

Nor is it true that the diabetic's body doesn't produce enough insulin, the hormone it must have to metabolize sugar. In fact, an early diagnosed diabetic has as much as two times the insulin of a normal person. At least that is the case in about 85 percent of all diabetics.

Still, not just diabetics, but all of us should restrict our sugar intake because the body is not used to sugar. It doesn't occur in a pure form in nature. The body was built to make its sugar from the digestion of complex carbohydrates, producing a couple of calories every minute or so. When you flood the blood with sugar; it rises in the blood and spills out through the kidneys. This sends a message to the pancreas to produce lots of insulin—as though this high sugar flow was going to last indefinitely. And so there is overproduction of insulin.

Unfortunately, when the insulin scavenges for sugar, it doesn't stop on time. This produces a low blood sugar condition. The scavenged sugar has been diverted into the fat reserves, or is stored as glycogen. With the absence of your normal sugar fuel, the body calls on free fatty acids once more, thereby raising your blood fat level. When blood fats rise high enough, they "desensitize" the insulin. What eventually occurs is a buildup of sugar in the blood, known as hyperglycemia. *Hyperglycemia* is the opposite of *hypoglycemia,* which is an abnormal decrease of sugar in the blood.

*What about hypoglycemia? I've heard a lot about that lately.*

No one can remain hypoglycemic on the Pritikin Diet for more than three weeks. With complex carbohydrates producing approximately 2 calories per minute, you have normal blood sugar levels—neither high nor low. There's an initial period of about five days when your blood sugar begins to stabilize, and then another week or two until the problem disappears altogether. Practically all of the hypoglycemics treated at the Pritikin Center have experienced this reversal of their condition.

*Is there any other reason for avoiding fat?*

There is a powerful argument for controlling both your intake and production of fat. Pesticides and other chemical pollutants find a home in fat cells and lodge there.

The actual concentration of pollutants increases upward in the food chain. As you can see in the graph, it is least concentrated in root vegetables, grains, legumes, fruits, and leafy vegetables. It is more concentrated in oils and fats and dairy products. It is most concentrated in the flesh and fowl that eat these things, reaching its ultimate concentration in man, who feeds on fat animals and fish that already have concentrated chemical pollutants in their tissues.

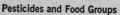

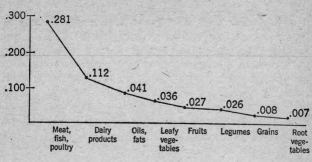

**Pesticides and Food Groups**

Source: *Runner's World*, February 1978.

# 3

## What Cholesterol Does

In the last chapter we mentioned cholesterol, which is not a fat, but is often associated with fats. It is a *sterol*—more like a wax than a fat or oil. But like a fat it does not dissolve easily in water or blood plasma.

Every cell in your body manufactures and contains some cholesterol, although the liver produces the greatest amount. It is also found in your nerve fiber sheaths and cell membranes. Cholesterol helps make bile acids for digestion and steroid hormones such as progesterone and the adrenal glucocorticoids.

We're mainly concerned with cholesterol because of its role in causing *atherosclerosis* and cardiovascular disease. When too much cholesterol gets into the blood, it settles into artery walls, hardening and narrowing them. But it can do other nasty things, such as cause enlargement of the prostate by lodging there in crystal form.

Atherosclerosis in the coronary arteries is called *coronary artery disease*. The coronary arteries, as you can see in any anatomy textbook, are the small blood vessels that feed the heart muscle. Atherosclerosis begins with a fatty yellow streak on the inner lining of these arteries, and ends with growing deposits of fibrous material rich in fatty cholesterol, or "arterial plaque." With plaque buildup, the flow of blood slows down. When the arterial bore becomes very narrow, only a tiny trickle of blood is able to nourish the heart.

*Arterial plaque* is made of fat, cholesterol, collagen,* possible calcium deposits, and cellular debris. Plaque has been seen in the arteries of three-year-olds!

---

* Collagen is a supportive albuminlike protein found in muscle, bone, cartilage, and other connective tissues in the body.

18

When plaque builds up and closes the vessel, the tissue dependent on the blood fed by that artery dies. When part of the heart begins to die from want of food and oxygen, a *myocardial infarction* occurs. When a section of brain is similarly starved, a *stroke* occurs.

## CHOLESTEROL AND CORONARY ARTERY DISEASE

Cholesterol-rich foods are at the very least a prime factor in coronary artery disease insofar as they contribute to high blood cholesterol levels. Many researchers, beginning with Dr. Ancel Keys at the University of Minnesota in 1947 and the Framingham Study, a continuing survey of 5,209 adults started in 1948, have confirmed the primacy of cholesterol as a contributor to atherosclerosis and coronary artery disease. Scientists since have found that they can cause and reverse arterial plaque disease simply by manipulating dietary fat and cholesterol levels.

To avoid cardiovascular disease altogether, a useful formula—and a valid one—is to keep your blood cholesterol level to 100 plus your age. A cholesterol level of 160 is *maximum*. The cholesterol levels given to you by laboratories after blood testing are in terms of so many milligrams per 100 milliliters of blood serum.

Any level over 165 can be *atherogenic*—meaning that it will encourage the growth of atheromas, or plaque, in the arteries.

Unfortunately, certain medical authorities have used cholesterol "norms" of from 150 to 330. While these may be the average or mean levels of various American communities, they are far too high for good health. They are the average levels of a sick population, abnormally high.

## LIPOPROTEINS

Since cholesterol—like fat—is not soluble in the blood, it must be carried by substances called *lipoproteins*. Of the lipoproteins that have been identified, three seem to have an important relevance to cardiovascular disease.

*Very Low Density Lipoproteins* (VLDLs) transport triglycerides (caused mainly by excessive intake of sweets, alcohol, and fats) from the liver to tissues where they form pockets of fat.

Once the VLDLs have dumped their load of triglycerides, they become Low Density Lipoproteins (LDLs) and begin carrying cholesterol from the liver to cells around the body.

Another kind of lipoprotein, called *High Density Lipoprotein* (HDL), is the apparent hero in this drama. The HDLs are thought to act as cholesterol scavengers, clearing out redundant cholesterol from the body's tissues and returning it to the liver for excretion.

You'll notice that we used the phrase "apparent hero." Indeed, the controversy about high- and low-density lipoproteins is an old, not a new one. Scientists have been debating the matter of lipoprotein density and coronary death risk since 1951. However, the popular press has publicized the "good" high-density lipoproteins only recently—and in the process has thoroughly muddied the waters and confused health professionals as well as laymen.

All that has been discovered only confirms the fact that your blood cholesterol level remains the best single parameter for estimating early coronary heart disease. Some doctors dispute this, but their arguments are unpersuasive.

## HDL VERSUS LDL

In 1977 W. P. Castelli, M.D., director of laboratories for the Framingham Study, reported that his data suggested that high HDL levels indicated a lower risk of heart disease.

People are born with equal amounts of HDL and LDL, in a one-to-one ratio. As we get older, however, our LDLs increase and thus create a greater risk of heart disease.

HDLs, however, are *not* necessarily good, nor are they

surefire protectors against heart disease. The HDLs of the Framingham men and Honolulu Japanese are roughly the same, according to Castelli, but the latter group have only half the coronary heart disease rate of the former.

Moreover, in the Multiple Risk Factor Intervention Trial (MRFIT)* study of 12,000 men, HDLs increased among men with higher diastolic blood pressure and were highest in men who had thirty-five drinks per week. Few responsible physicians would recommend increased alcoholic intake or higher blood pressure as protection against heart disease!

I consider LDL more meaningful than HDL. LDLs invade the artery wall and initiate plaque formation. When C. J. Glueck, M.D., studied people with very low levels of LDLs, he found they had one-fifth the death rate from heart disease of those with higher levels.

Most significant of all is the ratio of HDL to LDL. Arriving Pritikin Center patients have, on the average, an HDL to LDL ratio of 1:4. When they leave, four weeks later, the ratio is 1:3.3. After a year or two, some patients have ratios of 1:1.7—approaching the 1:1 ratio of a healthy newborn.

Interestingly, during our program, *both* HDLs and LDLs are lowered—the LDLs much more than the HDLs. With continued lowering of total cholesterol levels, the HDL fraction slowly rises.

I have been on my diet for eighteen years. My HDL to LDL ratio is 1:.5, with an HDL of 77. Dr. Castelli called it a most impressive HDL:LDL ratio.

As J. Stamler, M.D., noted in the Archives of Surgery in 1978:

It is worth noting that estrogen treatment of male survivors of myocardial infarction is associated with a considerable rise in HDL levels; however, this had proved ineffective in preventing recurrent coronary events and prolonging life.

The amassed data demonstrate incontrovertibly that

* The MRFIT is an ongoing study of 12,000 subjects, in which 6,000 are modifying their cardiovascular risk factors, cholesterol level, blood pressure, and smoking, and the other 6,000 are not. The study will run for six years.

there is a steady increment in premature atherosclerotic disease as the level of serum cholesterol rises, at least from levels of 220 mg./percent on up for middle-aged men. As the cholesterol concentration increases, the risk increases. The relationship is continuous.

The lesson to be taken from these facts is crystal clear: Keep cholesterol intake to the lowest possible level in order to keep serum cholesterol low. The HDL and LDL levels need not concern you. They are misleading and confusing. *Total cholesterol level* is what you ought to worry about.

## QUESTIONS AND ANSWERS

*Which foods are rich in cholesterol?*

*Only* foods from animal sources. You can't find a speck of cholesterol in grains, fruits, and vegetables—the foundation of the Pritikin Diet. Most Americans eat about 800 milligrams of cholesterol every day. On the Pritikin Diet you'll be eating less than 100 milligrams per day.

To keep this intake low, avoid shrimp, caviar, all organ and gland meats, and eggs. Lean meats, fish, chicken, and turkey are preferred for your limited ration of 1½ pounds per week of meat, fish, or fowl. The differences are tremendous. For example, 3 ounces of liver contain 300 milligrams of cholesterol; of kidney, 375 milligrams; of brains, 2,675 milligrams! Three ounces of chicken to turkey contain less than 65 milligrams.

*Is cholesterol found only in the fat?*

No, it's found in equal amounts in the fat and lean parts of any piece of meat. Peak concentrations of cholesterol are found in the organs and glands: heart, kidney, liver, sweetbreads. The brains have the most cholesterol of all the tissues.

Trimming fat or chicken skin or buying nonmarbled meat, as many people advise, *does* do some good. It reduces the amount of *fat* you'll be eating. But if you trim fat and then eat just a bit more lean meat to compensate for what you've trimmed, you'll be eating just as much *cholesterol!* Some authors maintain that there is just as much cholesterol in the ruby-red lean beef in steak tartare as there is in the greasy, white fat rim of a T-bone steak.

Incidentally, the few studies that have been done suggest that *cooking* does not affect the amount of cholesterol in meat.

### Do all eggs have huge amounts of cholesterol?

Yes, which is why they're not on your new diet.

And, by the way, egg substitutes usually have 50 percent more fat than eggs. Moreover, a glance at their contents tells you that you're involved with a "chemical feast." We do not recommend these products. The same goes for margarine. Margarines are made from plant fat, which contains no cholesterol, but they have as much fat as butter!

### What effect can the Pritikin Program have on cardiovascular disease?

Adopted early in life, it can prevent it. When the disease process has begun, it can virtually eliminate or at least alleviate the symptoms, depending upon how advanced the disease is. It does this by reducing all blood lipid levels (including cholesterol), eliminating cigarette smoking, reducing obesity and blood pressure, controlling diabetes, and providing an effective program of isotonic exercise.

Many people think cardiovascular disease is simply a part of growing old. It isn't. It is a natural consequence of a bad diet—period. People who eat right don't get it— with very, very rare exceptions. People on high-fat and high-cholesterol diets *do* get it. The American Heart Association says 29 million Americans have some kind of heart and blood vessel disease, and about 1 million of us die from it every year. Cardiovascular disease is the leading cause of death in the United States, taking 872,278 lives in 1974 from heart attack and stroke combined.

Nor are surgery or drugs a satisfactory alternative to diet in controlling cardiovascular disease. Remember that about one-fifth of all coronary bypasses (which cost about $10,000 to $20,000 each) close up within a year. The most recent Veterans Administration studies indicate that statistically they fail to extend their patients' survival times. As for drugs, a five-year double-blind test on the 8,000 men participating in the Coronary Drug Project* showed that men on placebos did as well as those on any of the drugs but without the side effects. Those side effects include gallstones, death from ventricular fibrillation, blindness, breast enlargement. Even nicotinic acid used at a 3-gram-a-day level showed toxic side effects, ranging from visual damage to irregular heartbeats.

*I've heard that lecithin can eliminate cholesterol. Is it true?*

Unfortunately, it is not. Nor does lecithin reduce arterial plaque. Yet many health magazines tout it highly—perhaps because many of their advertisers are lecithin vendors, or they believe in their products.

*Where did the idea begin?*

One of the earliest mentions of lecithin as a cardiovascular cure is found in Dr. Lester Morrison's book *The Low-Fat Way to Health and Longer Life,* published in 1958.

Morrison had good ideas, but lecithin was not one of them. He recommended that the bland soybean-powder extract be taken at breakfast as a food supplement. He credited Dr. Meyer Friedman of San Francisco as demonstrating "in a most convincing and dramatic manner how injections of lecithin remove the cholesterol plaques that were deposited in arteries."

In fact, Friedman was quite suspicious about any such use of lecithin. In his book, *Pathogenesis of Coronary Artery Disease,* Friedman allowed that lecithin might remove cholesterol from tissues, but warned that it would raise the serum cholesterol even higher. This, he said, could "lead to the deposition of excess cholesterol in tissues already atherosclerotic."

There are very few other studies of lecithin around.

* In the Coronary Drug Project, 8,341 men were given various drugs (or a placebo) to lower their cholesterol levels for five years. It was a double-blind study, i.e., neither the men nor their physicians knew what drug or placebo was in the capsules. (*JAMA*, May 15, 1972, vol. 220, #7, p. 996.)

One shows that when lecithin was given to several men between the ages of nineteen and twenty-five, it actually *raised* their blood lipids, *lowered* lung function, and created red-blood-cell clusters that lasted several days! Another shows that lecithin was ineffective in helping prairie dogs suffering from cholesterol gallstones. When cholesterol was removed from their diet, though, the gall-stones vanished.

### Does a high cholesterol diet cause cancer?

High cholesterol diets do nothing to prevent cancer. My basic criticism of high cholesterol diets is that they are practically guaranteed to close arteries and create diabetes and precancerous states. As a means of avoiding breast cancer women should shun high cholesterol diets.

Over the years some well-known nutritionists, including Adelle Davis, have advocated the high cholesterol diet to which I am opposed. This is not to say that nutritionists in general, and Adelle Davis in particular, don't deserve a great deal of credit for many of their accomplishments. They called attention to nutrition in the United States and got a lot of people interested in the subject for the first time.

It's good when someone like Adelle Davis brings the country's attention to the problem of chemical pollution of food and water. These are certainly important con-tributions, but they may account for less than 5 percent of the problem. Let's deal with the 95 percent first—our high fat and cholesterol diet—and then we can get to that 5 percent.

The millions of dollars our nation spends annually in heart-disease research are badly spent. Stress! Prescribing polyunsaturates! Additives! Pesticides! The focus is on the noncauses when we should be working on the elimination of dietary fats and cholesterol, the *known* causes of heart disease!

This brings us to another substance that is as much misunderstood as cholesterol—protein.

# 4

## What Protein Does

The Pritikin Diet does not emphasize protein, as most of the popular diets do, for two reasons. The first is that the body's need for protein has been grossly exaggerated. The second is that excessive protein is quite harmful. You will find that the Pritikin Diet challenges many of the most sacred assumptions about the role of protein.

Human beings do, of course, need protein—but much less than we're getting. What we need are protein's components, the *amino acids*. They are needed for life. As protein is digested it breaks down into these organic acids, which play an important role in growth, metabolism, and repair and maintenance of our body tissues. And eight of the twenty-two amino acids can *only* be obtained from food. That is, the body cannot manufacture them as it can the other fourteen.

### THE BEST PROTEIN FOODS

You may be surprised to learn that the best food sources for protein are grains, roots, vegetables, and fruits in an unrefined, minimally processed form—in other words, the substance of the Pritikin Diet. These are much better sources of protein than animal proteins such as meat, fish, eggs, and milk, which usually have very high—and often unacceptable—levels of fat and cholesterol.

You have doubtless heard the claim that animal protein is "superior" to vegetable protein. But this is absolutely untrue. *All* natural food grown contains *all* of the amino acids, "essential" and "nonessential," in sufficient quantities to satisfy human requirements. To speak of "superior" and "inferior" protein is nonsense.

You have probably also heard animal protein called the "complete" protein. This belief dates from 1916, when two investigators named Osborne and Mendel were experimenting on rats with different protein foods. These scientists described certain foods as "complete"—which really meant that they were adequate by themselves to maintain life and promote growth *in rats*. If *rats* did not grow well on a diet of any single food, the food was designated "incomplete." Eggs were considered complete, plant foods incomplete.

But our nutritional needs are different from rats'. If they were the same, then mother's milk should not be given to babies. After all, rats do not fare very well on human milk—since it is only 1.2 percent protein, compared with rat's milk's 9.5 percent protein. But babies do very well indeed on a milk one-eighth as protein-rich as rat's milk.

So it is just as incorrect to talk of "complete" and "incomplete" protein as it is of "superior" and "inferior" protein.


## PROTEIN DEFICIENCY

We have all heard stories about protein deficiencies among children in underdeveloped countries. But today we know that the problem with those children—and adults—is not one of too little *protein* but of too few *calories*.

When malnourished children were studied by the National Institute of Nutrition in Hyderabad, India, their protein consumption was shown to be 10 percent *higher* than the U.S. recommended level on a body weight basis! The children's problems were resolved when an extra 300 calories of low protein (4 percent) content were added to their daily 700-calorie diet.

The conclusion of the investigators (all members of India's Council of Medical Research) was that malnutrition among poor, rural Asian children should be attacked simply by giving them more *food*—rather than by giving them more protein.

## NITROGEN BALANCE

We do, of course, need a basic minimum of protein. We need enough to keep ourselves in what scientists call "positive nitrogen balance." This is a measure of the amount of protein the body retains from the diet in excess of its needs. Since protein is mostly nitrogen, scientists measure the nitrogen income versus the nitrogen outgo. If more nitrogen comes into the body than leaves it, you are in positive nitrogen balance. If you have a negative nitrogen balance, then you are losing protein from your muscles. And that's bad.

## MINIMUM PROTEIN REQUIREMENT

Tests have been made on adults eating white rice as their principal protein source. Six percent of total calories in protein from this white rice kept them in positive nitrogen balance. The Pritikin Diet gives between 10 and 15 percent of total calories in protein, with far better nutrition than is obtained from white rice.

If you think that you'll lack strength and endurance on a diet with 10 percent protein, consider the diet of the Mexican Tarahumara Indians. This diet is roughly the equivalent of the Pritikin Diet (10 percent protein, 10 percent fat, 80 percent complex carbohydrates). On this diet, the Tarahumaras can and do:

- Perform a 500-mile round-trip run in five days.
- Carry a 100-pound pack for 110 miles in seventy hours.
- In their national kickball game, run continuously for forty-eight hours and cover 175 miles. Playing this game, the Tarahumara Indian *women* are known to run continuously for fifty miles at a time!

These Indians eat animal protein about a dozen times a

year. Their diet comprises mainly corn, peas, beans, squash, and other native plants and fruits.

Physicians who have examined these people find them free of cardiovascular disease, hypertension, diabetes, and obesity!

## CALCULATING YOUR PROTEIN CALORIE REQUIREMENT

On the Pritikin Diet, it generally isn't necessary to estimate the number of calories one should have. Since carbohydrates are low-calorie foods (half the calories of fats and the same as proteins), you can eat more of them and not gain weight. Indeed, many people on this diet find gaining weight very difficult.

Nor do you have to estimate the number of calories in protein that you need on the Pritikin Diet. Even if you have little variety in your vegetables and grains and fruits, you'll automatically keep to within your minimum and maximum.

Counting calories, moreover, is an individual question, since every person's thyroid function and activity level are different. A Rocky Mountain lumberjack can eat 5,000 calories in a day and not gain an ounce; a housewife watching TV all day long can put on weight with only 1,400 calories.

However, once you know at what caloric level you should be, all you have to do is multiply that figure by 10 percent to calculate your minimum protein requirement, and by 15 percent to calculate your maximum protein requirement. Thus, if you require 2,000 calories a day, no less than 200 of them and no more than 300 should be in protein.

I repeat, there's no need to worry about having a variety of foods to fulfill this requirement. On the Pritikin Diet, you run no risk of any protein or amino acid deficiency whatsoever!

## QUESTIONS AND ANSWERS

*Would I run a risk in doing without meat altogether?*

Theoretically, you *might* run into a vitamin $B_{12}$ deficiency after five or ten years on a strict vegetarian diet. But remember, the Pritikin Diet allows you almost a quarter pound of meat or fish a day—many times the amount necessary to avoid a $B_{12}$ deficiency.

*Aren't there special cases—pregnant women, growing children, burn victims—where heavier protein intake is indicated?*

There are no exceptions that I am aware of. The Pritikin Diet formula is the best one for all of the categories you've mentioned. In fact, heavier protein intake can be *counterproductive.*

It is true that a burn victim throws out protein, in the same way that a diabetic throws out sugar. But it makes as little sense to treat a burn victim with extra protein as it does to treat a diabetic with extra sugar (which once upon a time was done routinely).

*How can a high-protein diet be harmful?*

When you exceed approximately 16 percent of your caloric intake in protein, on an average caloric intake of about 2,300 calories, you go into negative mineral balance. *Almost everyone* on the average American diet is in a negative mineral balance situation!

A negative mineral balance means that your body is actually losing its precious stores of important minerals such as calcium, iron, zinc, phosphorus, and magnesium. And, unfortunately, the mineral supplements taken by some people to remedy this loss generally do not do so.

*Isn't it widely believed that a high-protein diet improves the body's absorption and use of calcium?*

Yes. But it isn't true. That myth dies hard. Those who continue to perpetuate it ignore even the old studies, which show just the contrary. That is, as you increase protein, there is almost always a higher level of calcium found in the urine.

One of the most recent studies was done on young men

by the University of Wisconsin's Department of Nutritional Sciences. It showed that significant calcium loss resulted on a high-protein diet—but *not* on diets with low and medium levels of protein. The researchers opined that actual bone loss by demineralization—to a state of porous bones or osteoporosis—would result after a decade or so on a high-protein diet.

Egg, cheese, and beef eaters, take note!

*Does it help to supplement protein with calcium supplements?*

That won't work either. There is a direct, hard-and-fast correlation between the amount of protein you eat and the amount of minerals you excrete—no matter how much calcium you take.

This has been tested on over 2,000 students at the University of California at Berkeley since 1965. Increasing protein intake from 0 to 90 grams of nitrogen per day produces an eightfold increase in calcium loss! The amount of calcium taken—ranging from 100 milligrams to 2,300 milligrams—did not stop this loss. These findings have been amply confirmed by studies elsewhere.

*But aren't we taller and more beautiful than our grandparents because we eat more protein?*

Not because we eat more *protein*, but because we eat more *fat*. But we pay a high price for our increased physical stature! Both men and women are more likely to develop atherosclerosis younger, and die of strokes and heart attacks earlier, and be fatter in their middle age— though some won't live that long.

It's the high-fat levels that explain why girls begin to menstruate at eleven and twelve when they used to menstruate at sixteen and seventeen. High-fat levels provide a favorable home for anerobic bacteria, which create estrogens from the bile that stimulate growth in the sex organs, and also carcinogenic substances, one of which is deoxycholic acid.

On a high-fat diet (which most high-protein diets also turn out to be), bile levels are ten times higher, anerobic bacteria 100 times higher, and hormone and co-carcinogen levels 1,000 times greater!

This probably explains why high-fat diets seem to correlate with a greater incidence of breast, uterine, ovarian and colon cancers.

*I'd like my kids to be tall and beautiful, though. Would it be safe to start them on high-fat, high-protein foods, then switch to the Pritikin Diet after they've gotten their growth?*

There are many people on low-fat, low-protein diets all of their lives who are tall and beautiful. So giving children a proper diet does *not* inevitably result in their being stunted. We simply do not know enough about the chronology or mechanics of fat- and protein-carcinogenicity. But I think it's safe to say that your children would be grateful to you if you did not gamble with their lives.

*Why do people on high-protein diets drink so much water?*

They really have to—or else. In protein metabolism, complex by-products are formed. Some of them, such as ammonia, which becomes urea nitrogen, can be very toxic. So, in burning protein, to dilute these poisons, the body uses seven times as much water per calorie as it uses in burning carbohydrates or fat.

The instant weight loss achieved on a high-protein diet is due to the large quantity of water pulled from the body tissues to dilute the poisonous by-products of protein metabolism in the urine.

*What other risks are there in a protein-rich regimen?*

Too much protein with simple carbohydrates like sugar or honey can raise insulin blood levels to dangerous levels, producing a low-blood-sugar condition. It can raise uric acid levels, too, creating a risk of gout.

It is noteworthy that when some animals' intake of protein is reduced, they seem to develop a greater resistance to certain breast and blood cancers. When the protein in rodent feed is cut from 26 percent to 4 percent, both rats and mice live significantly longer and healthier lives.

*Can people die on high-protein diets?*

They can. As the number of liquid-protein dieters

reaches into the millions, the grave is already beginning to claim victims by the score. Many people are not even protecting themselves with a physician's monitoring of their diet, which, with dangerous gimmicks like liquid (or any other kind of high-level) protein, is an absolute must.

*What advice can you offer in regard to the liquid-protein diet?*

One of the innovators of the liquid-protein diet is Dr. George L. Blackburn, director of Nutritional Support at New England Deaconess Hospital. Dr. Blackburn, commenting on the first reports of fatalities linked to the predigested protein diets, said that such "nutrition" ought to carry a warning "as strong if not stronger than those for cigarettes."

At best, people on high-protein diets are often tired, irrational, logy, and unable to concentrate.

# 5

## What Carbohydrates Do

In Chapter 1, I probably surprised you by stating that carbohydrates are the best foods you can eat. But I also said that this does not apply to all kinds of carbohydrates. Starch-rich natural foods as they are grown are good for you. Simple, refined carbohydrates like sugar are not.

### WHY SUGAR IS BAD FOR YOU

Simply put, sugar has many deleterious effects and no good effects—except perhaps that of satisfying your sweet tooth. Being highly refined, it lacks vitamins, minerals, and fiber. It tends to make you fat, raise the level of your blood triglycerides (fat), and stress your pancreas—with pernicious consequences for the stability of your blood-sugar levels. It is very effective in making you hypoglycemic.

Sugar also seems to contribute to atherosclerosis. Sugar raises the level of blood fats and cholesterol, both of which crowd their way into diseased arteries and help make plaque.

Please understand, I am not against sugar because of its calories. I'm against sugar because it is an unnatural, highly concentrated food stripped of its fiber and nutritional components. If you were to eat the five ounces of sugar you normally eat in one day in the form of a three-pound sugar beet, you'd be getting some excellent nutrition and fiber—*and* you'd be satisfying your appetite as well. Herbivorous animals in a field never eat too much grass—simply because natural, unprocessed carbohydrates unfailingly signal the appetite when satiety has been

34

reached. There are no fat wild animals. Alas, there are all too many fat housewives and businessmen whose appetites are never satisfied by their candy bars, dry martinis, and white bread!

Almost *any* amount of sugar is too much. Most Americans eat about two pounds of sugar a week—which comes to about one-fourth of their total calories. Three-fourths of the sugar we eat comes in processed foods. Only one-fourth is eaten as sugar.

# WHY OTHER CARBOHYDRATES ARE BEN-EFICIAL

While simple carbohydrates like sugars and honey (monosaccharides and disaccharides) require no digestion and therefore quickly flood the system and then disappear, the more complex carbohydrates, including starches, take much longer to metabolize. In general, the more unrefined the carbohydrate, the longer the time required. These carbohydrates release a slow, constant stream of glucose into the bloodstream (about two calories per minute). This is an optimal rate for the body.

Glucose is the brain's only food; the brain uses about one-fourth of all the glucose in the body. Unlike the muscles, the brain cannot burn either fat or protein, except after an extended fast—though neither fat nor protein is burned by any body cells as efficiently as carbohydrates. Only carbohydrates burn 100 percent clean—converting into energy, carbon dioxide (which is breathed out), and water (which is excreted in urine, feces and sweat).

With a constant, slow supply of glucose provided by a diet of complex carbohydrates, mainly unrefined, there is rarely a blood sugar problem. You've always got something cooking on your alimentary burner, and you always have some glucose in the blood. Generally, people find that their hypoglycemia disappears in about two weeks on the Pritikin Diet and doesn't return as long as they stay on it, since there is never a deficiency of blood sugar. On the other hand, hypoglycemia is perpetuated by a high-protein, low-carbohydrate diet. The symptoms of fatigue and lightheadedness are a result of large amounts of toxins in the blood from the digestion of excessive amounts of protein, and the insufficient glucose for fuel for the brain.

## QUESTIONS AND ANSWERS

*Is honey better for me than sugar?*

No. *All* sugars are bad for you, and that includes all colors and brands of table sugar (cane or beet or corn), molasses, syrups, and honey. *Brown sugar* and *turbinado sugar* are the same as *white sugar*, but with insignificant levels of some nutrients. *Brown sugar* is table sugar with caramel coloring; *turbinado* is table sugar with some molasses; *"raw" sugar* is table sugar with beet pulp or cane fiber added to mime the taste of true raw sugar (authentic raw sugar is so impure it cannot be sold commercially).

*Is saccharin an answer to the sugar problem?*

It might be, but I don't recommend it. The studies showing that it can cause bladder cancer in animals are not conclusive, but they do raise suspicions about possible long-term, heavy-use effects. There is also a Canadian study showing a 60 percent higher incidence of bladder cancer in men who use saccharin than in men who do not. Since it is not a food and there is a risk, we steer clear of it.

*Do you regard sugar as an addiction?*

Yes, as do others who have investigated the problem. Sugar acts slowly to raise insulin levels and triglycerides and to create hypoglycemia and the feelings of lightheadedness, fatigue, weakness, and so forth, associated with it. What relieves those feelings is—more sugar. So it causes the problem, and resolves some of the symptoms of the problem—causing an addiction like cigarettes. It effectively makes you feel not quite well. You never really feel optimal.

*Suppose you had to choose between saccharin and sugar?*

I'd feel very uncomfortable. If you have to flavor your

water or Perrier water, spike them with fruit juices. Even fruit juices can raise your triglycerides, but not as much as sugar will. I wish we knew more about saccharin. Until we do, I avoid it.

*Are raw carbohydrate foods important in the diet?*

No question about it. We need to include plenty of raw carbohydrate foods in our diet. Two salads of raw vegetables a day, together with several pieces of fresh fruit, are not too much. In general, the less food is processed the better. However, it is difficult to eat enough calories on a diet of raw foods (which is why raw foods make an excellent weight-reducing diet), so that the major source of calories on our diet comes from cooked foods.

*If high-carbohydrate diets are so healthy, why are most popular diets low in carbohydrates?*

Low-carbohydrate diets have been around for at least 150 years. Like any low-calorie diets, such diets can promote weight loss, but in the case of low-carbohydrate diets, the weight loss is mainly temporary, mostly due to loss of water, and they can be deadly in the long run. During World War II, the Canadian Army made dehydrated beef their emergency ration, with nothing to drink but tea. Within three days the men's performances deteriorated so badly they chucked it. When a diet is not only high in fat, but high in protein as well, you have a very bad situation—because now you have to find a way of getting rid of the toxic breakdown products of protein. As you will learn as you read this book, both rapid and slow weight loss are best achieved by the Pritikin Diet—a diet you can live with happily and healthily the rest of your life.

A high-carbohydrate diet also comes with a bonus, one important enough for a chapter of its own—fiber.

# 6

# The Importance of Fiber

Food fiber consists of those parts of plant cells that cannot be digested by our enzymes or other digestive secretions. Basically, fiber comes from the structural and stabilizing parts of plants. Because of its importance to human health, it is still another benefit from a diet high in complex carbohydrates.

Perhaps its most important service is moving feces through the system at a faster speed. Fiber soaks up liquids like a sponge and gives bulk to human waste. People on the Pritikin Diet, which is high in fiber, almost never complain of constipation, owing to the laxative effect of fiber.

Fiber seems to help prevent colon-rectal cancers, diverticulosis, hemorrhoids, appendicitis, hiatus hernia, and other conditions. It is also known to reduce appetite by giving the dieter a feeling of fullness in the stomach. The addition to the diet of a highly concentrated source of fiber, such as wheat bran, is helpful in normalizing many body functions in people who have not eaten a diet sufficiently rich in fiber for many years.

## WHY WE DON'T GET ENOUGH FIBER

Anyone on a so-called "normal American diet" doesn't get enough fiber. Over a century ago, some genius made it possible to mill a new low-fiber flour and bake pretty new white breads and pastries. While these new products may have looked more elegant, they had less fiber. With less fiber came an assortment of pathologies, such as a virtual epidemic of diverticular disease, appendicitis, and hiatus hernia.

Since people eat about one-tenth as much bread today as they did a hundred years ago, they've lost even most of the fiber that's found in white bread. We do eat more fruit and vegetables, but not enough to compensate for the loss of grain fiber.

## THE REDISCOVERY OF FIBER

Before the turn of the century, men with names like Kellogg and Post popularized cereal products rich in "roughage." People had vague ideas about the value of roughage (or fiber) for laxative, prophylactic, and therapeutic purposes. Today, thanks mainly to fascinating epidemiological research, we know that many African peoples on high-fiber diets have an almost negligible incidence of coronary artery disease, colon-rectal cancer (which ranks second only to lung cancer in frequency among Americans), diverticulosis, varicose veins, gallbladder disease, and constipation. We are largely indebted to two British physicians, Denis Burkitt and Hugh Trowell, for this research which has made us aware of the importance of fiber to human health.

Research of this type has profoundly affected the treatment of diverticulosis, which is extremely common in this country. Two out of every five Americans over forty suffer from some form of the disease. Until very recently, most sufferers from diverticulosis disease were treated with bland diets almost devoid of fiber. Today, most experts prescribe just the contrary: high-fiber diets.

## QUESTIONS AND ANSWERS

*Why is it important to get rid of feces rapidly?*

It means less strain while moving the bowels, therefore less risk of hemorrhoids and diverticular disease. In diverticular disease the intestinal wall becomes pouched and, often, infected. Greater speed of elimination also reduces the time that carcinogens and poisons have to attack the gut wall.

## Would fiber help me to lose weight?

Yes, in the sense that fiber-rich complex carbohydrates are more filling than candy or sugar, yet contain fewer calories. For instance, you'd have to eat about three pounds of apples to equal the calories you get in one five-ounce chocolate bar.

## Are there risks in eating a high-fiber diet?

Flatulence is one, and it can last for weeks or months while your intestinal flora adapt themselves to their new nutritional environment. You may also feel bloated. Some people claim that yogurt seems to help speed the floral transition and terminate the flatulence.

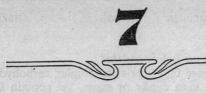

# 7

# Food Balancing

In addition to a diet that is low in fats, cholesterol, protein, and sugars and high in good starches and fiber, you need a *balanced diet* to assure yourself of getting all the vitamins and minerals you need for proper nutrition and good health. On the Pritikin Diet, balancing foods to get proper nutrition is remarkably uncomplicated. It isn't even necessary to eat at least one item from each of the major food groups every day. People whose palates have become adjusted to the Pritikin Diet often can balance their nutrition naturally by following their appetite preferences. Here's how it works.

## BASIC PRINCIPLES

To get all the essential vitamins, minerals, and roughage you require, as well as the correct amount of amino acids, you should follow these basic principles:

- *Eat two kinds of whole-grains daily,* such as wheat, oats, barley, brown rice, or buckwheat, every day.
- *Eat some raw vegetable salad and some raw or cooked green or yellow vegetables every day.* Potatoes may be eaten daily if desired.
- *Eat a piece of citrus fruit and up to three additional pieces of fresh fruit daily.*
- *Add beans or peas three times a week* if you like them. Once a week will do if you don't like them.
- *Eat sweet potatoes or hard yellow squash once or twice a week* if you like them.
- To provide needed vitamin $B_{12}$, *eat six ounces of low-*

*fat, low-cholesterol animal protein per week*—but not more than one-and-one-half pounds. Or, if you prefer a completely vegetarian diet, grow your own garden and eat some unwashed, unpolluted produce (rainwater contains vitamin $B_{12}$) or start taking vitamin $B_{12}$ supplements in a couple of years. (Your present body store of vitamin $B_{12}$ will last for five to ten years if you have been on a high-animal-protein Western diet.)

- *Add some unprocessed wheat bran flakes to your diet* (starting with one or two tablespoons a day) *if your bowel elimination is not yet normal.* Otherwise, the diet itself provides all the fiber that you need. (I don't use added wheat bran, and never have.)

- *Eat three full meals daily.* Don't go hungry between meals; eat snacks of whole-grain bread or crackers (ones that are free of oil, fats, added wheat germ, or sugar, honey, or other sweeteners), your fruit allotment, or some raw salad vegetables.

- *Maintain your ideal weight.* This you can do merely by using more or less of the permissible foods according to their calorie values. To lose weight, emphasize the low-calorie raw and cooked vegetables, by themselves or in combinations (as in salads and low-calorie soups); deemphasize the higher calorie foods, e.g., grains, grain products, and beans. To gain weight, do the reverse. Once weight has stabilized, most people on the Pritikin Diet don't bother watching calories, since their optimal weight is usually maintained by their appetite.

## FOLLOWING THE RULES

These are good rules, but they're not hard and fast. If your triglycerides are under 100, for example, you could safely eat up to eight pieces of fruit every day. But you actually don't *require* fruit or vegetables every single day of the week. Skipping a day or two isn't going to make a great difference, although having vegetables often will help keep your bowel movements regular.

On the other hand, limiting amounts of certain foods is important. You can, for instance, have trouble with beans and peas if you overdo them. They can raise your protein intake, which should be no more than 15 percent of your total calories. That's why I recommend eating no more than three large servings of *either* beans or peas a week. On the other hand, you can eat potatoes till kingdom come, every day or even at every meal. The potato is a splendidly balanced food. Avoid the skins though, which contain solanine, a toxic substance.

And, by the way, we counsel against weighing yourself daily. It can be an extremely frustrating and misleading experience. Weigh yourself twice a week. There are daily variations—due to bowel movements, timing, quantity of meals, water intake, and so forth—of up to four pounds daily. If you weigh yourself at night, you may be cheating yourself of two pounds (which you lose merely in water vapor in breathing).

As you can see, the Pritikin Diet has once and for all done away with the classic "balanced diet." It was feeble and ailing anyhow—and never very useful. Balancing meals probably began with the American Diabetic Association's system of insulin regulation. Later, during World War II, doctors urged people to eat from each of the seven food categories.

## QUESTIONS AND ANSWERS

*Will I need any vitamin or mineral supplements on the Pritikin Diet?*

None whatsoever—which eliminates the risks involved in taking supplements. At very high levels, vitamins and minerals may have a druglike, rather than nutritional, effect. Vitamin D and vitamin A can be extremely dangerous at high dosages.

*How much vitamin E will I get on the Pritikin Diet?*

About ten international units per day. Others may tell you that it isn't enough, or that the government recommends fifteen as a minimum, or that many people are taking much higher amounts. But just remember: the main role of vitamin E is to protect you from the dangers of oils. When you eat polyunsaturated oils, you run a real risk of creating a severely oxidizing condition. This sort of lipid peroxidation seems to poison the body and accelerate aging. The answer, however, is not to use vitamin E to put out the fire. The answer is not to start the fire in the first place. You do this by *reducing your fat intake.*

*How much milk should I drink every day to get enough calcium?*

None at all, if you don't care for milk. You get all the calcium you need from vegetables. In fact, the World Health Organization has been unable to document a single case of calcium deficiency!

As for the calcium requirements of growing children, on a diet with adequate but low protein (10 to 14 percent of total calories), even one glass would be adequate. Few children around the world drink milk after they are weaned, unless they are on the Western diet.

The same holds for pregnant women. African Bantu mothers on a daily calcium allotment of 350 milligrams per day (one-third of the American standard) bear and nurse, as an average, nine children, and have no calcium deficiencies. One glass of milk per day (320 to 350 milligrams of calcium) will provide double the Bantu intake, since there will be calcium available from other foods in the diet as well.

*Will I be getting enough nutrients even if I'm on the fast-weight-loss program?*

Yes. If you're trying to lose weight, you're still getting all the essentials. You're merely focusing on the low-calorie end of the spectrum. Low in calories, that is, but high in vitamins and minerals.

*Are there any problems with camping trips?*

On camping trips be sure to get some vegetable greens every day. Cabbage is a good bet, by the way, since it stays fresh for a long time and has high vitamin C content. Rolled oats are convenient since they can be eaten raw, having been steamed in their manufacturing process already.

*Can I be on your diet and suffer from constipation?*

It's almost impossible—in view of the high-fiber content of the foods you'll be eating. When someone complains to me of constipation, it's a sure sign that he or she has gone off the diet. If you drink a few glasses of water and just add up to four tablespoons of bran a day to your food, constipation becomes almost an impossibility.

*I'm following the diet but don't have any energy. Could I be eating too much or too little of certain foods?*

Probably neither. More likely you're not getting enough sleep. This is a common problem among our dieters, since the burst of energy most people experience early in the day sometimes convinces them that they can dispense with sleep. It's true that you may be able to cut down your sleep budget by an hour or two—but no more. Count your sleeping time and make sure you get enough.

A second possibility is that you're not exercising properly. To maintain a feeling of well-being you need at least two half-hour walks a day. Every day you don't walk regularly, your circulation will slow down and de-energize you. The exercise chapter discusses this and alternate forms of exercise.

A third possibility is that you may be coming down with a cold. In this case, sleep an extra hour or two and don't strain yourself.

*I have insomnia. What do you think is causing it?*

Worry, probably. If you solve your problems, or just stop worrying about them, you'll most likely lose your insomnia. Also, try to eat nothing three hours before bedtime and drink nothing but water. I often recommend taking a fifteen-minute walk a half hour before retiring. It has the soporific effect of a strong tranquilizer.

Even a perfectly balanced diet, however, can be ruined by what you add to it. And one of the worst offenders is a substance most of us take for granted—salt.

# 8

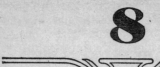

# What Salt Does

Salt is highly restricted on the Pritikin Diet. Although Americans on the average take in from six to eighteen grams of salt per day, we advocate no more than two to four grams. (Four grams of salt measure approximately one-half teaspoon.) Your body needs some salt, but the natural salt present in varying amounts in almost all foods more than suffices for most of us.

## SALT AND HYPERTENSION

For four decades now, we have known that dietary salt contributes mightily to hypertension. By the same token, removing salt from the diet reduces hypertension.

Just how salt creates hypertension, we're not exactly sure. But excess salt upsets your natural water/salt balance, forcing the body to hold onto extra amounts of water to make up for the salt you've eaten. Just a little salt can add extra pounds of retained water in your body. With all that additional water weight, your heart has to work harder because your tissues are flooded in the spaces between the blood capillaries. Salt-caused edema (swelling) can cut down your capillary blood oxygen transfer to the cells between the capillaries—and create extra pressure against the vessel walls.

In general, salt eaters have much more hypertension than people who don't eat salt. The Northern Japanese, for instance, eat three times as much salt as we do—and 40 percent of them have hypertension. Low-salt eaters have low rates of hypertension; witness the Greenland

Eskimos, aboriginal Chinese, Panamanian Cuna Indians, and Australian aborigines.

## SALT AND THE PRITIKIN DIET

There is *some* added salt permitted in the Pritikin recipes. For instance, some recipes use canned tomatoes, tomato sauce, prepared mustard, or mild soy sauce. All of these products contain some salt. What we do *not* permit is adding salt from a shaker to the cooking pot or the serving plate. And even the amount of salt that is introduced into the diet through the use of the various permitted ingredients can become excessive for some people if very many canned or frozen foods are used. Incidentally, there are varying amounts of salt naturally present in almost all foods.

People need to monitor the amount of salt they can tolerate for themselves. Less is better for everyone, and some people are almost exquisitely sensitive to even a little salt, and really need to be on a "salt-free" diet. (There is no such thing as a *totally* salt-free diet, of course.)

In general, lowering the fat content of the diet is enough to bring people with hypertension into a normal blood-pressure range very quickly, so long as salt intake is restricted. For some people, however, salt intake needs to be restricted even more by eliminating commercially packaged, canned, and frozen foods which have added salt.

## QUESTIONS AND ANSWERS

*Is salt the main cause of hypertension?*
No. Excessive fats and insufficient complex carbohydrates are equally as important causes of hypertension. You can reduce hypertension by lowering fats and raising carbohydrates in the diet—and keep on eating nine or ten grams of salt per day.

*What is the main reason you restrict salt then?*

The main reason is the edema it causes in the human body. The edema tends to deprive tissues of oxygen—thus creating a host of circulatory problems, including arthritis, reduced visual, auditory, and tactile sensations, and so forth. If you have joint and muscular stiffness on awakening in the morning, you may be suffering from salt-caused edema.

Just as some people err by adding table salt to foods that naturally contain this mineral, others are in the habit of adding a substance with practically no food value—alcohol.

# 9

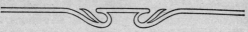

# What Alcohol Does

Basically, I consider alcohol a drug, not a food. It has practically no nutritive value outside of its calories. In that respect, its calories resemble the practically empty calories of sugar and honey. As a drug, alcohol only causes havoc within the body.

## THE EFFECTS OF ALCOHOL

Alcohol's bad effect on the liver is too well known to require explanation.

Less well known is the fact that alcohol causes platelets to stick together and sludges the red blood cells, reducing their oxygen-carrying capacity and the blood supply to the heart. This has a devastating effect on brain cells and brain function as well.

Alcohol also inhibits mobilization of lymphocytes from the lymph into the blood when they're needed to fight infection. This is why alcoholics, for instance, have a much higher rate of pneumonia—and spend so much more time incapacitated by it—than nonalcoholics. Alcohol depresses your immunization system.

Alcohol seems to make arthritis worse, too. To simplify considerably, let me explain that arthritis pains can be induced by blood-cell sludging—which alcohol stimulates. When the red blood cells sludge, capillaries get blocked and the watery part of the blood is forced through the capillary walls. This creates an edema which reduces the amount of oxygen available to the cells in the tissue spaces. Without oxygen, the affected tissues become inflamed and can be quite painful.

**FURTHER BAD EFFECTS**

I could go on and on saying unkind things about alcohol, but let me just make a few more points:

- Even a little bit of alcohol destroys judgment, as is amply demonstrated by the fact that nearly half of all automobile fatalities involve drinking drivers. In one study of professional bus drivers, even several who had drunk less than would normally be considered an intoxicating amount stubbornly tried to perform the impossible—such as drive their bus through a space more than a foot narrower than their vehicle!

- Alcohol loads the liver with triglycerides and other fats, forcing a rise in those levels in the blood as well. (We've described the mischief all *that* can cause in Chapter 2.)

- Irritation of the entire urinary tract, from the urethra to the bladder, is a common consequence of alcoholic overindulgence. It also irritates the prostate.

- Alcohol is a disaster for pregnant women. Nearly one out of every six babies born to alcoholic women dies and some 44 percent have at least borderline mental retardation.

- The emotional distress to a close family member or other person intimately concerned with an alcoholic's problems is considerable.


**QUESTIONS AND ANSWERS**

*I know that alcohol is bad for me, but I find it's the only escape I have from a nagging spouse.*

I can't argue with you—except to suggest that you probably could find an escape in something far less self-destructive.

*I find I don't have angina pains when I'm drinking, and I'm assuming this is because of a beneficial vasodilating effect. I also find that Jack Daniel's bourbon tastes better than nitroglycerin pills.*

Well, there's no arguing with taste. But there *is* another side to the myths you've been taken in by.

In the first place, alcohol *reduces* your heart's working capacity. If you have angina, just two cocktails will cut it by about 20 percent for about twenty-four hours! So, if you're a two-drink-a-day person, you've already deprived yourself of one-fifth of your heart.

Then why don't you feel this cardiac deficiency? Because the alcohol anesthetizes your body, that's why. It's lucky you don't do any hard manual labor while you're drinking, because then you'd get very dramatic proof that alcohol does not relieve angina*—much less prevent it. It most certainly would make your angina pains far worse and occur far more often.

Alcohol *does* have a vasodilating effect, that's true. But *on the skin*—not on the large arteries. This means that when you have angina pains, your suffering arteries have to fight for blood that's congested the little capillaries in the skin—where the blood is not needed.

*Alcohol not only relaxes me, it puts me to sleep.*

I don't doubt it. So will ether. But neither ether nor alcohol represents an ideal sleeping potion. Exercise works much better, gives you a better sleep, and gives you more energy for the next day.

*I enjoy a glass of wine with my dinner—and I have no intention of giving it up.*

If you are otherwise in excellent health and get a lot of exercise, a glass of wine with dinner may not harm you. The rise in blood triglycerides may be resolved during your morning jogging.

But there is a great difference between the half-ounce of alcohol you drink in one four-ounce wineglass and the full ounce you drink with *two* glasses. There's also a *world* of difference between a glass of wine and hard liquor, which has seven or eight times as much alcohol per volume!

* Angina customarily occurs during physical exertion or severe emotional stress.

By all means, don't chuck the rest of the diet because
you have a weakness for a glass of wine with your meals.
Every part of the diet you observe will help you that
much. (Although lapsing by smoking cigarettes, or ignor-
ing fat restrictions or cholesterol levels, may obliterate *almost all* of the benefits this diet gives you.)

At this point it should be clear why alcohol has no
place in our diet program.** Now for some other undesirable beverages.

** Small amounts of alcohol used as a cooking liquid are permitted, since most of the alcohol evaporates anyway.

# 10

## What Caffeine Beverages Do

Coffee and tea are not permitted on the Pritikin Diet. While the final verdict on beverages containing caffeine is not in yet, the research available raises grave suspicions about the wisdom of drinking either coffee or tea regularly. The entire area of caffeine toxicity, however, is quite controversial.

### WHAT'S WRONG WITH COFFEE AND TEA

People drink coffee and tea because both these beverages have perk-up qualities that people on "normal" high-fat diets seem to require. Along with caffeine's cousins theophylline (found with caffeine in tea) and theobromine (in cocoa), the group is known as the xanthines. The xanthines stimulate the central nervous system, act as diuretics, stimulate the heart muscle, relax smooth muscles (particularly the bronchial), and stimulate the cerebral cortex (alleviating drowsiness and fatigue, sharpening thoughts). None of these would be necessary on a healthy, low-fat diet. And eliminating coffee and tea means eliminating the main culprit—caffeine.

Caffeine is a drug known to produce peculiar and rapid heartbeats, insomnia, high free-fatty-acids levels in the blood, high blood glucose levels in diabetics, increased gastric acid secretion, and high blood pressure. The raising of blood lipids is suspected to be a factor in atherosclerosis.

The actual quantity of caffeine depends on the amount

53

of water used, the brand of coffee or tea, the method of brewing, and so forth. In general, the longer you brew, the more caffeine you extract from leaf or bean. Coffee, brewed or instant, contains between 90 and 120 milligrams per five-ounce serving; decaffeinated coffee between 1 and 6 milligrams; leaf tea, 30 to 60 milligrams; bagged tea, 42 to 100 milligrams; instant tea, 30 to 60 milligrams; cocoa, up to 50 milligrams; and cola drinks, 15 to 40 milligrams.

Few doctors even recognize caffeinism when they see it. Dr. John F. Greden, former psychiatric research director at Walter Reed Army Medical Center, reported that none of one hundred psychiatric outpatients spot-checked had even been asked about their coffee- or tea-drinking habits. This despite diagnoses of anxiety neurosis in forty-two of them!

Nutritional causes of illness and nutritional therapies are frequently ignored altogether—even when they are obviously indicated. Consider the case of a Reno, Nevada, state prison inmate suffering from severe anxiety. He was unsuccessfully treated with tranquilizers and other drugs—until somebody thought to suggest that he stop drinking the whopping fifty cups of coffee he was imbibing daily. (When he switched to decaffeinated, his condition improved.)

## CAFFEINISM

Caffeinism is a problem for people of all ages—particularly children. Kids get huge quantities of caffeine from chocolate, cocoa, and cola drinks. Consider that a small chocolate bar has about 25 milligrams of caffeine, a Coke about 40 milligrams. *A seven-year-old boy who drinks three Cokes a day—since he weighs only sixty pounds—is actually drinking the equivalent of eight cups of coffee that a 175-pound man would drink.* Physicians, particularly pediatricians, are extremely concerned about widespread caffeine-caused symptoms of irritability, nervousness, and insomnia among children.

The Food and Drug Administration is conducting an investigation into the possibility that the caffeination of nearly 65 percent of the six billion gallons of soda produced annually in the United States may be contributing to growth and development disorders among children.

## OTHER POSSIBLE HARMFUL EFFECTS

There is evidence that death in acute myocardial infarction may be triggered by caffeine in susceptible people. Free fatty acids can give rise to sudden ventricular tachycardia and fibrillation.

It has been said that coffee can cause ulcers. So far, the evidence is statistical. That is, researchers have not established a *direct* cause-and-effect relationship. But a study by Dr. Ralph Paffenbarger, Jr., at the University of California School of Public Health showed that former male college students who reported drinking coffee daily had 1.4 times the risk of developing peptic ulcers that noncoffee-drinkers did. If gastric acid secretion is the culprit, then decaffeinated coffee is no improvement on regular coffee, since it is every bit as potent a stimulator.

Caffeine has also been suspected of contributing to birth defects. Once again, the evidence is anything but conclusive. Still, many physicians are advising mothers-to-be to avoid caffeine-containing beverages while pregnant. Caffeine is so configurated, molecularly, that it can cross the placenta and enter the fetal gonad. At the very least, according to Dr. John J. Mulvihill, head of clinical genetics in the National Cancer Institute epidemiology branch, caffeine is highly mutagenic and possibly even teratogenic. This would imply that caffeine might cause chromosomal changes and abnormal babies.

## QUESTIONS AND ANSWERS

*Is decaffeinated coffee safe?*

I neither recommend nor ban decaffeinated coffee. Not enough is known about its physiological and psychological effects. What raises my suspicions are the slightly toxic substances that have not been removed.

*Is tea an improvement on coffee?*

Only to the extent that it generally contains about one-half the caffeine equivalent.

Some scientists suspect that tea may be *more* dangerous than coffee in some respects. The high rate of gastric and esophogeal cancers among tea-drinking populations (particularly those which do not bind the tannin in the tea by adding milk) is a source of concern.

*What about herbal teas? Surely they're safer than regular tea.*

According to the University of Miami's Dr. Julia Morton, who has made a comprehensive study of teas, "In turning to 'herb tea' . . . a person . . . may be leaping from the frying pan into the fire, especially since many seem to feel that if a little 'herb tea' is good, a large quantity will produce the wished-for miracle of sound sleep, renewed health, vigor, and longevity."

Almost all of the herbal teas seem to have problems. Remember, Dr. Morton's warnings are based on hypotheses—not actual cause-and-effect proof. But I have been impressed with the seriousness of her survey as well as her clinical suspicions. Sassafras, for instance, contains a carcinogen called safrole, which is now banned as a food additive. Shave grass tea—like so many other herbal teas sold in health food stores—was originally a medicinal tea, *not* a refreshment beverage. It was used to treat venereal disease. Sheep, cattle, and horses are poisoned by it. Rose hips contain substantial quantities of tannin, as do peppermint, South American maté, Comfrey, Lady's mantle, and Yellow Dock teas.

*Aren't there any safe teas?*

Yes. *Linden* tea, according to Dr. Morton, is apparently safe. So are most *Chinese* teas that contain little or no tannin. (That includes teas from both mainland China and Formosa, by the way.) Many Chinese restaurants serve a safe Chinese tea. You can often tell by the astringent effect on the tongue whether it has tannin. If your tongue feels fuzzy after drinking large amounts of the tea, you got the wrong kind. Tannin is responsible for that highly touted "brisk" sensation of orange pekoe teas.

If you drink tea as the English do, with a healthy amount of milk in it, you bind the troublemaking tannin. But even if the tannin issue is resolved, the caffeine problem is not.

*Should I add whole milk or nonfat milk to tea?*
Nonfat milk will bind the tannin as well as whole milk, since it's the milk *protein*—not the fat—which neutralizes the toxicity. Whole milk for *anything* is a big no-no because of its high fat content. And *don't* follow the English custom of adding sugar to your tea, because that opens up another Pandora's box which we've already peeked into.

We now come to what is probably the worst anti-health habit there is. Do I have to name it?

# 11

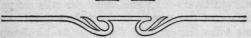

# What Smoking Does

Smoking can nullify practically all of the benefits that you would receive by adherence to the Pritikin Program.

Lung cancer has been touted as the principal smoking risk. It is *one* of them, certainly. (High cholesterol levels also seem closely linked with lung cancer.) Smoking appears to be a powerful factor in bladder cancer, too. Since the many carcinogens in cigarette smoke have up to ten hours to loll around in the body's tissues before being excreted in the urine, the cancer risk is clear-cut.

However, in terms of numbers affected by smoking—and in terms of deaths—I am more concerned with another of its evils: carbon monoxide.

## CARBON MONOXIDE

While health officials seem obsessed with cigarettes' nicotine and tars, the carbon monoxide (CO) is probably the most devastating element in smoke's grisly collection of chemical assassins.

One reason is that no filter traps CO. Filters, in fact, tend to increase the CO intake by as much as 28 percent, according to one study. The filter paper, it seems, blocks the pores in the cigarette paper from its air intake.

Blood cells seem suicidally drawn to carbon monoxide. They are two hundred times more attracted to this toxin than to oxygen. When CO and the red blood cells' hemoglobin bind together, they form a stable compound, carboxyhemoglobin, which can tie up the red blood cells' oxygen-carrying capacity for up to twelve hours.

Of course, if you *really* want to put a contract out on your red blood cells, just combine a high-fat diet with smoking. The net result is oxygen starvation. The oxygen-starved layers react and cause the cells lining the inside surface of the arteries to open their tight boundaries to allow more oxygen in. This permits betalipoproteins (made up of fat, cholesterol, and protein) to invade the layer, cause artery inflammation and initiation of the deadly plaque growth.

All this means that smokers have a much higher risk of heart disease, stroke, hypertension, angina, and all the other atherosclerosis-related diseases.

Statistics bear this out. They show that the actual risk of dying of a heart attack increases the earlier you start smoking, the more you smoke, and the more you inhale.

In a war veteran study, heavy smokers between thirty-five and fifty-four had a fivefold to tenfold greater risk of death from coronary heart disease than nonsmokers. An investigation of smoking doctors in Britain showed similar results: a five times greater chance of dying of heart attack.

## OTHER SMOKING HAZARDS

Meanwhile, nicotine makes a heart patient more liable to ventricular fibrillation. By increasing the stickiness of platelets, nicotine raises the danger of blood clots. Enough has been written by everybody else on the cancer-causing properties of cigarette tars. It's true and it's ghastly and it's well known. If what you've heard already hasn't given you a healthy fear, *nothing* will.

Smoking accelerates aging by speeding up many of those pathologies that seem to begin to get worse with old age. Osteoporosis is an example. Normally symptoms of this bone-eroding disease don't appear until the later years. When they do show up early, chances are overwhelming that the victim is a heavy smoker.

In one study of seventeen women with premature osteoporosis at three hospitals near Redding, California, fifteen of them turned out to be heavy smokers and one a moderate smoker.

Smoking changes bone tissue, making it easier for minerals to leave the bone in solution.

We've mentioned heart disease, stroke, cancer, but we haven't mentioned emphysema and the gamut of bronchial diseases worsened by smoking.

Many dermatologists also warn that smoking makes both men and women look older by increasing deep skin wrinkling* and reducing skin elasticity.

There are other dangers you might not know about. If you've got heartburn, it might well be your cigarettes— and not your food. Also, if you're a driver, your field of vision is much less than it otherwise would be. A new smoker loses 26 percent of his field of vision; a smoker who gives up the habit finds that his field of vision expands 36 percent.


## STOPPING SMOKING


Once the damage has been done, there is one thing you can do—stop smoking. The earlier the better. A University of Southern California team of physicians, headed by Dr. David H. Blankerhorn, showed that cessation of smoking can produce actual diminishing of arterial plaque in heart-attack patients. One of the forty male executives studied had smoked two packs of cigarettes a day for thirty years. After his heart attack, he stopped. Digital image processing of his angiograms showed that plaque regression had happened within eighteen months after he had stopped smoking. The thinking is that young plaque is more easily eroded than older, harder plaque.

Stopping smoking can actually reduce the risk of getting heart disease, according to expert interpretation of

* Dr. Harry W. Daniell of Redding, California, reported in 1971 that a study of 1,100 patients between the ages of thirty and seventy showed far more pronounced "crow's feet" around the eyes as well as other facial wrinkling. Why? Daniell believes that smokers' nonblushing, yellow-gray complexions may stem from the contraction of small blood vessels in the skin caused by nicotine. "Over a period of time," he noted, "this mechanism might cause a progressive deterioration in skin tissue that could result in wrinkling."

the Second Report of the Combined Experience of the Albany and Framingham Longitudinal Studies. Other studies too numerous to mention suggest that your risk decreases as your nonsmoking time lengthens. Some experts believe that after a decade of nonsmoking, a former smoker's risk equals that of a lifelong nonsmoker in many areas of risk.

But if you give up smoking you'll get a feeling of increased well-being within days!

## QUESTIONS AND ANSWERS

*How can I tell if smoking is giving me arterial plaque?*

Sometimes you can't tell. Angiograms are not always reliable. In one-fourth of older victims of coronary artery disease, the first clinical symptom they have is—death! It's called the "sudden death syndrome." Heavy smoking increases the chance of sudden death in both sexes.

*Is smoking the major factor in lung cancer?*

It is not the only one, certainly. Serum cholesterol is another. Dr. Jeremiah Stamler did a long-term study on 876 male employees of the Peoples Gas Company in Chicago, dividing them into three groups of low, medium, and high serum cholesterol levels. There was a dramatically positive correlation between serum cholesterol levels and nine-year cancer death rates.

*Aren't there people who smoke who don't get heart disease?*

Some smokers have very low heart-disease rates. They include inhabitants of Crete, Corfu, parts of Japan, and Yugoslavia. These people exercise heavily, don't get fat, and don't eat fat and cholesterol in significant quantities.

What this shows is that smoking works together with other risk factors to create a much greater danger than the mere sum of those factors.

Just eliminating one or two of the major risk factors is not enough. To make the most of your years—and stretch them out as long as possible—you ought to reduce all of them.

This is precisely what the Pritikin Program is designed to do for you.

*I understand you have tremendous success in getting your patients to stop smoking.*

That's true. We have about an 85 percent success rate. Our follow-ups a year later show that this may decrease to about 75 percent. A few go back to smoking.

*That's still impressive. How do you do it?*

With the facts, peer pressure, quick positive benefits, the investment they've made in the program, and the fear of returning to their old condition.

*Which facts do you emphasize?*

The connection with calcium loss in the bones; calcified aortas and loss of arterial elasticity; earlier menopause for females; reduction of estrogen production and all the problems of skin wrinkling, dehydration, etc., that go with it; basically, all the consequences of plaque formation: hearing and vision impairment, taste impairment, general loss of physiological and mental functioning.

*Tell me about peer pressure.*

That may be the most important feature of our anti-smoking program. We tell them that they can't slow down and stop. We tell them they have already smoked their last cigarette. If they smoke another, they'll probably never stop. They have to throw away *every* cigarette—then and there—and avoid being near a smoker for the next four days. They also have to avoid places where they might buy cigarettes. That problem is solved at the Pritikin Center. It's more difficult if they're at home.

*Why four days?*

It takes four to six days for withdrawal symptoms to subside. After that, 90 percent of their problem is gone. They begin to taste things they haven't tasted in years. The coughing stops, especially the morning cough. To get them over those first four days is the hard part. We sometimes suggest that their physicians prescribe a tranquilizer. The important thing is for them to understand why they've stopped. If they do, chances are they'll never go back. And they don't like the idea of spending several thousand dollars for a stay at the Pritikin Center, and then blowing it all up with a puff of smoke.

And now for the second—and equally basic—aspect of the Pritikin Program, something Americans haven't been doing enough of for years!

# TWO

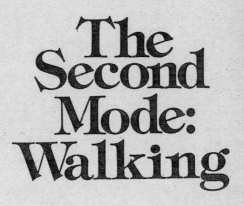

# The Second Mode: Walking

# 12

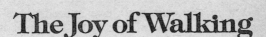

# The Joy of Walking

> The sovereign invigorator of the body is exercise, and of all exercises walking is the best.
>
> —Thomas Jefferson

How much would you pay to feel younger and live longer? What do you think it would cost you to be able to reassert control over your life and your energies, recharge your batteries, and improve your health, happiness, and outlook on life?

Such benefits are without price, although fortunes have been paid over the years to charlatans and alchemists who have purported to produce them with magic elixirs and pills and potions.

I will give them to you for free, as a gift. All you have to do is stretch your legs and start walking. That's right. Just walk.

Although the simple pleasure of walking has been overshadowed by glamorous sports such as tennis, skiing, and scuba diving, its rewards for most people equal those of any other form of exercise.

Walking helps to:
- Control your blood circulation
- Prevent heart disease
- Keep your bones from weakening
- Maintain your weight at a proper level

Walking also:
- Relaxes you better than a tranquilizer

- Improves your looks
- Burns off fat
- Suppresses your appetite
- Reduces anxiety and depression
- Increases general fitness

In recent months, you may have noticed a new phenomenon in your neighborhood: small armies of lightly clad people of all ages jogging or walking unnaturally fast—and doing it every day.

At the crack of a muggy summer's dawn, a potpourri of regulars begins to jog around the mile-and-three quarters cinder track engirdling Manhattan's Central Park reservoir.

Their skins glisten with sweat as their lungs heave forth staccato huffs and grunts. Their grim faces mask a unique "high" blended of transcendental joy, brimming health, muscular tautness, fatigue, and serenity.

Each keeps his or her own pace. For some it is a run. Others alternate jogs with breath-catching walks. Still others churn the track with their own sort of shuffle.

They come in all shapes, colors, and ages. They file around the reservoir in velour warm-up suits, embroidered gym pants, cutoff Levis, windbreakers. A septuagenarian in long johns and brown pinstripe trousers does a slow-and-steady pace with his shirt clutched in his fist. A very fat young woman clips the bottom sector of the track in her cross-the-park trek to buy the morning paper at a distant newsstand.

This corps of exercisers is not unique to New York. You see them all over the country, making do with available footpaths to put in their daily walking and jogging stints. You may be lucky enough to live in the vicinity of one of the several score *Parcourses* round the country. The *Parcourse* is a Swiss idea involving a two-mile jogging circuit with twenty different stations that provide opportunities for cardiovascular-stimulation exercises such as log jumping and chin-ups. Generally, however, one must make do with high school cinder tracks, city blocks, and rather perilous country roads with narrow shoulders.

Despite the dearth of jogging and walking routes, these exercises have swept the country in the past two or three years. Some ninety million Americans are now actively involved in regular athletic activities, the healthiest being walking and its variations: jogging, running, tennis, soccer, racketball, squash, basketball, and handball—all of which use the long leg muscles, pump blood from the feet to the heart, build new little vessels that skirt blockages and clots.

Walking does the body enormous good. A benefit that ranks high for most people is its rapid beautifying effect. Fat people—both men and women—have considerably more trouble establishing satisfactory relationships with the opposite sex than the bellyless. Regular exercise removes excess pounds and unsightly lumps and improves the complexion. It also minimizes aches, pains, tension, sleeplessness, and depression.

What else? Exercise lengthens blood-clotting time, preventing spontaneous blood clotting. It lowers blood pressure and helps prevent gout by lowering uric acid levels. It makes your arteries more elastic, your body more flexible and strong. It increases the blood's oxygen-carrying capacity, and quite dramatically, too. This means you get more oxygen where you need it, faster and more efficiently. Because of that new efficiency, your heart learns how to work less. You also recover faster from illnesses and accidents—and have fewer of both.

When combined with the Pritikin Diet, the walking variations do far more. Together they constitute your best possible defense against degenerative aging conditions—as well as the best therapy if you're suffering from them. Atherosclerosis and all of its nasty results respond best to the combination of diet and exercise. Of course, of the two, diet is the most important. Only diet, for example, can reduce cholesterol levels.

*Caution!* Before starting anything more than a comfortable walking program, you ought to get yourself checked out by a physician with a stress-treadmill electrocardiogram. If your arteries are "clean" (i.e., relatively free of plaque) your endurance will surprise you. The healthy human on a natural diet has fantastic stamina. Australian aborigines, for example, can stalk a kangaroo day and night until *it* gets tired. The Tarahumara Indians in Mexico keep in shape by running footraces as long as one hundred fifty miles!

Much of what follows will refer to jogging and running, which are the exercises of preference for healthy people bent on improving cardiovascularity. But walking can produce similar improvement among those unable to jog.

The basic idea is to create an insufficiency of blood to the heart, in order to create tiny new blood vessels. If you're in top shape, creating such an insufficiency requires considerable effort. But for those suffering from intermittent claudication or angina, for whom just walking can be painful, this insufficiency can be created just by walking.

But first, a few words about the benefits of exercise in general.

# 13

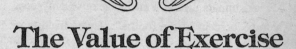

# The Value of Exercise

Exercise, its proponents say, will help you to live longer. It would require several generations of controlled clinical tests to prove it. Some evidence, however, strongly suggests that exercise—particularly when coupled with the Pritikin Diet—vastly improves the quality of life. That is, you feel better, look better, perform better, and enjoy life more. And it is not unreasonable to suppose that living better might contribute to living longer.

## THE BEST KIND OF EXERCISE

The best kind of exercise, I believe, is that which helps your heart and circulation. This is called *isotonic* (dynamic) exercise. It involves moving your arms and, more important, your legs. Any exercise that puts a constant stress on your legs and involves walking and running is a good one.

Another popular kind of exercise is called *isometrics*. Weight lifting is an example. Isometrics involve muscular contractions without much motion. *These exercises do not help the heart.* In fact, they stress the heart and raise blood pressure. People with weak hearts would do well to avoid isometric exercises.

There is corroboration for this in research that has been done to determine whether athletes live longer than nonathletes. *Some* athletes seem to live long, but *others* don't live even as long as the average man or woman. There seems to be an interesting correlation between the type of physical activity and the longevity of the athlete.

In a study of the life spans of athletes listed in *Who's Who in American Sports,* it was found that:

- Football players died at a mean age of fifty-seven.
- Boxers died at a mean age of sixty-one.
- Baseball players died at a mean age of sixty-four.
- Track runners died at a mean age of seventy-one.

Only 65 percent of the football players lived more than fifty years, compared with 87 percent of the runners. Why? It might be because running is a sustained, long-muscle, isotonic exercise. The others are stop-and-go, with substantial periods of layoffs and nonexercise.

## FINDING THE RIGHT AMOUNT OF EXERCISE

There seems to be a minimum time for warming up before the body begins to accrue benefits from exercise. The President's Council on Physical Fitness says you need at least a half hour per day to create any trace of physical fitness. That half hour, incidentally, should involve exercise which pushes your heart to operate at between 70 and 80 percent of its heartbeat capacity. A rough estimate of your heartbeat capacity can be made by subtracting your age from 220 (for instance, a twenty-year-old person would subtract 20 from 220, for a heart rate of 200).

At the minimum, I would recommend a half hour to an hour of walking, twice a day. Two half-hour walks are more productive than a single one-hour walk. If your health is excellent (especially your heart), then ideally you should be jogging. But to jog you must build up your capacity slowly with brief periods of jogging laced with walking. With jogging, the minimum should be a half-hour a day, five days a week.

## HOW EXERCISE BENEFITS THE HEART

Exercise benefits the heart by making it work more efficiently. With regular exercise, the heart can pump blood with less effort. It has more time to rest between beats. And you can exercise for longer periods without getting tired, and respond to physical or emotional crises without racing your heart or raising your blood pressure.

Inactivity is also bad for the heart, as are smoking or high blood pressure. This fact emerged from the famous study of 3,686 active and inactive California longshoremen by Dr. Ralph S. Paffenbarger, Jr., and other investigators. They also found that the combination of inactivity, smoking, and hypertension could raise a person's susceptibility to a fatal heart attack by a factor of twenty! Over a twenty-two-year period, 395 of the inactive longshoremen who were studied died from heart attacks before reaching the age of seventy-five. Dr. Paffenbarger concluded that none of those heart attacks might have happened if all those victims had not smoked, had lowered their blood pressure, and had worked at physically demanding jobs.

Exercise seems also to *prevent* heart disease. Hard, regular exercise develops valuable collateral circulation. This is something the body does even while resting—but the process is speeded up with exercise. Sometimes the new vessels provide enough circulation to replace that blocked by a plaque-choked artery. Statistics show a strong positive relationship between exercise and patients' survival following their first heart attack.

Two studies illustrate this. One was done on 20,000 railroad employees. Office-bound clerks had twice the rate of heart attacks as switchmen. The basic difference was that the switchmen walked around all day and the clerks did not. The second is the longshoremen study we've mentioned. The men suffered fatal heart attacks in direct proportion to the lack of physical effort required to do their work. Office clerks (pity these poor clerks!) had the highest number. Arduous, muscle-tugging chores seemed to protect the toters, pushers, and pullers from heart attacks. Owing to such studies, the noted cardiologist Dr. Paul Dudley White insisted that his famous patient, President Dwight D. Eisenhower, give priority to his golf game—even over affairs of state!

## OTHER BENEFITS

In addition to benefiting the heart, exercise is good because it *burns off fat*—although not all. For instance, it does *not* burn off cholesterol (which is customarily, but erroneously, lumped together with the fats). Only diet can reduce serum cholesterol. But exercise does burn up triglycerides. Just reducing triglycerides is important because they tend to raise uric acid levels which produce gout.

Exercise is also good for mental health. By making the heart more efficient, it improves brain circulation and functioning. A Purdue University researcher, A. H. Ismail, put sixty unfit, older men on a four-month exercise program. At the end of the program, these previously sedentary men appeared to be far more self-confident, emotionally stable, and imaginative than before.

By the same token, *no* exercise is *bad* for your brain. Researchers have found that freshmen coeds who exercise regularly have very few physical complaints. Those who don't flood the medical office with complaints about digestive upsets, fatigue, menstrual discomfort, backaches, colds, and allergies.

Exercise can even dramatically improve your appearance. It gives you better posture. As unsightly fat melts away from hips and buttocks and thighs, and as muscles begin to ripen and ripple where you thought they'd vanished for good, you begin to look better, healthier, and younger. You also develop a rosier complexion because of better circulation. In point of fact, I have found exercise far more beautifying than any surgical face-lift.

Exercise can also relax you. Inactive muscles build up strong electrical charges that can keep you awake. If you exercise and move around a lot, you can discharge these voltages and relax the muscles. Dissipating those electric charges in the muscles is precisely what tranquilizers do. One investigation showed that fifteen minutes of walking lowered those charges more effectively than a popular tranquilizer.

Finally, exercise improves general fitness by providing a smoother flow of energy to the muscles. Good exercise gives your body twice as much glycogen (a starch stored in the muscles and liver) as usual. Glycogen is the athlete's chief fuel. If you have glycogen stored in the muscles, it does not have to be summoned from the liver. That is why athletes have greater endurance and stamina.

## LACK OF EXERCISE

Just as exercising is healthy, not exercising is unhealthy. In one experiment on active young athletes who spent twenty days in bed, it was found that their oxygen intake capacity was reduced by more than a fourth. Their hearts' pumping capacity dropped by the same amount, too. Bed rest has also been shown to deprive the body of up to 15 percent of its red blood cells. The good news is that exercise reverses these lowered levels.

And remember, in our sedentariness, many of us get little more exercise than we would if we were bound to our beds. A group of young men in their twenties who went to bed for between thirty to thirty-six weeks promptly went into a negative calcium balance—and stayed there for the whole of their time in bed. Their loss reached a little over 4 percent of their total calcium supply. This is even worse than it sounds, because in critical weight-bearing areas, such as the heel, the loss ran from a fourth to a half of the total amount of bone!

Incidentally, exercise can correct some calcium loss. Physical activity actually increases the density of the bones used. This is why runners have higher femur bone densities than swimmers.

## QUESTIONS AND ANSWERS

*Which does more for you, walking or jogging?*
All other things being equal, jogging does more for you because it stresses the heart more and makes more demands upon your heart. But people with diseased arteries or bad hearts cannot jog right away. For them, even a walk produces stress—and thus collateral circulation development. Significant physiological improvement may derive from both walking and jogging.

*What happens if I stop exercising?*

It is a mistake to think of the exercise you do today as a capital investment giving you quarterly benefits as long as you live. When you stop exercising, the benefits stop too. Twelve twenty-year-old men embarked on an intensive six-month army physical-training program involving vigorous gymnastics and running four or five times per week. The regimen put them in superb condition. When these men left the army, however, they all stopped exercising. Tested twenty and thirty years later by doctors, the men were found to be no healthier or in better shape than comparable men who had *never* exercised so vigorously.

If you do have to stop exercising for a while, however, remember that you've lost the benefits you had built up and act accordingly. When you resume your exercising, start slowly to reach the level of exercise you left off at. *Do not begin where you left off.* You're probably not ready for it. Warm up for five or ten minutes before you walk or jog vigorously. Then plan for a five- or ten-minute cooling-off period afterwards.

*Is it true that you shouldn't exercise in smog?*

It is true that you're better off exercising vigorously in a smog-free environment than in a polluted environment. It's also safer to *live* in a smog-free environment. Smog contains dangerous carcinogens and threatens the entire respiratory system. Strenuous activity raises your respiratory rate and your smog intake. I would suggest you tone down your exercise in thick smog—but not eliminate it.

*Is it best to walk or jog on an empty stomach?*

Not if you can help it. You should always have *something* in your stomach when you exercise. If you generally exercise at the crack of dawn, then you ought to have a piece of fruit and/or a couple of crackers before leaving home. After eating a full breakfast, some people may find it necessary to wait up to an hour before exercising.

If you jog *without* eating, you throw free fatty acids into your blood. And that's not good. Free fatty acids irritate your muscles—particularly your heart muscle, the myocardium—and are capable of producing ventricular fibrillation and even death. While the risk is small in people with healthy arteries, it is a very real one when there is substantial blockage in the coronary arteries.

### Can't exercise produce a heart attack?

Yes, it can. This seems to happen most often when part of the heart is well nourished and another part is not. The line between the part that is glowing pink with oxygen-rich blood and the part that is turning blue from oxygen starvation, due to plaque narrowing the small arteries feeding that part, is called an "oxygen differential" line.

This differential causes variance in electric potentials of the two parts of the heart. The blue part lessens its potential, causing its voltage to drop well below that of the healthy pink part. This can cause the heart to flutter or fibrillate. A fluttering heart is unable to pump blood effectively. If the flutter is not corrected within six minutes, the possibility of death is great.

To a great extent this can be corrected with exercise—which, as you know, produces collateral arterial growth to enrich the blood supply to starved portions of the heart.

But don't make the mistake of believing that exercise alone can prevent plaque from forming in your arteries. It can't. Only exercise plus diet can do this. I know of two runners, both of them marathonists, who died after marathons. Neither had the right nutritional habits.

### Can exercise rejuvenate old people?

In a very real sense it can. A study by Kenneth H. Sidney of the University of Toronto shows that older people can—after as little as seven weeks of exercise—acquire fitness levels of those ten to twenty years younger. Regardless of their health before starting their exercise programs (walking and calisthenics), these Canadians, all over sixty, began to resemble people a decade or two younger. Both men and women, for example, increased their respiratory power by about 15 percent. That is the normal level for much younger people.

Enough about exercise in general. Now let's get down to the dos and don'ts of the best exercise you can get—and a *dynamite* high.

# 14

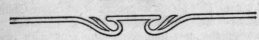

# Walking and Jogging

Man is naturally a walker. In walking, the body becomes more efficient in delivering oxygen to its cells. New circulation is formed which allows the heart to deliver more blood to each muscle with every heartbeat. The constant movements of the legs in walking puts to work the calves, which are powerful pumps. When they contract, the blood inside gets squeezed and pushed upward. When they relax, they suck up more blood from the feet, like a siphon, and move it up to that other superpump, the heart.

## STARTING OUT

One who hasn't walked for a long while should start slowly. If you are out of shape, walk the distance you feel comfortable with. Do this for three days. On the fourth day, increase that distance by 10 percent. Four days later, increase *that* distance by another 10 percent. And so on. This way, you'll be doubling your walking distance in forty days. And it's a safe and effective way to increase your distance.

The speed at which you walk is less important than *distance*. Increase your walking speed only after you've had about forty days of conditioning—and only then. When you do speed up, do it only to the extent that you feel you can manage comfortably.

If you are walking four or five miles at a time, and can maintain a brisk pace, you could be ready for jogging. Anyone over thirty years old should have a stress-treadmill test to ascertain if the heart can tolerate jogging.

If you pass the test, the transition from walking to jogging is easy. Walk sixty seconds, then jog ten seconds at a slow rate. Follow this pattern during your exercise for three to four days. Then increase the jogging time ten seconds, decreasing walking time ten seconds. Changes should be made every two weeks. In a few months, you will be jogging continuously for perhaps twenty minutes—and now you can increase your speed, if you feel the urge.

## THE BEST WAY TO JOG

You'll have to discover your own jogging method for yourself with a little experimenting. You may find that you're accident prone in the morning, and want to schedule your jogging for the afternoon. Your knees may tolerate a smooth asphalt surface better than cinders. You won't know till you try both. You may tire more easily with a shorter stride than a longer one. Preheating (with hot-water bottle or heating pad) the knees in cold weather can make jogging less painful. You may prefer stretching exercises to warm up—or just walking. If you're big, you may need a heavier shoe. If you get pains in the shins or knees or legs, you may need corrective inserts for your shoes.

A poll of 1,000 serious joggers produced this list of ailments, in order of frequency:

1. Runner's knee (cartilage inflammation)
2. Shin splints (pain and tenderness of the lower muscles and tendons between the leg bones)
3. Swollen Achilles tendon
4. Heel bone spurs
5. Small foot-stress fractures

Incidentally, jogging won't increase your appetite unless you're putting in the long, strenuous hours of a professional athlete. Inactivity increases appetite; moderate exercise suppresses appetite. In fact, a good time to exercise is just before dinner. You'll find yourself hungering less and eating less.

## JOGGING STYLE

If you think you'd feel foolish parading around in gym clothes, that problem is easily overcome. If you look around you today, you'll see more and more bright people of both sexes giving their jogging the priority it deserves and outfitting themselves appropriately. If you join them, you will have the satisfaction of knowing you're part of an elite who are doing the best thing to preserve and enrich their lives.

Metropolitan Opera baritone Robert Merrill, who jogs between flights in an airport baggage room, on a landing strip, or even in his hotel room, says: "I just listen to my legs and feet, turn everything off, and my mind becomes very clear."

Dr. Kenneth Cooper, director of the Aerobics Center in Dallas, puts in three miles a day *wherever* he is: on a Pacific atoll or in downtown Tokyo.

Once you perceive how important jogging is to you, you'll have no trouble dressing for the occasion. Nor will you give a second thought to what anyone else is thinking.

In fact, look at it this way: If you're going to be uncomfortable walking or jogging, you might just decide to chuck the whole program. So spoil yourself. Get the very best running shoes you can find to cushion and support your feet. Make sure you won't be too hot or too cold. A light windbreaker or cardigan or zippered jacket you can remove when you get hot often does the trick.

And speaking of shoes, don't fall for the "negative heel" pitch. Had you been wearing negative heels all your life, they might do. But since you haven't, they can cause a stretching of your Achilles tendon in the heel—and cripple you.

Nor are plain old sneakers tough enough for daily jogging. You need cushioned arch support, more than you get from ordinary shoes or sneakers. Each running step you take throws three times your body weight onto each foot—and shoe. Without adequate protection, you risk harming your feet.

One precaution: *Don't* order running shoes by mail. You simply must try them on before buying. Shoe sizes tend to be a bit helter-skelter in the running styles. Your shoes ought to fit like gloves, with just a mite of space at the toe end. You'll want enough heel width for impact spread space; a stiff, hard-leather heel counter on the upper back; no middle cut-out parts; and a padded, raised heel for shock support. The shoes ought to bend naturally and easily to about one-third the way up.

The only big problem with jogging clothes is that often they have no pockets, making it impossible to carry money or housekeys or, as I do, an expired driver's license for identification. The manufacturers seem not to understand that their clothes are being used on country roads and city streets—and not just in school gymnasiums.

## A DYNAMITE HIGH

Jogging seems like a lot of hard work, but joggers say it gives pleasure that cannot be matched. It is an addiction with a dynamite "high." In fact, when a runner is unable to run, he often goes through withdrawal symptoms, becoming unhappy or restless. Experts say that it takes about six to eight weeks before the addiction takes hold. San Diego Mercy Hospital's chief of psychiatry, Dr. Thaddeus Kostrubala, believes running is an addiction that may allow other addicts, such as alcoholics and heroin users, to transfer their allegiance from harmful to healthful peak experiences.

Joggers use words like *ecstasy* and *ethereal* to explain their "high." It arrives in a veteran jogger after a half-hour workout. About ten minutes later, your thoughts begin to organize the disarray of your mind. Insights and concepts and ideas rush through your consciousness. After an hour, you seem to enter a joglike trance of exquisite awareness and sensitivity.

It's not certain just how jogging works on mood. It may work by the increased flow of *epinephrine*, which is sometimes mistakenly referred to as "adrenalin" (actually the synthetic hormone). Epinephrine levels double after only ten minutes of jogging—and much of the supplemental hormone persists even after you've stopped jogging. That may explain why it's hard to worry when you're jogging.

But people don't jog just to reduce depression or anxiety. They do it for many reasons. Deborah Szekely Mazzanti, whose Golden Door spa clients begin and end their day with a run, has a good answer to this question. "What makes people run is that they like themselves very, very much," she says. "*That's* the motivation."


## WALKING WISDOM

Here are some suggestions on walking from former patients at the Pritikin Center.

### *On establishing an exercise priority*

- The problem is one of priorities. *Exercise must have top priority*, one that supersedes everything except your spouse, your children, and the food you eat.
- *The excuse of not being able to find the time is a cop-out.* We find time to sleep because it is mandatory. So is exercise. I get up early enough to run at daybreak. Any other exercise I get is a bonus.
- *You'll never "find the time" for exercise.* You *make* it. You must say, "I am the most important person in the world, and nothing is more important than my life and my walking."
- If it seems silly to give walking top priority, then what can deserve that esteemed position? How about *your life?* But only walking can keep you alive, loving, and functioning at your peak.
- *If your life doesn't mean that much to you, it probably does to those in your family and among your friends who love you.* If you don't owe daily exercise to yourself, you owe it to them.
- *It is unfair to think of exercise taking extra time.* It simply doesn't. With the new energy you've got, you're probably sleeping an hour less per night. Your exercise does not eat into your working, playing, or leisure time at all.
- The way to do it is to *schedule your walks the day before,* and then fit your work schedule into them.

*On getting back on your feet*

- *Company can make a big difference.* Arrange with a friend to take turns waking each other up for a morning walk. It should always be the first item of the day's business with top priority.

- *Arrange a simple schedule* that works well for you. Walk from 6:30 to 7:00 every morning of the week. On weekends take a five-mile walk, starting at 1:00.

- Since *resolve to walk tends to weaken in the afternoon and evening,* make sure that you get a good long walk in before work every morning.

- *Stop driving the car!* For variety, alternate between a bicycle and walking. But remember that walking is a far better exercise.

- *Scale down your wheels.* Use the bike for errands wherever you can and your feet where you used to bicycle. Save the car for blizzards, floods, hurricanes, tornadoes, and warfare!

- Make a point of *parking farther from your destination.*

- *Take longer and more vacations.*

- If you're out for a short stroll, *choose a route with inclines.* That will get your pulse rate up faster.

- *Walk to work.*

- *Save your weekends* for interesting cultural, historical, nature, or just plain fun walks.

- *Get a dog.* (If you have any humanitarian impulses at all, that will get you out walking three times a day.)

- Walking can be terrific fun if you occasionally *go bargain hunting* through markets, department stores, malls, esplanades and shopping centers.

- *Watch out for erratic drivers,* especially on blind turns where there are no sidewalks.

- *If* you're in shape, *sweep the snow* from porches, walks, and the car. That will help get your circulation going.

- If you've nothing better, *walk up and down your driveway or around the yard.* But calculate the distance you're walking. Remember that 750 steps equals ¼ mile.

- If it's impossible for you to get up much before leaving for work, at least strive for a half-hour morning walk. Then save your longer walk for the afternoon.

- You can use a swimming pool deck as a promenade or jogging track. But pace it off so you know how far around it is.
- *Walk or jog around the local school cinder track early in the morning.* If you time yourself, you can monitor the improvement.
- If you're only going to have one walk a day, plan to make it *at least an hour.*
- Eventually, if you're in the pink, shoot for making at least *three ten-mile strenuous walks* each week. But tailor your schedule for yourself and, above all, *don't make invidious comparisons* with others. Increase your distance *gradually.*
- *Vary your routes.*

### On jogging and running

- If you're vacationing at a *higher altitude,* remember that your body has to work harder to do the same amount of work. So *take it easier.*
- Use the foot stroke that many runners find *the least traumatic:* coming down with the full flat of the foot in order to distribute the weight over the greatest area.
- Keep your *head erect, arms down, body loose, legs straight up and down and parallel to your motion.*
- The best surface for either walking or jogging is *grass.* The worst is *cement or rocks.*
- The best shoes are long-distance running shoes that *fit well,* have considerable *cushioning* where the foot strikes the ground, and *do not slip* around.
- *Attend to any redness or blisters* that pop up—immediately.
- *Don't run in oppressive heat or after large meals.*
- *Avoid very hot showers* after a session.

### On bad weather and indoor exercise

*If you use your head, you can always* figure out a way of getting in your daily walk(s), no matter what kind of weather prevails. Here are some ideas:

- Find the *largest indoor space* you can for inclement weather. This might be a barn, warehouse, department store, shopping mall, subway interchange, building concourse, or your own basement.
- Get a *stationary bicycle.*
- Get a *treadmill.* Your speed can be controlled, your incline and distance can be measured, and there are no space limitations or traffic hazards.
- *Walk around a TV set* in your basement.
- Listen to *music* while you're walking indoors.
- If you're housebound by the weather, *vary your walking route* by doing circles and figure eights and taking different routes.
- *Measure off a block on your terrace or in your basement.* That way you can walk with complete informality, nude or all dressed up, watching TV or listening to music, and know just how far you've walked.
- Dip your toe into the exercise pool by starting off with nothing more complicated than *using the stairs instead of the elevator.*

## HOW TO TELL IF YOU'RE OVERDOING IT

It is important not to walk or jog faster than you should. This adaptation of the internationally used Harvard Step Test may help you to find out if you are overdoing it.

- After a walk or jog, stop and rest for a full minute.
- Count your pulse. (Multiply a thirty-second count by two.)
- If your pulse exceeds 130, slow down for the next time out and thereafter.
- When you're really in shape, your one-minute pulse should be about 100—even if you've been exercising strenuously.

Now that you've learned how simple the Pritikin Program really is, you may want to know more about its effectiveness. If the next part of the book won't convince you, nothing will!

# THREE

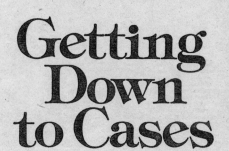

# Getting Down to Cases

# 15

## Histories

*. . . If I feel any better, I will
have to consider additional surgery—
a vasectomy!*
Everett Ramsay, after
leaving the Pritikin
Center in 1977

The following case histories demonstrate the kind of results that may be obtained on the Pritikin Program. Each participant has a great story to tell, and the history of the Pritikin Program boasts many similar success stories.

The Pritikin Program is more than a method of tapering chins and fannies. It transforms sick people into healthy people. And it keeps them healthy.

There is a similarity of story line for most of the histories. It runs like this: Patient suffers for years; patient becomes critically ill; doctors try surgery, drugs; surgery, drugs fail; patient discovers Pritikin Program, tries it as last resort; patient gets better, stays better.

These stories make it clear that the program is greater than any of its parts. Several of these patients had been assiduous followers of one or another health regimen. Some had been Weight Watchers. Others had followed the American Heart Association and other low-calorie, low-fat diets. Some had been joggers. Yet none succeeded in solving his or her major complaints before embarking on the Pritikin Program.

Most of these people had been treated at the first Pritikin Center in California. Any seriously ill person (i.e., anyone on medication) ought to be monitored by a physician while on the program—as those at the Pritikin Centers are.

Although spectacular reversals of serious illnesses have been achieved independently, the Centers offer certain advantages. They make dieting easier for most people, since they control nutritional intake and exercise, eliminate temptations, indoctrinate the dieter, compute daily progress, and apply the magic of peer pressure and enthusiasm.

But when you come right down to it, the good results come from just two factors: *consistently* eating the right food and *consistently* performing the right exercise.

There is a school of opinion that holds that case histories prove nothing; that only double-blind, controlled testing produces irrefutable "proof."

I disagree. While I cannot isolate the precise factors in my program that cause dramatic reversals of serious illnesses, I know that nothing else known to medical science or nutrition performs as well as the diet and exercise we offer. And controlled, blind testing is impossible for a diet-exercise regimen taking place in an intimate setting such as ours. In a blind test, the investigators and subjects are supposed to be unaware of who is a control and who is an experimental subject. At the Center, however, it would be very difficult to conceal whether or not one is eating meat, smoking a cigarette, using salt, or drinking liquor.

Near the end of this book you will find an evaluation of the results obtained with the first 900 patients at the Pritikin Center.

## CASE HISTORY 1: AUTHOR

     *Name*:   Nathan Pritikin
      *Age*:   Sixty-three
*Indications*:   Hypercholesterolemia, atherosclerosis, posterior wall myocardial ischemia

Years before discovering my own health problem, I had become intrigued with nutrition. During World War

II, I saw classified documents showing European deaths from heart disease and diabetes dropping dramatically. This struck me as peculiar, because I had always been taught that atherosclerosis-related conditions like heart disease were caused by stress. What could produce more stress among the civilian population than war itself with its food rationing, fire bombings, and anarchy?

Equally paradoxical was the fact that by 1958 cardiovascular deaths in Austria, for instance, leaped to a level seven times higher than during the war. Nutritionists wondered if the end of food rationing (particularly of foods high in animal fats, cholesterol, protein, and sugar) might not explain those figures. They also began to ponder the conventional medical wisdom on the origins of heart disease.

I was not alone in my fascination for these wartime mortality data. Dr. Lester Morrison thought they could be useful, too. He placed fifty of his heart-attack patients on a diet mimicking the low-cholesterol, low-fat wartime fare Europeans survived on, and another fifty on the conventional American diet.

The study was to last twelve years. But in 1955 I learned that the experimental group's cholesterol levels had already dropped from an average of 312 mg./percent to 220 mg./percent, while the control group's levels stayed the same. Over half (56 percent) of the experimental group's patients were still alive, compared with 24 percent of the controls. By 1960, all of the control group had died, while 38 percent of the low-fat, low-cholesterol group were still alive.

Mainly out of curiosity, I visited Morrison in California. As he described his work, I asked him if he would do a cholesterol test on me. He did. My first reading was in the neighborhood of 300—which Morrison described as in the "high normal" range.

From then on I did nothing but *watch* my cholesterol level. *Doing* something about it was out of the question. How could I possibly give up my pint of ice cream after dinner? I ate bread with my butter, not the other way around. I devoured bowls of whipped cream, crammed several eggs down my gullet for breakfast. I estimate that

my cholesterol level was probably 300 or more for at
least twenty years.

"A 300 cholesterol?" said Morrison. "Nothing to worry
about. But don't let it get any higher than that." Then he
had me do a Master's Two-Step stress electrocardiogram
test. It showed some coronary insufficiency. Nothing to
worry about. It, too, was "normal." Morrison suggested,
nonetheless, that I have another cardiogram—just to be
safe.

Two years later, after moving to Santa Barbara, I finally consulted a cardiologist at the Sansum Clinic and
had another stress test. The cardiologist told me I had
"substantial coronary heart disease," according to the
same Master's Two-Step I'd taken in Morrison's office.
"Posterior wall myocardial ischemia" was the exact diagnosis.

What should I do? I was told to stop all exercise, stop
climbing stairs, take it easy. I began to nap in the after-
noons. I became a typical cardiac case. When they put me
on drugs, I really got scared. Sure, they were the doctors.
They ought to know what was right. But it was *my* life.

My readings of population studies had convinced me
that dangerous arterial plaque would form at any cholesterol level over 160. If I could just get my high cholesterol level down, I figured I might have a chance of
surviving. But what diet would lower serum cholesterol?

I visited the UCLA medical school's department of nutrition and talked to a woman in charge. Would she
recommend a graduate student who could help me design
a diet to lower my blood cholesterol? "Ridiculous!" she
snapped. "You *can't* control your cholesterol level. The
one you have is what nature *intended* you to have."

"Still, I'd like to try," I said.

"Absurd! If you did succeed, you'd probably get very
sick. For one thing, you will run into vitamin deficiencies,
mineral deficiencies, and you won't be getting essential
animal protein."

Since I couldn't get professional help, I decided to start
the diet changes on my own. I was frightened. But I was
also obstinate. Out of caution, I had every imaginable test
done on me while I went about my experimenting: for vitamin levels, mineral levels, fat levels, liver function—you

name it. These were repeated regularly. The problem was that there was no accurate information on what would happen to me on a low-cholesterol diet. Since I was operating on no authority but my own, I was prepared for the worst.

By April 1958 I had become a practicing vegetarian. By May, my cholesterol had fallen to 162. Still my stress tests failed to show any improvement in heart function.

I had long before stopped eating *all animal protein,* even ice cream and milk and eggs. This time I seemed to hit pay dirt. With my vegetarian diet, my cholesterol plummeted to 120 by January 1960. Even more important, I was rewarded with my first normal electrocardiogram! Admittedly, it was taken while I was sitting down—not during stress. (In the two decades since then, by the way, my cholesterol level has stabilized between 100 and 125. As of this writing it is 107.)

Now I was ready for increasing my coronary circulation. In 1960 I started to increase my walking, and gradually started to jog. Proceeding very slowly, I was running for an hour continuously by 1965.

The news that I had outfoxed the Grim Reaper's cardiac division came home to me in 1966. I took a stress treadmill test, which is a far more rigorous and exacting measure of heart condition and performance than the old Master's Two-Step. When I stepped onto the treadmill, I felt confident. After all, by now I could run about eight miles without stopping. For twenty minutes I ran at a rate of 177 beats per minute—with not a trace of coronary insufficiency.

I felt then, and feel now, that I had found a solution for reversing coronary artery closure. Remember, only six years earlier my coronary arteries were closing up. I was not getting enough blood into the heart even when I was sitting motionless. Now, with maximum physical exertion, I was developing no coronary insufficiency at all.

## CASE HISTORY 2: CO-AUTHOR

*Name*:       Patrick M. McGrady, Jr.
*Age*:        Forty-five
*Indications*:  Obesity, mild arthritis, chest pains, hypertension

The dinner party was enjoyable until a woman sitting across from me said with a saccharine smile, "How can a man who writes about staying young let himself go as you have?"

She was not the first to comment on my blossoming paunch and jowls, but her remark exposed the yawning gap between my preoccupation with the subject of "youth" treatments and my reluctance to try anything that might stave off the ravages that time was working upon me.

As a medical writer, I was well aware that diet and exercise can strongly influence how quickly or how slowly a person ages. But which diet was best? What kind of exercise? Even the experts couldn't seem to agree. And I had yet to come across a nutritionally sound diet that guaranteed sufficient rewards to convince me to abandon the joys of indulgence for the agonies of food skimping. What's more, I had always hated *dutiful* exercise.

As a result, I had grown fat and sluggish. At age forty-three, I was carrying around at least thirty pounds more than my six-foot, one-inch frame should have had to support. I napped often and felt anything but energetic.

Moreover, I suffered chronic arthritis pains in the elbows, fingers, shoulders, and knees. Also vague chest pains. These were not angina, because they did not get worse when I exercised. But they were scary. A cardiologist I consulted handed me several sets of pills: amphetamines for weight loss, nitroglycerin pills for the chest pains, and some tranquilizers. The pills were frightening and I decided to chuck them.

It was a phone call from my friend Paul Glenn, a philanthropist who had sponsored several research projects on aging, that prompted me to look into a new diet and exercise program. "This call may just save your life," he said. "You're overweight and you probably have high blood pressure. Nathan Pritikin is the brightest nutritionist I've ever met. In time, he'll probably change the eating and exercise habits of the world. Take some time off to try the four-week program he's giving in Santa Barbara. I've been on the Pritikin regimen for a couple of years now, and I've never felt better."

Four weeks! It seemed like an eternity. Everything else I was doing seemed so much more important than my health: my writing, my kids (I'm a bachelor father), my consultations, my radio and TV guest appearances, my lectures.

Two things convinced me to go. One was that I could regard the trip to the coast as business and do a magazine article. (Only business seems to have top priority in the American male's scheme of things.) Second was the fact that Paul would not get excited about anything but a first-rate idea. He was too sharp. We were part of a founding group that launched the American Aging Association and were familiar with quackery and fringe medical ideas. Both of us were hardnosed enough not to recommend any program until it had proven itself.

I checked Nathan Pritikin out with another friend, the gerontologist-biochemist Johan Bjorksten, whose name I noted was on Pritikin's advisory board. Bjorksten felt that the ultimate rejuvenation-life-extension treatment would be some biochemical agent that would reverse the bonds of molecular cross-linkage that wreak havoc with our cellular and organic functioning as we age. In the meantime, though, nutrition and exercise that could suppress formation of those cross-linkages would be extremely important, he felt. He himself, he said, abided by a Pritikin style of living. And he suggested that such a life-style could mean anywhere from twenty to thirty extra years of good living for me.

I enrolled in the four-week program. Within four days, I began to feel exuberant. I definitely didn't want to lose that feeling, so I behaved myself. I even (with occasional brief lapses) gave up cigars and coffee—difficult habits to overcome since for years I had needed them at my side in order to write.

Within those four weeks, I dropped twenty-three pounds, from 252 to 229. It was delightful! I could bend from the waist without effort, with no paunch to block the motion! Just walking on my newly muscular legs, feeling the spring in my feet, was a thrill.

A strong sense of competition developed among the members of our group as we strove to lose weight, reduce our blood pressure, improve our blood profiles, increase our walking distances, and get off drugs. The motivation to stick to the program was provided by those early, eye-opening benefits and the evening lecture by Nathan Priti-kin, explaining every aspect of the diet and exercise program and answering patients' questions.

A year and a half later, I am still on the diet. I now jog for thirty minutes every morning and walk for another thirty later in the day. My blood pressure has stayed normal (except for two or three weeks when I went off the diet) and I've lost still another fourteen pounds.

The chest pains seem gone for good. The arthritis returns only when I go off the diet. And I have a new optimistic outlook—I know I can feel and act younger thanks to the *certainties* of this program. No small part of the optimism has been due to the fact that women, even the ones I'm interested in, look at me longer and harder.

## CASE HISTORY 3: PHYSICIAN

*Name*:  Ben Zimmerman
*Age*:  Fifty
*Indications*:  Severe coronary heart disease, angina, blocked coronary bypass

George Bernard Shaw regarded a sick doctor as the most tragic thing in the world, and Dr. Ben Zimmerman's case was at least pathetic.

He had had angina for fifteen years, worsening over the past three. Sometimes it took several nitroglycerin pills to get him across a room or a street. In July 1975, following an abnormal treadmill test, he had the plaque removed from his carotid artery.

Zimmerman is a barrel of a man, a robust five foot, nine inches, and an active general practitioner. For years he had been known as a gourmet. Now suddenly he was another cardiac cripple who smeared his chest with Ni-tro-Bid Ointment and took at least fifty nitros orally to combat the angina attacks. His practice just limped along, too.

After four episodes of coronary heart failure following his customary high-fat meals, he had a coronary angiogram and, in August 1975, scheduled himself for bypass surgery.

For a short time, the bypass seemed to have solved some of his trouble. In six weeks he was walking two miles a day. But four days later his limit plummeted to two blocks. Every few steps, he found himself reaching for a nitro. After meals the angina became almost intolerable.

A new angiogram confirmed that his bypass had clogged completely and the atherosclerotic plaques seemed to be proliferating elsewhere. Since the last pictures, taken nine months earlier, blockage of his right coronary had risen from 30 to 50 percent.

The Fort Worth surgeons told him that another operation was out of the question. He grasped at a straw—the chance that he could be helped by the Pritikin Program.

On arrival at the Center, Zimmerman weighed in at 219 pounds and lasted only four minutes on the treadmill and a half mile on the walking paths. His heartbeat was irregular with many preventricular contractions. His drugs included Inderal, Catapres, Zyloprim, Atromid, Lasix, Ni-tro-Bid Ointment, and nitroglycerin pills. Thanks to medication, he was keeping his blood pressure to 170/100.

Although he had never been able to lose weight before, in his first week at the Center he lost five pounds. His after-dinner bouts with angina diminished considerably—enough for him to call attention to the fact. In his impatience to cut down his drugs, however, he went off them too fast and suffered a setback the next weekend.

His second week was a good one. He was now walking eight to ten miles per day, and made a 400 percent improvement on the treadmill by lasting sixteen minutes. The walking had provoked some problems: shin splints, blisters, ankle sprain, pulled ligaments, and low-back problems. But he was delighted with the reduction in irregular heartbeats, the increased exercise tolerance that enabled him to increase his heart rate from 94 to 110, and the better blood picture.

By month's end, Dr. Zimmerman had lowered his blood pressure to 110 or 120 over 70. He was climbing real hills and averaging only four nitros on good days. He was walking thirteen to fifteen miles a day with no trouble and had lost twenty-two pounds. To say that he was thrilled with the results is to understate his excitement.

Seventeen months later, during a follow-up interview, the doctor said he has returned to a bustling, full-time general practice, spending two days a week in surgery. (He was even well enough to attend the Orange Bowl game and root raucously with little or no pain.)

His blood pressure has stabilized at 115/90 with no medication. He spends at least a half hour to an hour daily walking or bicycling.

He adheres to the Pritikin Diet with about 95 percent fidelity, thanks to the elimination of all meat, save fish and chicken, and the fresh garden vegetables he keeps in his office refrigerator. His most recent lab tests showed a cholesterol hovering around 200 and a triglyceride level under 100.

Incidentally, Dr. Zimmerman has introduced nutrition counseling into his practice. It's a case of preaching what he learned to practice the hard way.


## CASE HISTORY 4: TV PERSONALITY

*Name*: Jack Barry
*Age*: Fifty-eight
*Indications*: Mild obesity, cardiac ischemia, hypertension

Since visiting the Pritikin Center six months ago, I've lost forty-five pounds. I've put back maybe two or three. To put them back, I eat like a horse.

On my annual physical, I had a poor treadmill result. I could have ignored it, but everybody said: "You've got to do something. Diet, exercise, something."

I'd heard about the Center from three former patients in Palm Springs. They had such glowing things to say about it that when my doctor said merely "some diet" and "some exercise," I decided to go whole hog and go to Santa Barbara. I'm very pleased that I did.

I lost about twenty pounds at the center, but the big weight loss came when I got home—maybe twenty-eight more pounds when I got back.

I had been a moderate drinker, and I stopped altogether.

Actually, the weight loss was sort of devastating to me. I had mixed emotions. If I were younger and trying to carve out a career for myself, I'd probably try harder to put *back* some weight. But I have a very successful show called *"The Joker's Wild"* which plays all over the United States and should play for years. So I'm not concerned. Nobody can take me off my own show.

It's hard for me to put weight back on now. I eat enough grains in the morning to feed a thoroughbred.

My last two EKGs showed some improvement in the duration of time on the treadmill and in my strength.

I feel just super—I say that without qualification! I jog two or three miles every morning. I have a very cooperative wife, and my food is very judiciously prepared. She's been super. My kids rebelled at the diet, but little by little—seeing me—they eat some of my stuff and find it isn't all that ghastly.

I've never felt this good in my life, but I don't know why. I felt well when I went to the Center, but I feel more alive, more alert now. Maybe it's just the weight loss.

It's a kind of *joie de vivre*. I hope you won't laugh when I tell you that I feel like laughing and singing a lot. I never felt this way before—except when I had some very good news. There's a correlation, I feel, between a feeling of well-being and mental and emotional stability.

My blood pressure? It's beyond belief! I just took it twenty minutes ago: 122 over 78 this morning. When I went to the Center, it was 160 over 95. I had been plagued with bad blood pressure all of my adult life, having had scarlet fever at fourteen, and high-blood pressure and rapid pulse ever since.

For the first time in my life, I am off *all* medication. When I went up there, I want to tell you that I was *loaded* with medication: Inderal, Aldomet, and all the other drugs they give you for high blood pressure, all the diazides.

I was apprehensive about going off them, but Pritikin's doctors said try. My doctor at home did not want me to go off them. But I did it on my own—with much trepidation. That was four months ago. My blood pressure is still down, and I feel no need for them.

All I know is that I've never felt better in my life.

## CASE HISTORY 5: NONAGENARIAN

|  |  |
|---|---|
| *Name*: | Eula Weaver |
| *Age*: | Ninety |
| *Indications*: | Intermittent claudication, angina, hypertension, advanced atherosclerosis, arthritis |

If you think you're too old to profit from the Pritikin Program, or that you can't work small health miracles on your own, consider the case of Eula Weaver.

As she rounded her eightieth year, Mrs. Weaver was ready to throw in the towel. Her circulation was so bad she wore gloves in the summer. After walking no farther than fifty feet from home, this one-hundred-pound, five-foot, three-inch woman would occasionally have to be carried back. Three blocks was a long walk, and if her calves didn't buckle from cramps, angina dissuaded her from walking more.

At sixty-seven, she began treatment for angina. At seventy-five she was hospitalized with a myocardial infarct. At eighty-one she suffered congestive heart failure.

She got by with drugs: aspirin for arthritis; Pro-Banthine for the GI tract; Arlidin as a vasodilator; Digoxin for the heart; nitroglycerin for her angina; Aldomet, Esidrix, and K-lyte for her high blood pressure.

But it was *just* getting by. She became bedridden and could barely shuffle across the room. It was the unpleasant specter of the bedpan, spoon-feeding, and being dressed by others for the remainder of her life that made her resolve to do something about her condition.

Under constant supervision, she began the Pritikin Program at home in 1970. In one year's time she had freed herself from all drugs. Her circulation improved. So did her walking performance.

Within two years (at eighty-two) she was walking three miles and riding ten miles daily on her stationary bicycle. She was also jogging a quarter-mile every day.

In 1975 she entered the National Senior Olympics in Irvine, California. In five years she won ten gold medals and a plaque running the half-mile and one-mile events.

At ninety she is faithful to the diet, jogs one mile daily, lifts light weights twice weekly, and feels fit as a fiddle. On occasional visits to the Pritikin Center, she inspires the patients with her vitality and enthusiasm.

## CASE HISTORY 6: AIRLINE PILOT

        *Name*:    R.P.
         *Age*:    Fifty-eight
*Indications*:    Diabetes, hypertension

On a routine physical, this TWA pilot from Clearwater, Florida, discovered that he had elevated blood sugar and a strikingly positive glucose tolerance test which was diagnosed as diabetes. He arrived at the Center on August 9, 1976.

His blood pressure, treated with drugs, was right at the top of the Federal Aviation Administration limit—and he was suspended from flying.

By the end of his month's stay, R.P. had a completely normal glucose tolerance test and a normal blood pressure—130/70—without medication.

When he returned home, he was permitted to resume flying. After one year, he was still flying, his diabetes and hypertension relics of the past. The only time he has trouble sticking to the diet, he says, is when he's flying.

Not all of his symptoms vanished immediately. An old leg pain diagnosed as intermittent claudication remained, but was more easily tolerated. He never had to stop jogging on account of it. And although the atherosclerosis was clearly present, the high blood pressure, blood fats, and cholesterol levels came down to normal by the end of his stay.

## CASE HISTORY 7: HOUSEWIFE

  *Name*:       M.C.
   *Age*:       Middle-aged
*Indications*:  Constipation

We have never found anyone who remained constipated for long on the Pritikin Program. M.C. was no exception.

For over twenty years she had bowel movements only by recourse to enemas and laxatives. Sometimes she would have to struggle for over three hours to succeed. This handicap made most of her life miserable.

Her diet before coming to the Center had been the average American diet: highly refined foods practically devoid of fiber. At the Pritikin Center she went on a diet of unrefined foods full of natural fiber. The natural fiber absorbs water, making the feces bulky, soft, and easy to eliminate. Dr. Denis Burkitt puts it well: "What goes in soft comes out hard; what comes in hard goes out soft."

Within ten days at the center, M.C. had her first natural, unassisted bowel movement—and ever since has been constipation-free.

## CASE HISTORY 8: HYPERTENSIVE JOGGER

  *Name*:       Charles McCullen
   *Age*:       Fifty-four
*Indications*:  Essential hypertension, atherosclerosis, intermittent claudication

On September 29, 1976, Charles McCullen checked into the Pritikin Center with little working in his favor aside from the fact that he was a jogger. His father and mother both had died of heart disease, at forty-eight and fifty-nine, respectively. One of his sisters had died of a heart attack at thirty-eight, a second of cancer at sixty.

His major complaint was pain in his left leg while jogging. His blood pressure, controlled by drugs, was 160/105. His diet included sausages, eggs, milk, cream, peanut butter and other nuts, margarine, mayonnaise, vegetable oils, coffee, and soft drinks.

Within a few days, McCullen stopped taking all of his medications, which included Aldomet, Atromid S, and Diazide.

When he left the Center, nearly a month later, his blood pressure had gone down to 120/70, without drugs; his weight from 175 to 163, a 12-pound loss; his cholesterol from 360 to 189; his triglycerides from 658 to 185; and his total lipids from 1,447 to 536!

## CASE HISTORY 9: A "DYING" MAN

*Name*:     Norman Rosenberg
*Age*:      Sixty
*Indications*:   Diabetes, clogging triple coronary bypasses, gallstones, angina

For a quarter of a century, I had been diabetic. I was on thirty-five daily units of insulin, 320 milligrams of Inderal, as well as antidepressants, tranquilizers, Demerol, and other pain-killers.

I also had a bad heart. In August 1972 I had a triple coronary bypass operation. This was followed by severe angina attacks that failed totally to respond to nitroglycerin pills or Isordil. Only Percodan and Demerol seemed to ease the anguish.

The pain, I was assured by my doctor, was merely a sign of "healing." I knew better. When I had my second angiogram, it showed that one of the bypass vessels had vanished altogether, a second was totally clogged, and only the third was working. They operated again—and again I felt chest pains.

This time the pain was due to surgical clips that had come undone and began to extrude through the skin. But more pain followed. A third angiogram showed much scarring of the heart muscle, adhesions, and enough of a mess to dissuade my surgeon from opening me up again.

I tried to get a more optimistic prognosis. In the winter of 1975, I had a fourth angiogram at the Mayo Clinic, plus an impressive battery of tests given cardiac patients.

The doctor's verdict was this (I remember his exact words): "Your way of life from now on will be this: You will walk, do whatever you have to do, and when the pain becomes too great, you will take Demerol."

And that's just how I did live. I became a vegetable. I refused to leave my bed. I'd wait for the pain to come, and it came more and more rapidly, then I'd pop a Demerol. I couldn't stand it.

"Either I find help," I told my wife, Beatrice, "or I put all my pills in a glass and swallow them all at once." In my youth I'd been an athlete at college and then in the service: I played and loved baseball, football, basketball. This life wasn't worth living.

That very day Beatrice had come across an article (by Benno Isaacs) in *New York* magazine about a Nathan Pritikin. He wasn't a doctor. What was he? A charlatan? A healer? Or what? She checked him out, and by the very next weekend I was on a plane bound for Santa Barbara.

I ought to add that before leaving for Santa Barbara I had my gallbladder removed. A so-called "common duct" takes over its function. Well, it turned out that I had, according to my X rays, a huge stone blocking the common duct. They postponed operating, since my doctors felt that I was dying.

I could hardly believe how fast I improved at the Center. By my fourth week, I was down to five units of insulin. Mr. Pritikin wanted my doctor to take me off the last five, which he did soon after I returned home. I haven't taken insulin since. That was December 1976.

I also took my last Demerol at the Center—and haven't touched the stuff since. In fact, I went off all of my other drugs. I take a Valium every now and then when I feel a bit uptight. But I have no pain whatever.

By the end of my stay there, I began to feel like an entirely new person. I was walking and jogging up to ten miles a day. My last cholesterol level was 142, my triglyceride 65 (that's within Pritikin's recommended limits, by the way). My glucose tolerance level is down to 95.

Only one thing worried me. A year later I began to

have pains where my gallbladder had been. My doctor at the New York University Medical Center looked at my old X rays and announced that he would proceed with surgery in five days.

Fortunately, I had engaged a nutrition-oriented doctor to monitor my progress and he insisted I have more X rays before being operated on.

I asked the surgeon if it wasn't possible for the stone to pass through and be dissolved.

"Yes," he said sarcastically, "that stone will pass through the same as you might open that window, jump out, fall sixteen floors, land on your feet, and walk away!"

New X rays were taken. When the surgeon saw them, he yelled "You did it again! I can't believe it!" The pain I had felt was the stone pushing itself through. And it *had* dissolved. Operation cancelled.

I am convinced if it weren't for the Pritikin Program, I wouldn't be here today. And I feel terrific. I'm now happily fulfilling a dream I've always had: buying and selling antiques. And I just made a trip to Europe and found it no trouble sticking to my diet 100 percent, just as I do at home.

### *Postscript from Beatrice Rosenberg:*

While accompanying Norman to Santa Barbara and following his diet, I went from a size 14 to a size 8 in one year. My blood pressure went down from 180/90 on medication to 112/60 on none. I feel so much better, too. My change wasn't the renaissance that it was for Norman, but I feel lighter, less frightened. And now, for the first time in my life, I no longer regard food as a devastating, killing thing. I actually enjoy eating!

### CASE HISTORY 10: NURSE

*Name*:  Major Jean Innes
*Age*:  Sixty-six
*Indications*:  Arthritis, claudication

This retired army nurse's main complaint was a serious intermittent claudication in her right leg. Because of reduced blood flow, caused by atherosclerosis, she experienced pain when she walked. Doctors were advising bypass leg surgery.

Arthritis had also clenched her hand and badly swollen the joints of her right little finger. To write Christmas cards, she had to stick a bunion pad under the finger to keep it from touching the desk. Any contact on the finger created pain.

During her stay at the Pritikin Center, the swelling in the little finger went down completely. After five years of impaired function, she was now able to use it effortlessly, without pain. In other parts of her body afflicted by arthritis, the pains have subsided dramatically, too.

The major benefit, to her mind, has been the eradication of the pains from claudication and of the prospect of surgery. She now walks five miles every other day.

"I don't feel good if I don't walk," she says. "It's improved the quality of my life, my mental brightness, my attitude, my sense of well-being."

At home, she sticks to the diet. In restaurants, she occasionally has salad dressing with oil. And although she scorns desserts, she still cannot resist penny licorice whips.

An inveterate camper, she always takes with her an icebox full of soups, lasagne, and frozen foods Pritikin-style.


## CASE HISTORY 11: THE EXPECTANT MOTHER

      *Name*:    E.P.
       *Age*:    Thirty-one
*Indication*:    Pregnancy

When she became pregnant six years ago, E.P. adopted the Pritikin Program as a means of assuring maximum health for her unborn child.

She was faithful to most of the program's principles, studiously avoiding medications, additives, preservatives, liquor, tea, and coffee. She did yield occasionally to several of the cravings pregnant women traditionally succumb to: ice cream, salted wheat crackers, and doughnuts.

She exercised vigorously during her pregnancy, jogging for the first seven months, riding a stationary bicycle the last two. She also performed appropriate exercises at a local gymnasium for the duration of her pregnancy.

The Lamaze Method worked perfectly for her: her labor was brief, the delivery smooth. Her son was born, as she put it, "supremely healthy."

According to the Apgar Score,* E.P.'s baby had an unusual, "perfect" rating of 10, which E.P. attributes in good part to the diet and exercise program she followed.

## CASE HISTORY 12: HEAVYWEIGHT

*Name*:        Julian L. Torgerson
*Age*:         Fifty-four
*Indications*: Obesity, atherosclerotic cardiovascular disease, intermittent claudication, hypertension

At 353 pounds, financier Torgerson had difficulty making his way about the walking routes of the Santa Barbara Center. His obesity was compounded by: edema in the feet and legs; a peculiar angina that struck during rest (and not with stress); gout in the left big toe; borderline diabetes; and hypertension.

Prior to admission, he got practically no exercise except summer swimming. He smoked four cigars a day and worked under considerable pressure.

In Santa Barbara, he began by walking a mile a day and slowly upped his distance to five miles. By day's end, the exercise had exhausted him. But the diet-exercise program paid off handsomely.

His blood pressure, which had been as high as 220/120 and for which he had taken various medications, dropped to a normal 120/70. His serum cholesterol dropped 40 percent, his triglycerides by half, and total lipids by 30 percent. He no longer smokes.

* The Apgar Score evaluates a newborn infant's condition by assigning a point system for heart rate, respiratory effort, muscle tone, reflex irritability, and skin color.

The loss of excess weight was perhaps the most dramatic benefit of his sojourn. His weigh-in poundage was reduced by 31 pounds to 322! Moreover, within the next month he lost another 17 pounds.

His attitude has also improved dramatically. Instead of delegating his many responsibilities to associates, he has begun to execute more detail work himself.

The case above is compelling testimony to the efficacy of the Pritikin Program for obese persons. Further testimonies come through our mailbox, as we shall see in the next chapter.

# 16

## Letters

For many people, the Pritikin Program is more than a diet-exercise plan—it is a new, challenging life-style. The impact on the new dieter is considerable, and we get letters to that effect. With the permission of the authors, we present a sampling of our mail.*

### January 15–February 10, 1977

My wife and I have been following the LRI diet since last February and both of us showed spectacular improvements in our annual physical checkups this year. We are particularly impressed because for quite a few years before last February we had been following the fat-controlled, low-cholesterol died recommended by the American Heart Association.

I am now sixty-two years old, run two miles (approximately sixteen minutes) daily, and walk briskly another one-and-one-quarter miles.

A brief summary of my blood values is contained in the following chart.

| Date | 11/5/71 | 3/19/73 | 10/22/74 | 5/17/76 |
|---|---|---|---|---|
| Age | 57 | 58 1/2 | 60 | 61 1/2 |
| Cholesterol | 260 | 245 | 240 | 170 |
| Triglycerides | — | — | — | 98 |
| Blood pressure | 130/65 | 130/65 | 120/70 | 110/70 |
| Resting pulse rate | 80 | 70 | 70 | 60 |

The 5/17/76 data were taken three months after starting the LRI diet on 2/14/76.

* In some of these letters authors refer to the Longevity Research Institute (L.R.I.) or L.R.I. Diet, which are earlier names used in connection with the Pritikin Centers and Diet.

My cholesterol intake had been somewhat limited for over twenty years (nonfat milk, margarine instead of butter, bacon and eggs for breakfast once a week). I started following the American Heart Association diet sometime in 1970.

In 1971 I stopped smoking and started a daily exercise program on a bicycle exerciser. A jogging program was substituted for the bicycle exerciser on 11/1/73. I am now running three days out of every four and taking a one-hour brisk walk on the fourth day. Needless to say, I am still following the LRI diet enthusiastically.

Ernest W. Pierce
Rolling Hills Estates, California

August 30, 1976

My daughter, a physical therapist, introduced me to your book, *Live Longer Now*. I have never been a health food addict and always believed that eating in moderation was healthy. Naturally I thought I ate in moderation.

I am fifty-two years old and after reading your book decided to follow your diet and exercise program in order to improve my general health. I began the day after Thanksgiving, 1975. Despite eating heartily, within a month or two I lost ten to fifteen pounds. I also noticed an unexpected dividend—a distinct decrease in the frequency of headaches, which, in varying degrees, I had been experiencing weekly during most of my adult life. After several months I was certain that my headaches had virtually disappeared. In addition to adhering to your diet (with minor exceptions) I am on a walking program consisting of a daily three-mile walk at a four-mile-per-hour pace.

No one in the medical profession or otherwise had been any help previously. I am now happier, feel better, am more productive in my profession and in general cannot express my appreciation enough for your book and its philosophy.

Eric Diller
Redondo Beach, California

Briefly my history was: February 1972, acute posterior infarction with complete recovery. April 1972, acute coronary insufficiency. January 1973, Cleveland Clinic reported 70 percent blockage of both main arteries. September 1976, hospitalized for severe angina pains. After release from hospital I was taking at least one nitro tablet per day and frequently three or four tablets.

Upon receipt of your letter of November 3, 1976, I immediately purchased a copy of *Live Longer Now* and began a no-salt, no-sugar, minimum-fat diet. Since starting on the diet I have taken exactly two nitro tablets. My weight loss has been thirteen pounds and is now holding steady. The improvement has been dramatic. I am now off all medication except two aspirin every other day.

At age seventy-two I think that *dramatic* is a mild term.

Loren G. Windom
Reynoldsburg, Ohio

March 7, 1977

Hail and kudos for the "Pritikin diet." As long as I can remember, going back to my teen years, I've been adjudged to be hypertensive and medicated and medicated with limited results. I even jogged for eight years rather regularly and still no results, in fact, a worsening of the situation, despite some initial results of feeling great. Then my cousin sent me a copy of the *New York* magazine article about the diet and I decided to try it along with the exercises—walking and bicycling. The results are dynamite—from readings as high as 160/110 I have come full cycle to a low of 112/72—*with no medication*. I've lost about ten pounds and I look and feel great, all in a few short weeks. My sons, nineteen and sixteen, who have monitored my BP these many years, are also so impressed with my results that they have switched to the diet.

I'm wondering when the medical profession will awaken and begin curing countless numbers of people who are not so hopelessly ill as the medical profession makes them out to be. Keep up your excellent work.

Eugene Kopacz
New Providence, New Jersey

October 3, 1977

As you know, I sold my business last year after I had two coronaries and the doctor told me that my coronary arteries were too bad to do a bypass operation on me. Then a year ago last June I had a session with loss of control of my arms and legs and with very bad headaches and was in the hospital for a week recovering, after which the doctor told me that I would rapidly lose my faculties and that I should get my affairs in order as I would be a vegetable in a short time.

Then I spent some seven weeks there in Santa Barbara and you have my record on this.

Since that time I have been traveling to Brazil and Mexico, doing consulting work with and for my old friends and customers, and also advising them from my office in my home. I am also planning a trip to South America again to see a customer and then go to Iran to see the pipe factory that I sold to the government.

There is one major problem in such traveling and that is staying on the reversal diet, as it is almost impossible to eat in hotels and restaurants and airplanes and eat a low-fat, high-carbohydrate meal, and it is not practical to fix your own meals all the time.

In spite of getting off the diet somewhat while traveling, I feel good. I did go back to my old family doctor for a complete checkup and he put me in the hospital for three days and ran every test that he could think of. He was amazed because they could find no trace of a heart or circulation problem, and he finally told me that in his opinion I had never had a heart attack at all, and, after a brain scan, that I had no circulation problem there either.

He frankly did not understand how my blood pressure was normal when I had been treated by him for high blood pressure for over twenty years with it being up to

230/140 for some periods. I did read the hospital chart where he had written his admittance comments after talking to me; he had written that I was rambling and confused about my condition because I tried to tell him that I had found a way to bring my blood pressure down without drugs, and could also control my cholesterol by diet. He just could not understand at all.

Now that I am functioning again I am fixing up my thirty-seven-foot cabin cruiser and getting it ready to use for offshore cruising and relaxing and living again. When that doctor told me that I would be a vegetable if I lived at all I lost interest in the boat and a lot of other things and it is good to be alive and aware again.

Charles A. Babbitt
Rolling Hills, California

Christmas, 1976

This has been a wonderful year for the Bonneys. Bonney's health has been a small miracle. Since his two heart attacks in 1970 and small stroke in 1975 he's been on a lot of heart medicine with all its side effects. He's done fair only.

Early this year we heard of a program at the newly opened Longevity Rehabilitation Center in Santa Barbara that was not only halting the degenerative diseases but was reversing them. Hardheaded Bonney didn't want much to do with it. He said his pills had kept him going since 1970 and he was getting along okay. Nevertheless, I was even harder-headed and we went to Santa Barbara for the month of April where they put us on an 80 percent complex carbohydrate diet, with only 10 percent fat and 10 percent protein, no sugars, and no salt. Well, after a month Bonney was off all his heart medicine, was walking six to seven miles a day, had the best control of his diabetes that he'd ever had and on 20 percent less insulin, no insulin shocks, etc. He was even jogging toward the end of the month. And he felt better.

Besides learning how to cook the diet, I lost eighteen pounds. Beautiful. Results in Wyoming, still following the same diet, were even better. Bonney began hiking at the higher altitude and never once needed the emergency oxygn we'd been carting around for the last few years. He hiked to a lot of mountain lakes he thought he'd never see again.

My mother and her sister, both with high blood pressure and on pills, came to stay with us for the summer, lived on the same diet and hiked a lot. By the summer's end both had regular blood pressure and were off their pills, and both looked so well. Both of them (eighty-one years old) also hiked to the lakes.

We were on the Santa Barbara diet, called the reversal or regression diet, very strict, for at least three months. Now we are on the maintenance diet—vegetables, beans, fruits, whole grains. The no-nos are cholesterol, fat, sugar, salt, nicotine, and alcoholic liquors. We sweeten our cereals with sliced bananas or fruit juices (like concentrated frozen apple juice).

I still can't believe my powerhouse sweet tooth hasn't had any sugar in over six months and I don't even want it. My figure sure shows the benefits. I've never been so sylphlike nor felt so good nor climbed so well as this summer. I easily outwalked the horses. And although I've eaten like a horse I doubt I'll ever have a weight problem again. I've whipped up several cooky and popsicle recipes which I fed the kids and family this summer and which they all liked. It's a whole new way of cooking.

Orrin and Lorraine Bonney
Houston, Texas

September 11, 1976

I was heading for disaster, then I reversed the process. I am a retired MD of eighty-four years and feel great. After two minor heart attacks, an abdominal aneurysm operated by Dr. DeBakey in Houston, Texas, and then angina pectoris (I could not walk a block without severe chest pains, relieved only by nitroglycerin), I realized that I was a fit subject for a fatal heart attack or stroke. The medicine I was taking gave me dizzy spells. So I was encouraged by the statement of the Longevity Research people that "degenerative processes can be reversed" by a program of diet and activity, without drugs!

I determined to test their theory. So, for six months I have been following their regime with marvelous results. I walk four miles a day without pain and without drugs. My blood pressure has dropped to a normal range, I have lost fifteen pounds of weight (without trying), and I have greater energy and bounce.

The diet may seem a bit drab. I am allowed no sugar or syrup, but only complex carbohydrates such as starchy foods, cereals, potatoes, and most fruits. These carbohydrates should make up 82 percent of the calories of the diet. Fats are reduced to 10 percent of the calories of the diet, where the average American diet has 42 percent fat. That means no butter or oleo, no mayonnaise, no cream, no shortening, or any rich food. Protein is 10 percent and is allowed in chicken or turkey, lean meats or fish (with fat removed).

Some train for the Olympics. I train for life. At eighty-four, I feel that I have extended my life span and the enjoyment of it.

Floyd O. Woodward, MD
Letter to the Editor,
*Santa Barbara News-Press*

August 6, 1977

I had been diagnosed as a borderline diabetic with a blood cholesterol of 190 and a triglyceride of 250. I am happy to report that after two months on your diet my cholesterol was 160 and triglyceride 72.

We are appreciative of the work all of you have done—and excited. Thank you.

Fredrick H. Marler, DDS
Rockford, Illinois

Since commencing your program, I have gone from 205 to 182 pounds. I am about six-feet, one-half-inch, and am thirty-eight. I was raised in a Seventh Day Adventist home, so much of your diet is a return to basics for me. I never smoked, but was using wine on a daily basis. Also, coffee was a regular and excessive habit. I was so inspired by your well-presented facts that I am totally off alcohol, with occasionally one cup a day of decaffeinated coffee, and a strong exercise program is part of my daily schedule. I am self-employed so I have the time to ride a bike here in Bishop at a 4,000-feet altitude. I have been riding in the area of thirty-two miles a day, five days a week, weather permitting.

I accompany this with a light workout with ten-pound dumbbells for upper-body development.

I just remarried a year and a half ago. It is clear to me that the person in your kitchen is either your enemy or your friend. In my case, she is my ally and I owe much to her. We now buy in bulk when in Los Angeles so as to have a good supply of peas, beans, rice, etc., on hand. All my adult life, I have been plagued with lower-back pain, which is now nonexistent. I had a hearing problem, medically treated with lecithin, that is greatly improved now, without lecithin.

E. K. Jensen
Bishop, California

# FOUR

# The Maximum Weight Loss Diet

# 17

## The Surest
## and Safest Diet

Even though it is the usual reason for dieting, we have scarcely mentioned weight loss.

Let's be perfectly clear: The Pritikin Diet is unbeatable for safe, effective, long-lasting weight loss. For a ten-pound loss or a two-hundred-pound loss.

Moreover, you achieve weight loss absolutely without hunger. You can eat from the permissible foods list all day long if you want to—and still keep your calories down to the point of automatic weight loss.

You have a choice. You can lose weight slowly or quickly. The slow route is with the regular Pritikin Diet by simply cutting back on the permitted higher-calorie foods; the fast route is with the Maximum Weight Loss Diet. Even though the Maximum Weight Loss Diet is much lower in calories, it does not require supplements.

There is considerable precedent for the use of a carbo-hydrate diet in producing weight reduction. One of the most remarkable was Dr. William Kempner's famous rice diet of the 1940s. At that time, he used a diet consisting almost entirely of rice and fruit to treat high blood pressure, heart disease, and kidney disease.

Using a lower-calorie version of that diet (420–800 calories daily), Kempner achieved weight losses among massively obese people to the tune of a half-pound per day until they had lost at least one hundred pounds.

# LOSING WEIGHT ON THE PRITIKIN DIETS

Let's get down to cases: How much can you expect to lose on the Pritikin diets—and how fast can you lose it?

Most overweight people at the Pritikin Center in Santa Barbara (where there are no quantitative restrictions on the low-calorie foods) eat six to eight meals a day and lose an average of 13.2 pounds. (The champion flesh-shedder lost 31 pounds during his month there!)

The entire group of dieters at the Center lose an average of 8.9 pounds their first month. Even those *not* trying to lose generally see 3 or 4 (water) pounds go. Indeed, a big problem often is controlling weight loss—since many people develop a preference for the low-calorie salads and soups that guarantee continued thinning.

The Maximum Weight Loss Diet was developed for those people who have to lose a lot of weight fast: an actress trying to make a comeback; an executive who has to qualify for an insurance program; the prospect of a job interview; a sweetheart or spouse who's been told to "take it off or else!"

This diet is considerably safer than the popular high-protein or high-fat diets, such as the Atkins, the Stillman, the Linn or Last Chance, the Save Your Life, and other similar diets.

There is no risk of electrolyte imbalance (loss of potassium or calcium or other minerals), no need to drink liquids to flush out the harmful protein metabolites to avoid kidney toxicity, no risk to the liver, no controlled ketosis producing a diabeticlike syndrome.

## HIGH-PROTEIN DIETS

The trouble with high-protein, low-carbohydrate diets is that they are too high in fat. While carbohydrates burn efficiently and cleanly, breaking down to safe water and carbon dioxide, fats do not. Fats are not 100 percent efficient (as are carbohydrates), since fats produce part of their residue in ketones.

True, ketones tend to decrease appetite. But ketones are also dangerous. Being acidic, they tend to change the nearly neutral pH of the blood. If they rise too fast in the blood, they can acidify it to the extent of producing a diabeticlike ketosis state. The ultimate danger of excessive ketones is ketoacidosis, which can be fatal.

Therefore, diets such as the Atkins and Stillman diets are risky. Although Atkins says his is "controlled" ketosis, experience with this diet makes it plain that ketones are sometimes far too elusive to control.

The high protein intake of these diets poses another problem. The body draws large amounts of water from the tissues to dilute to safe levels of toxic breakdown products of protein digestion. Seven times as much water is required in protein digestion as in carbohydrate or fat digestion. The dehydration produces an instant temporary weight loss, but if at least some of the water is not replenished, a serious state of dehydration can result.

An example of extreme dehydration from a high protein intake has been shown in infants on soy-milk diets exclusively who died from dehydration.

## OTHER DIETING METHODS

Another way to lose weight quickly is to stop eating altogether. But even if you wanted to run the considerable risks attendant upon a total fast, you would lose at most seven pounds per month more than you would on the Pritikin Maximum Weight Loss Diet.

You also lose weight, but less rapidly, on the regular Pritikin Diet. People on either of our diets reduce to their lean muscle mass and stay there. In fact, it takes a concerted effort to regain weight (unless, of course, you go off the diet). But the main point is that the Pritikin Diet is one you can stick with, happily, safely, effectively, the rest of your life.

I emphasize the *happily*. The latest fad in diet is behavioral modification, in which dieters are subjected to various contortions of their natural responses to food. To my mind, this is a don't-raise-the-bridge-lower-the-water approach—awkward, self-defeating, and painful.

I'm not pretending that embarking on the Pritikin Diet is easy. It isn't. And there *is* behavioral modification to the extent that you're well advised to throw out harmful foods, just as you might empty a medicine chest of dangerous and out-of-date medications that might tempt a small child. But that's *it*.

The accompanying table will give you an idea of how other diets strain to maintain adherence (and none too successfully, either, I might add). In compiling it, I've borrowed various authors' suggestions, which our dieters regard as irksome and unnecessary.

| Behavioral Modification Suggestion | Pritikin Response |
| --- | --- |
| Keep a diary of everything you eat, noting time of day, what you ate, how much, where you were, whom you were with, and how well you were feeling. | Nonsense. All that takes time away from eating. |
| Read this diary. | Clean the basement instead. |
| Restrict all eating to one room. | If you have only one room. |
| Put knife and fork down between bites. | So you can use spoon. |
| After every four bites, wait two minutes before taking another bite. | Only if it takes two minutes to chew each mouthful and if you like three-hour meals. |
| Eat a small portion, then set timer for twenty minutes. If still hungry, eat a second helping. | See above. |
| Reward yourself by giving yourself gold stars for good eating behavior. | . . . and paste on your Snoopy blanket. |

| | |
|---|---|
| Eat like a bird, not like an animal. | All arguments to the contrary notwithstanding, man is an animal. |
| Use a small plate and fork, to make less look like more. | . . . and a large table to catch spillovers. |
| Always leave something on your plate. | Only at McDonald's. |

| **Behavioral Modification Suggestion** | **Pritikin Response** |
|---|---|
| Throw any scraps away right after the meal. If you keep them around, you might eat them. | On the other hand, in time they may become valuable. |
| Imagine yourself eating until you're ready to throw up. When you get hungry, recall the feeling of vomiting. | Not in my house. |
| Keep foods out of sight. | By carefully placing on tongue, crushing with teeth, and concealing in stomach. |

About the only thing that can be said for diets requiring such behavioral modification is that they're a cut better than some other diet aids, such as intestinal bypass surgery, wiring the jaw shut, or taking amphetamines and other appetite depressants.

Basically, the Maximum Weight Loss plan involves careful monitoring of low-calorie foods. The next two chapters are your operating manual for success on the Maximum Weight Loss Diet. They provide the necessary guidelines and recipes.

# 18

# Following the Maximum Weight Loss Diet Plan

To follow the Maximum Weight Loss plan, select a menu for the day from the sample menus given later in this chapter, or improvise your own one-day menu. This entails choosing breakfast, lunch, afternoon snack, and dinner from among eight calorie food groups, according to the following guidelines:

1. Choose one food serving only from food group 1 (Grains).
2. Choose one food serving only from food group 2 (Dairy Products).
3. Choose one food serving only from food group 3 (Fruits). The reason for this limitation is that, calorie for calorie, the foods in the food groups 4–8 tend to be more filling than fruits.
4. Choose any additional foods desired from food groups 4, 5, 6, 7, and 8 to bring the combined total caloric intake for breakfast, lunch, afternoon snack, and dinner to approximately 600 calories.

All foods marked with an asterisk (*) in food groups 4, 5, 6, 7, and 8 are especially low in calories and are considered "unrestricted." While they are to be included in the 600-calorie daily total, being so low calorically, they can be eaten in relatively unlimited amounts.

To keep from being hungry, it is important to nibble *all day long* on raw vegetables from food group 6. Constant eating of these unrestricted foods helps the dieter avoid the temptation to deviate by providing a satisfying sense of bulk while adding very few calories. A half pound of zucchini, for instance, has only 39 calories.

Occasionally, when the dieter feels a change is necessary or in order, up to 400 additional calories may be chosen from the 1000-calorie diet suggestions. This could bring the combined total for breakfast, lunch, afternoon snack, and dinner to a maximum of approximately 1,000 calories.

For most dieters at most times, weighing of foods should not be necessary. Satisfactory weight loss of 10 pounds and more per month will be achieved by simply eating each day mainly unrestricted asterisk-marked foods in food groups 4–8 and only one food serving each from food groups 1, 2, and 3. Only if your weight loss is under 10 pounds per month following these guidelines will it be advisable to monitor your caloric intake more closely by weighing your portions.

---

### Summary of Maximum Weight Loss Diet Rules

*Rule #1:* EAT ALL DAY LONG TO LOSE WEIGHT. This is the most important rule. If you don't eat all day long from the lower-calorie foods that are on this diet, you run the risk of going off the diet. So the first thing you must do is CARRY A PLASTIC BAG FILLED WITH RAW VEGETABLES AND EAT THEM ALL DAY LONG.

*Rule #2:* RESTRICT YOURSELF TO ONE PORTION PER DAY FROM FOOD GROUPS 1, 2, AND 3. Groups 4–8 are not restricted, but the combined total calories for breakfast, lunch, afternoon snack, and dinner should be around 600. The all-day-long raw vegetable snacking will add some additional calories, but not many, since they are very low-calorie foods. On occasion, when there is a need, you are permitted to choose up to 400 additional calories from the foods in the 1,000 Calorie Diet.

## DIET STRATEGY

▪ Provide plenty of diet interest by eating a variety of vegetables. Using our vegetable combination suggestions and recipes as a starting point, you can invent a clutch of new interesting low-cal dishes. On the other hand, you may find it simpler to rely on a few standby dishes that you particularly like.

▪ To eat so many vegetables in one day requires a great deal of preparation: peeling, slicing, chopping. You may wish to purchase a good eight-to-ten-inch chef's knife and/or a food processor (Cuisinart or the like) to help you in your efforts.

▪ You can cut down the time spent in the kitchen by cooking in quantity for the freezer. Two or three batches of different soups can be cooked on a Sunday evening, for instance, and frozen in containers that will feed you for several days. If you were planning to eat a soup twice on the same day for two days, you could freeze a quart (four-to-eight-ounce servings) in one container and defrost it, for example on Wednesday for Thursday and Friday. You can even make up salad dressings in quantity and freeze them in four-ounce containers, which will give you a few days' supply when defrosted. Dishes like *Ratatouille\**, *Cole Slaw, Green Bean Marinade, Vegetable Casserole, Chinese Vegetables and Chicken, Cabbage Rolls,* and *Stuffed Eggplant* will keep refrigerated after cooking for several days, so make up a large batch.

▪ Even by estimating approximate portions, you should be able to lose ten pounds per month. If you do not attain this weight loss, you may need a scale with a capacity of one to three pounds for a more accurate determination of portion amounts.

## 600-CALORIE DIET—FOOD GROUPS

The 600-calorie diet contains 30–35 grams of protein which should be adequate because high carbohydrate diets

---

\* Recipes for all dishes in italics here and in the pages that follow can be found in Chapter 19, Maximum Weight Loss Recipes.

are protein-sparing. If more protein is desired, 3 oz. of uncreamed cottage cheese each day will add 17 grams of protein, bringing the total protein intake to 50 grams and the calorie intake to 680.

| *Group 1: Grains* | *Calories* |
|---|---|
| 4.5 oz. cooked *cracked wheat cereal* | 100 |
| 4.5 oz. cooked *oatmeal* | 100 |
| 3.0 oz. cooked *brown rice* | 100 |

(2 Tbs. of bran, not counted as a grain serving, may be added to cereal or other foods, as desired. If used, add 15 calories per Tbs.)

### Group 2: Dairy Products

| 4 oz. skim milk | 40 |
|---|---|

### Group 3: Fruit

| ½ orange | 50 |
|---|---|
| ½ banana | 50 |
| ½ grapefruit | 50 |

(Foods marked with an asterisk (\*) are "unrestricted"; that is, they are especially low-calorie and can be eaten in relatively unlimited amounts.)

### Group 4: Soups

| 8 oz. *Latin Belle Soup\** | 35 |
|---|---|
| 8 oz. *Southern Vegetable Soup\** | 47 |
| 8 oz. *Garden Potpourri Soup\** | 50 |
| 8 oz. *Tomato-Vegetable Soup\** | 50 |
| 8 oz. *Sweet and Sour Cabbage Soup\** | 67 |
| 8 oz. *Italian Vegetable Soup\** | 70 |
| 8 oz. *Gazpacho\** | 70 |
| 8 oz. *Special Vegetable Soup\** | 70 |
| 8 oz. *Beet Borscht* | 75 |
| 8 oz. *Cabbage-Beet Borscht* | 80 |
| 8 oz. *Tomato-Rice Soup* | 90 |
| 8 oz. *Tomato-Okra Soup* | 95 |

## Group 5: A. Cooked Vegetables

| | | |
|---|---|---:|
| 4 oz. | tomato juice* | 22 |
| 8 oz. | bok choy* | 32 |
| 4 oz. | hubbard squash, boiled* | 35 |
| 4 oz. | pumpkin, boiled or canned* | 37 |
| 4 oz. | acorn squash, boiled | 39 |
| 4 oz. | tomato sauce | 46 |
| 4 oz. | butternut squash, boiled | 47 |
| 16 oz. | zucchini* | 54 |
| 4 oz. | hubbard squash, baked | 57 |
| 4 oz. | acorn squash, baked | 63 |
| 16 oz. | celery* | 63 |
| 16 oz. | summer squash* | 64 |
| 16 oz. | crookneck squash* | 68 |
| 8 oz. | dandelion greens | 75 |
| 4 oz. | butternut, baked | 78 |
| 16 oz. | bell pepper* | 82 |
| 16 oz. | eggplant* | 86 |
| 16 oz. | cabbage* | 91 |
| 16 oz. | asparagus* | 91 |
| 16 oz. | cauliflower* | 100 |
| 8 oz. | canned tomatoes* | 48 |
| 8 oz. | turnips* | 52 |
| 8 oz. | kohlrabi* | 55 |
| 8 oz. | snap beans* | 57 |
| 8 oz. | broccoli* | 59 |
| 8 oz. | tomatoes, fresh cooked* | 60 |
| 8 oz. | okra | 66 |
| 8 oz. | onions* | 66 |
| 8 oz. | carrots* | 70 |
| 8 oz. | rutabagas | 80 |
| 8 oz. | Brussels sprouts | 82 |
| 8 oz. | leeks | 93 |
| 8 oz. | artichokes (The fresher the artichoke, the fewer the calories.) | 20–100 |

## Group 5: B. Cooked Vegetable Combinations

| | | |
|---|---|---:|
| 8 oz. | zucchini, crookneck, scalloped squash* | 31 |
| 8 oz. | celery, zucchini, and mushrooms* | 34 |
| 8 oz. | zucchini, bell pepper, eggplant* | 37 |

8 oz. shredded cabbage, onions, and tomatoes*     57
8 oz. cauliflower and carrots*                    60
8 oz. broccoli, carrots, and green beans*         61
8 oz. carrots, turnips, and rutabagas             66

### Group 5: C. Cooked Vegetable Specialties

8 oz. *Zucchini Stew**                            47
8 oz. *Ratatouille**                              60
8 oz. (2) *Chili Rellenos**                       63

### Group 6: Raw Vegetables

8 oz. Chinese cabbage*                            30
4 oz. chives*                                     32
4 oz. mushrooms*                                  32
8 oz. cucumbers*                                  34
8 oz. zucchini*                                   39
8 oz. celery*                                     39
8 oz. radishes*                                   39
8 oz. lettuce (Bibb, romaine, iceberg, etc.)*     41
8 oz. summer squash*                              46
8 oz. crookneck squash*                           46
8 oz. endive*                                     47
4 oz. carrots                                     48
8 oz. scalloped squash*                           48
8 oz. bell pepper*                                50
4 oz. sunchokes, "Jerusalem artichokes"
      (The fresher the sunchoke, the fewer
      the calories.)                            8-86
8 oz. tomatoes*                                   50
4 oz. rutabagas*                                  52
8 oz. green cabbage*                              55
8 oz. savoy cabbage*                              55
8 oz. cauliflower*                                60
8 oz. chayote (squash)*                           64
8 oz. onions, Spanish*                            65
8 oz. turnips*                                    68
8 oz. red cabbage*                                71
8 oz. broccoli*                                   73
8 oz. green onions*                               82

## Group 7: Salads and Dressings

| | |
|---|---:|
| 8 oz. *Green Bean Marinade*\* | 35 |
| 8 oz. *Cauliflower Marinade*\* | 44 |
| 8 oz. *Cole Slaw*\* | 56 |
| 2 oz. *Herb Vinegar Dressing*\* | 3 |
| 2 oz. *French Dressing*\* | 10 |
| 2 oz. *Italian Dressing*\* | 10 |
| 2 oz. *Russian Dressing*\* | 10 |
| 2 oz. *Tomato-Lemon Dressing*\* | 10 |
| 2 oz. *Tillie Lewis Dressing*\*† | 10 |
| 2 oz. *lemon juice*\* | 14 |
| 2 oz. *Capers Dressing* | 40 |

## Group 8: Entrees and Sauces

| | |
|---|---:|
| 8 oz. *Vegetable Cutlets* | 62 |
| 8 oz. *Stuffed Eggplant* | 70 |
| 8 oz. *Cabbage Rolls* | 93 |
| 8 oz. *Chinese Vegetables and Chicken* | 95 |
| 8 oz. *Stuffed Zucchini* | 96 |
| 3 oz. *"Little Beef" Patties* | 108 |
| 8 oz. *Breaded Eggplant* | 160 |
| 8 oz. *Vegetable Casserole* | 170 |
| 2 oz. *Salsa I*\* | 18 |
| 2 oz. *Salsa II* | 25 |
| 4 oz. *Enchilada Sauce* | 41 |

# SAMPLE MENUS FOR THREE DAYS

| *Sample Menu: Day 1* | *Calories* |
|---|---:|

Breakfast:

| | | |
|---|---|---:|
| Group 1 | 4.5 oz. cooked *Cracked Wheat Cereal* (plus bran) | 130 |
| Group 2 | 4 oz. nonfat milk | 40 |
| Group 3 | ½ banana | 50 |

† A commerical dressing. Dilute in half with water to reduce the salt content to a more acceptable level. You may wish to add extra vinegar, garlic, or dillweed to diluted mixture to improve flavor.

Lunch:
Group 4   8 oz. *Tomato Vegetable Soup*               50
Group 6   8 oz. lettuce                              41
          2 oz. radishes                             10
          2 oz. cucumbers                             9
          4 oz. tomatoes                             25
          2 oz. alfalfa sprouts                       —
          2 oz. shredded carrots                     24
Group 7   2 oz. *Italian Dressing*                   10

Afternoon Snack:
Group 4   8 oz. *Southern Vegetable Soup*            47

Dinner:
Group 8   16 oz. *Chinese Vegetable and Chicken*    190
                                          Total     626

## Sample Menu: Day 2

Breakfast:
Group 1   3 oz. cooked *Brown Rice* (plus bran)     130
Group 3   ½ grapefruit                               50

Lunch:
Group 4   8 oz. *Tomato-Okra Soup*                   95
Group 7   8 oz. *Green Bean Marinade*                35

Afternoon Snack:
Group 5   8 oz. *Ratatouille*                        60

Dinner:
Group 4   8 oz. *Special Vegetable Soup*             70
Group 5   8 oz. (two) *Chile Rellenos*              63
Group 8   8 oz. (one-half) *Stuffed Zucchini*        96
                                          Total     599

## Sample Menu: Day 3

Breakfast:
Group 1   3.5 oz. cooked *Oatmeal* (plus bran)      130
Group 2   4 oz. nonfat milk                          40
Group 3   ½ orange                                   50

Lunch:

| | | | |
|---|---|---|---|
| Group 4 | 8 oz. | *Latin Belle Soup* | 35 |
| Group 6 | 4 oz. | raw bell pepper | 25 |
| | 4 oz. | raw carrots | 48 |
| | 4 oz. | raw cauliflower | 30 |
| | 4 oz. | raw cucumbers | 17 |

Dinner:

| | | | |
|---|---|---|---|
| Group 4 | 8 oz. | *Tomato-Rice Soup* | 90 |
| Group 5 | 8 oz. | shredded cabbage, onions, and tomatoes | 57 |
| Group 8 | 8 oz. | *Stuffed Eggplant* | 70 |
| | | Total | 592 |

## 1,000-CALORIE DIET—FOOD GROUPS

Use the 600-Calorie Diet as a basis for the 1,000-Calorie Diet. Another 400 calories can be added in a variety of ways. Some suggestions follow:

Calories

1. 1 6-oz. baked potato (without peel)     145
   1 5-oz. potato, boiled and then peeled   105
   1 5-oz. potato, peeled and then boiled    90

2. Some possible fruits:
   8 oz. casaba                              75
   8 oz. cantaloupe                          80
   4 oz. grapes                              80
   1 medium apple                           100
   8 medium strawberries                    100

3. One serving** of fish or fowl every other day, not to exceed 1½ lbs. per week. You might choose from:
   4 oz. cod                                 90
   4 oz. sole or flounder                    90
   4 oz. red snapper                        105
   4 oz. pink salmon (if canned, remove all visible fat)                          135
   4 oz. tuna (water-packed)                145

** Calorie values are given for raw foods except tuna.

| | |
|---|---|
| 4 oz. halibut | 165 |
| 4 oz. lean chicken, light meat | 135 |
| 4 oz. lean turkey, light meat | 115 |

All fish or fowl should be served without skin and should be broiled, boiled, or poached.

4. Additional grains approximating 100 calories per day. These could include:

| | |
|---|---|
| more breakfast cereal or brown rice (see Group 1) | 100 |
| 1 slice whole wheat bread (see Index) | 100 |
| 1 small bran muffin (see Index) | 100 |
| Whole-grain rice, wheat or rye crackers (acceptable varieties) | 100 |

In addition to the entrees available on the 600-Calorie Diet, here are two other choices:

| | |
|---|---|
| 8 oz. lasagne (see Index) | 195 |
| 8 oz. spaghetti, plus 4 oz. spaghetti sauce (see Index) | 220 |

# 19

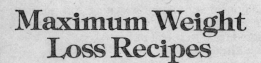

# Maximum Weight
# Loss Recipes

## GRAINS

### CRACKED WHEAT CEREAL

½  cup cracked wheat
2  cups water

Bring the water to a rolling boil; stir in the cracked wheat. Lower the heat so that mixture cooks slowly. Cook approximately 20 to 25 minutes, stirring from time to time, until mixture thickens sufficiently. (Cover near end of cooking time if a softer texture is desired.)

Serve plain, or with a light sprinkling of cinnamon, and bran, if desired, and/or sliced fruit.

*Note:* 1¾ level tablespoons of raw cracked wheat = 3.5 ounces (100 calories).

*Serves 1 to 2*

### OATMEAL

1  cup "old-fashioned" rolled oats
2  cups water

Bring 2 cups of water to a rolling boil; stir in the oats. Lower the heat so that the mixture cooks slowly. Cook approximately 12 to 15 minutes, stirring from time to time, until mixture thickens sufficiently. (Cover near the end of cooking time if a softer texture is desired.)

Serve plain, or with a light sprinkling of cinnamon, and bran, if desired, and/or sliced fruit.

*Note:* 5 level tablespoons of dry oatmeal = 3 ounces cooked oatmeal (100 calories).

*Serves 1 to 2*

## BROWN RICE

1 cup brown rice
2 cups water, if using long-grain rice, or 1¾ cups water, if using short-grain rice

Bring water to rolling boil. Add rice; bring back to boil. Turn flame low, cover pot tightly, and cook for 35 to 40 minutes (or cook in covered ovenproof casserole in a preheated 350 degree oven for 40 to 45 minutes).

*Note:* 3¼ level tablespoons of raw rice = 3 ounces cooked brown rice (100 calories).

*Serves 3 to 4*

## SOUPS

### LATIN BELLE SOUP

½ cup chopped turnips
½ cup chopped rutabagas
½ cup chopped onions
½ cup chopped celery
½ cup chopped carrots
¼ cup chopped green pepper
½ cup chopped crookneck squash
⅔ cup chopped zucchini
2¼ cups frozen green beans
6 to 7 cups water
3 ounces canned tomato paste
3 ounces canned salsa (or substitute Salsa I, see Index)
½ teaspoon garlic powder
½ teaspoon onion powder
¼ teaspoon ground cumin (optional)
½ teaspoon oregano

Bring the water, tomato paste, and salsa to a boil. Add all the vegetables except the squash. Reduce heat. Simmer until vegetables are half-done, then add the squash and the seasonings. Continue cooking until done.

*Serves 10*

## SOUTHERN VEGETABLE SOUP

½  cup diced turnips
½  cup diced rutabagas
½  cup chopped onions
⅓  cup chopped carrots
⅓  cup cauliflower buds
½  cup chopped broccoli
⅓  cup halved Brussels sprouts
⅓  cup chopped tomatoes
¼  small head cabbage, shredded
¼  cup chopped summer squash (zucchini, crookneck, or
       scalloped)
¼  cup chopped mustard greens (optional)
¼  to ½ teaspoon each oregano, basil, and garlic powder
 1  teaspoon grated sapsago (green) cheese (optional)
 8  cups water (approximately)

Bring about 2 cups of water to boil in the bottom of the soup pot and add the root vegetables—turnips, rutabagas, onions, and carrots. Cook for a few minutes, adding more water as required to keep vegetables almost covered, until vegetables are partly done. Add the other vegetables to the soup pot and cover with water. Bring to a boil, then turn heat down to a simmer. Add oregano, basil, and garlic powder and continue cooking until vegetables are tender. If sapsago cheese is used, add when soup is finished cooking. Add additional water if thinner soup consistency is desired.

## GARDEN POTPOURRI SOUP

1⅓ cups chopped onions
1¾ cups chopped celery
 ¾ cup chopped carrots
1¾ cups chopped turnips
1¾ cups chopped rutabagas
 ¾ cup chopped zucchini
 ¾ cup sliced mushrooms
 ¾ cup sliced crookneck squash
 ¾ cup cauliflower florets
 6 cups water
 ¾ cup canned diced tomatoes
 ¾ cup tomato purée
 ¾ teaspoon onion powder
 ¾ teaspoon garlic powder
 ¾ teaspoon Italian seasoning
 1 bay leaf

Bring the water and tomato products to a boil. Add all the vegetables except the squash. Reduce heat. Then simmer until the vegetables are half-done. Now add the squash and the seasonings. Continue cooking until the vegetables are done.

*Makes about 16 servings*

## TOMATO-VEGETABLE SOUP

1 cup chopped onion
1 cup chopped celery
1 cup chopped carrots
½ cup chopped green pepper
1 cup shredded white cabbage
⅓ cup diced potato
½ cup frozen "mixed" vegetables
7 cups water
1 cup canned tomato juice
1 cup canned diced tomatoes
2 tablespoons lemon juice
¼ teaspoon marjoram
¼ teaspoon basil
½ teaspoon onion powder
½ teaspoon garlic powder
½ teaspoon dried parsley

Bring the water and the tomato products to a boil. Add all the vegetables and the seasonings. Reduce heat and simmer until the vegetables are tender.

*Serves 8*

## SWEET AND SOUR CABBAGE SOUP

2 to 3 potatoes, peeled and diced
1 head cabbage, shredded
4 diced carrots
1 onion, chopped
2 cups chopped celery
3 whole tomatoes, canned or fresh, diced
1 16-ounce can sauerkraut
¼ cup undiluted frozen apple juice concentrate, thawed
½ cup cider vinegar
  Garlic powder and celery seed, to taste
10 cups water

Bring water to a boil. Add all the ingredients and bring to a boil once again. Turn down heat and simmer covered for about 40 minutes, thinning with water as required to maintain desired consistency.

Serve hot or cold, garnished with Mock Sour Cream (see Index) and chopped green onions.

*Makes about 16 servings*

## ITALIAN VEGETABLE SOUP

1¼  cups chopped onions
 ½  cup chopped celery
 ½  cup chopped carrots
1¾  cups chopped turnips
 2  cups diced zucchini
 3  sliced mushrooms
 ½  cup sliced green beans
 2  28-ounce cans diced tomatoes
 ½  15-ounce can tomato paste
 4  cups water
 2  bay leaves
 ½  teaspoon onion powder
 ½  teaspoon garlic powder
 ½  teaspoon Italian seasoning
 1  teaspoon dried parsley

Heat the water and the tomato products to a boil. Add all the vegetables except the zucchini. Bring to a boil once again, turn down heat and simmer until vegetables are half-done. Add the zucchini and the seasonings. Continue cooking until done.

*Makes about 16 servings*

## GAZPACHO

2  medium ripe tomatoes
1  medium zucchini
1  celery stem
1  small red onion (or 1 bunch green onions)
1  clove garlic
4  cups well-chilled canned tomato juice
   Juice of 3 limes and lime slices for garnish

Finely chop vegetables. Put about ⅓ of the chopped vegetables in a blender with a little of the tomato juice; blend until puréed. Stir puréed vegetables and the rest of the vegetables into a bowl. Add lime juice and the balance of the tomato juice. Chill mixture well. Garnish with lime slices.

*Serves 4 to 6*

## SPECIAL VEGETABLE SOUP

½  cup frozen lima beans
½  cup frozen corn
½  cup frozen green beans
¾  cup chopped carrots
¾  cup chopped celery
¾  cup chopped onions
¾  cup chopped potatoes
¾  cup chopped broccoli
¾  cup crookneck squash
¾  cup cauliflower florets
¾  cup sliced mushrooms
1½  cups canned diced tomatoes
1½  cups canned crushed tomatoes or tomato purée
10  cups water
2  bay leaves
½  teaspoon oregano
¼  teaspoon dill seed
1  teaspoon celery seed
½  teaspoon marjoram
¼  teaspoon cumin (optional)
1  teaspoon garlic powder
1  teaspoon onion powder
½  teaspoon Italian seasoning

Bring the water and the tomato products to a boil. Add all the vegetables except the squash. Reduce heat. Simmer until vegetables are almost done, then add the squash and the seasonings. Cook until done.

*Makes about 16 servings*

## BEET BORSCHT

3 medium-sized beets
1 16-ounce can diced beets, undrained
1 16-ounce can sauerkraut
1 16-ounce can tomato juice
2 teaspoons lemon juice
2 teaspoons vinegar
  Dash of allspice
  Dash of cloves
  Water as required

Scrub the beets clean and boil them until they are done. Run them under cold water and remove the skins. Dice the beets and add with the other ingredients to a soup pot. Bring the soup to a boil, then simmer it slowly until the flavors are well blended (about 25 minutes), adding water as needed to maintain desired consistency.

Serve hot or cold. Pass a bowl of chopped green onions as a garnish.

*Serves 8 to 10*


## CABBAGE-BEET BORSCHT

7 cups diced cooked beets, fresh or canned
1⅓ cups shredded cabbage
¾ cup canned sauerkraut
1⅔ cups chopped onion
1½ cups canned tomato juice
2 teaspoons lemon juice
⅓ cup unsweetened apple juice
¼ to ⅓ cup apple cider vinegar
2⅓ cups beet juice
4 cups water, or more for a thinner soup
¼ teaspoon ground allspice
¼ teaspoon cloves

Heat the water, tomato juice, and beet juice (if using canned beets) to a boil. If using fresh beets, boil the beets with their skins on, washing them thoroughly so you can use the juice in the pot after they have been cooked. Remove the beet skins under cold water when they are done. Then dice them. Add the sauerkraut, onions, and cabbage and simmer for about 30 minutes or until the vegetables are tender. Add the beets, lemon juice, apple juice, apple cider vinegar, and spices. Let this mixture simmer for a few minutes more. (If a thicker soup base is desired, remove some of the soup to a blender and blend, then return the purée to the soup pot to mix with the rest of the soup.)

Serve either hot or cold.
*Serves 10*


## TOMATO-RICE SOUP

*Fresh vegetables are ground to provide a flavor base for this delicious soup.*

 1 onion, chopped
 2 small carrots, chopped
 3 stalks, celery, chopped
 1 large green pepper, chopped
½ head cabbage, chopped
 1 28-ounce can whole-pack tomatoes, chopped, with juice
 3 cups canned tomato juice (or tomato paste blended with water) and additional water, if a thinner soup is desired
 1 15-ounce can salsa (or substitute Salsa I, see Index)
 3 cups brown rice, about half-cooked
   Suggested seasonings to taste: bay leaf, garlic powder, oregano, chili powder, celery seed

Place the onion, carrots, celery, green pepper, and cabbage in a blender for grinding, together with some of the tomato juice to make blending easier. Transfer the ground vegetables to a soup pot. Add the rest of the juice and the chopped canned tomatoes with juice and salsa. Bring the contents to a boil and simmer gently for 15 minutes.

Add the partially cooked rice and seasonings and continue simmering until the rice is done. If more liquid is required to keep the soup at desired consistency, add additional water or tomato juice or a combination of water and juice.

*Makes about 16 servings*

## TOMATO-OKRA SOUP

1 7-ounce package frozen Chinese pea pods
2 cups shredded green cabbage
2 cups chopped mixed vegetables (carrots, celery, onion, or others of your choice), fresh or frozen
3 cups canned tomato juice
½ teaspoon cumin or other desired seasoning
3 cups water
1 7-ounce package frozen chopped okra

Bring water and tomato juice to a boil. Add all the ingredients, except the okra. Reduce heat and gently simmer the soup for about an hour. Add the okra during the last 10 to 15 minutes of the cooking period. Add more water if a thinner soup is desired. Serve hot.

*Makes 6 to 8 servings*

## VEGETABLE SPECIALTIES

### ZUCCHINI STEW

6 cups diced zucchini
2 cups chopped onion
2 cups chopped green pepper
2 cups diced fresh or canned tomatoes
1½ tablespoons tomato paste
1 cup canned salsa (or substitute Salsa I, see Index)
½ teaspoon oregano
½ teaspoon basil
1 teaspoon chili powder (optional)
2 teaspoons garlic powder

Combine the vegetables, tomato products, salsa, and a little water in a skillet. Add the seasonings. Water-sauté the vegetables, stirring occasionally, until tender.

*Serves 8*

### RATATOUILLE

½ eggplant, peeled and cut into chunks
1 cup sliced zucchini
1 green pepper, cut into chunks
1 large onion, cut into chunks
2 stalks celery, cut in diagonal slices (Chinese style)
2 shallots, finely chopped (optional)
1 clove garlic, minced
2 to 3 tablespoons chopped fresh parsley
⅛ teaspoon ground pepper
2 cups fresh tomatoes, cut into chunks, or diced canned
   tomatoes

Combine all the ingredients (except the fresh tomatoes) in a large pot or skillet. Cover and cook over low heat for about 20 minutes. Uncover and cook 15 minutes more over moderate heat, stirring with a spoon to prevent scorching. Add the tomatoes, heating through, but not permitting tomatoes to become mushy. Serve hot.
*Note:* This dish is easily varied by adding additional seasonings as desired, such as canned salsa, Italian seasoning, oregano, basil or any combination of the above.
*Serves 8*


### CHILI RELLENOS

1 28-ounce can whole green chili peppers
1 medium sized Bermuda onion, diced
½ cup grated sapsago cheese
1 tablespoon chopped parsley
1 teaspoon oregano
½ teaspoon garlic powder
2 cups hoop cheese, mashed (or other uncreamed cottage cheese)
3 egg whites, stiffly beaten
½ cup canned tomato sauce
2 to 3 tablespoons bread crumbs (permissible variety), matzo meal, or bran for topping (optional)

Rinse and drain the chili peppers. Combine the

chopped onion, sapsago cheese, seasonings, and mashed hoop cheese, mixing well. Carefully fold the egg whites into the hoop cheese mixture. Cut each pepper down the center (taking care to keep chili in one piece), then fill it with the hoop-cheese mixture. Lay the filled peppers in a pan with the cut-side up (with filling showing), pinching the ends together so they look like little boats. Pour some tomato sauce over the top of each filled chili pepper, and, if desired, sprinkle some bread crumbs, matzo meal or bran over the tomato sauce. Bake the peppers, uncovered, in a 350 degree oven for about 20 minutes.

*Serves 6 to 8*

## SALADS and SALAD DRESSINGS

### GREEN BEAN OR CAULIFLOWER MARINADE

¾ cup apple cider vinegar
1 tablespoon prepared mustard
1 teaspoon dillweed
1 tablespoon finely chopped celery
⅓ cup finely chopped onion
1 tablespoon chopped parsley
5½ cups cut, cooked green beans (canned, fresh, or frozen), drained, or partially steamed cauliflower

Blend the vinegar, mustard, dillweed, and chopped vegetables in a blender. Pour the marinade over the drained beans or cauliflower and marinate for several hours in the refrigerator. Serve chilled.

*Makes 6 servings*

## COLE SLAW

1½  cups chopped green onion
2½  cups shredded red cabbage
 6  cups shredded green cabbage
 1  cup finely chopped dill pickles
 1  cup chopped red pepper
 3  cups grated carrots
 2  cups peeled apple slices
 ½  cup undiluted frozen apple juice concentrate, thawed
 ¼  cup apple cider vinegar or lemon juice
 1  teaspoon ground ginger
 ¼  teaspoon garlic powder
 1  tablespoon celery seed
 1  teaspoon dry mustard

Chop and shred the vegetables and pickles as directed.
Place the apple slices in a blender together with the apple
juice, vinegar, and spices; blend thoroughly. Pour the
mixture over the chopped and shredded vegetables, mixing well. Refrigerate the cole slaw for several hours or
overnight to blend the flavors. Serve chilled.
*Makes about 1 gallon*

## HERB VINEGAR DRESSING

 1  cup wine vinegar
 ¼  cup fresh dill (or ½ teaspoon dried dillweed)
 ¼  cup snipped fresh chives
 ⅓  cup snipped fresh mint
 1  clove garlic, finely chopped

Combine all the ingredients. Let the dressing stay in
the refrigerator for at least 4 days (to get maximum flavor). Strain to remove herbs.
*Makes about 1¼ cups*

## FRENCH DRESSING

1 onion, chopped
1 cucumber, chopped
½ green pepper, chopped (optional)
2 cups water
2 cups vinegar (cider, wine, or rice vinegar)
  Juice of 2 lemons and some of the pulp
½ teaspoon garlic powder
½ teaspoon ground black pepper
1 teaspoon ground celery seed
1 teaspoon dillweed
3 teaspoons chopped parsley

In a blender, grate the chopped onion, cucumber, and green pepper, if used, together with water. Add the other ingredients; continue blending until all is well blended. Chill and serve.

*Note:* To make Tomato French Dressing, substitute tomato juice for part of the water in the above recipe.

*Makes about 5½ cups*

## ITALIAN DRESSING

¼ cup lemon juice
¼ cup cider vinegar
¼ cup unsweetened apple juice
½ teaspoon oregano
½ teaspoon dry mustard
½ teaspoon onion powder
½ teaspoon garlic powder
½ teaspoon paprika
⅛ teaspoon thyme
⅛ teaspoon rosemary

Combine all the ingredients in a blender. Blend well. Chill and refrigerate overnight or better yet, two days—to permit flavors to blend.

*Makes about ¾ cup*

## RUSSIAN DRESSING

¾  cup cider or rice vinegar
¾  cup water
⅛  cup lemon juice
¼  medium onion, chopped
½  tablespoon dry mustard
½  tablespoon garlic powder
   Dash of white pepper
   Dash of paprika
 2  small carrots, grated

Blend all ingredients, except carrots, in blender, until well mixed. Float grated carrots in dressing. Chill before serving.
*Makes about 2 cups*


## TOMATO-LEMON DRESSING

¾  cup canned tomato juice
¼  cup lemon juice
¼  cup unsweetened apple juice
⅓  cup chopped celery
½  cup chopped onion
½  clove garlic, minced

Combine all the ingredients in a blender and blend well. Chill and serve.
*Makes about 3½ cups*


## CAPERS DRESSING

1¾  cups hoop cheese (or other uncreamed cottage cheese)
¼   cup apple-cider vinegar
 1  tablespoon lemon juice
 1  tablespoon unsweetened apple juice
 2  teaspoons capers, rinsed and drained
1½  teaspoons prepared mustard

Combine all ingredients in a blender. Blend well. Chill and serve.

*Note:* The addition of ¼ teaspoon of curry powder makes an interesting version of tartar sauce.

*Makes about 2½ cups*

# ENTREES AND SAUCES

## VEGETABLE CUTLETS

1 cup chopped onion
½ cup chopped celery
1 cup grated carrots
½ cup fresh or frozen green beans
½ cup frozen green peas
2 egg whites, stiffly beaten
¼ teaspoon ground black pepper
4 tablespoons matzo meal

Bring ¾ cup of water to a boil in a skillet. Add the onion, celery, and carrots and cook until half-done. Add the beans and peas (and more water, if necessary) and continue to cook until all the water is gone and vegetables are tender. Add the egg whites and combine the vegetables, pepper, and matzo meal. Shape into patties and place on a nonstick baking pan. Bake in a 400 degree oven for 20 minutes.

*Serves 6*

## STUFFED EGGPLANT

 1 celery stalk, finely chopped
 ½ carrot, finely chopped
 ¾ cup chopped onion
 ¼ cup canned tomato sauce
 1 cup chopped mushrooms
1½ cups water
1½ teaspoons soy sauce (salt-reduced variety)
 ½ teaspoon cornstarch
 ¼ teaspoon onion powder
 ¼ teaspoon oregano
 ¼ teaspoon garlic powder
 ¾ cup ground whole-wheat bread (permissible kind),
    leftover corn bread, or whole-wheat pita bread, or
    any combination of the three
 1 eggplant, sliced
    Spaghetti Sauce (see Index for Our Favorite Spa-
    ghetti Sauce), or substitute canned tomato sauce

Bring a few tablespoons of water to a boil in a skillet.
Add the celery, carrot, and onion and cook until almost
tender, stirring as required. Add the tomato sauce, water,
mushrooms, soy sauce, cornstarch, and seasonings. Add
the ground bread last (you may use a blender to grind).
Put the eggplant slices in a nonstick baking pan and
spoon the vegetable mixture on top. Bake in a 350 degree
oven for 45 minutes.
  Serve with the spaghetti sauce.
*Serves 8*

## CABBAGE ROLLS

 2 large cabbages

*Filling*

 1 cup brown rice
 1 bay leaf
 1 cup chopped onion
 1 cup chopped celery

1 cup chopped green pepper
¼ teaspoon onion powder
½ teaspoon garlic powder
½ cup canned salsa
1 tablespoon soy sauce (salt-reduced variety)
¼ cup unsweetened apple juice
¼ cup lemon juice

Cook the rice in 2 cups water with the bay leaf until the rice is done (about 45 minutes) or until all the water has been absorbed. Place the whole cabbages in a large pot with 1½ to 2 cups water; cover the pot and steam the cabbages until they begin to separate—about 20 minutes —adding more water if it becomes necessary.

Chop the vegetables and combine them with the rice and the seasonings. Separate the cabbage leaves. Place 2 to 3 tablespoons of the filling in the center of each leaf. Fold the sides of the leaf over the stuffing and roll up to enclose securely. Place the rolls seam-side down in a shallow, nonstick pan.

Cover and bake the rolls for 45 minutes in a 350 degree oven.

*Makes 18 rolls or 9 portions*

## CHINESE VEGETABLES AND CHICKEN

2½ cups cooked chunks of boned breast of chicken (about 3 medium-sized breasts)
¾ pound bean sprouts
½ medium Chinese cabbage, shredded
2 large onions, cut into chunks
4 to 5 stems celery, in 2-inch diagonally cut chunks
1 medium head bok choy, in 2-inch diagonally cut chunks
2 large green peppers, cut into strips
½ pound Chinese pea pods, (remove outer "string" from pods)
1 cup sliced mushrooms
½ cup canned bamboo shoots, drained (save liquid for sauce, if needed)

⅔ cup sliced water chestnuts, drained (save liquid for
    sauce, if needed)
⅓ cup fresh pineapple chunks

*Sauce*

    3 cups fat-free chicken broth (see Index)
1½ tablespoons undiluted frozen apple juice concentrate,
    thawed
    2 to 3 tablespoons soy sauce, salt-reduced variety (op-
    tional)
    2 to 3 tablespoons cornstarch
    ¼ teaspoon garlic powder, or more, to taste
    1 tablespoon grated fresh ginger

Bring 2 cups of the chicken broth to a boil. Add the
onions, celery, and bok choy. Cook quickly, over a high
flame, stirring continuously until the vegetables are partly
cooked, though still crisp. Add the Chinese cabbage, pea
pods, green pepper, and mushrooms. Continue to cook
quickly, stirring frequently for a few more minutes.

*The sauce:* Make a paste of the cornstarch, garlic powder, ginger, apple juice, and soy sauce with a few tablespoons of the chicken broth. Stir the paste into the
cooking vegetables. Continue stirring until the mixture
thickens.

Add the bean sprouts, water chestnuts, bamboo shoots,
and cut-up chicken to the vegetables. Cook and stir the
mixture for a few more minutes. If the sauce becomes too
thick, thin it with some liquid (using the broth, or the liquid from the canned bamboo shoots and water chestnuts,
or just plain water). If a thicker sauce is desired, prepare
some more cornstarch paste and stir it into the cooking
vegetables.

Stir in the fresh pineapple just before serving.
*Serves 8*

## STUFFED ZUCCHINI

4  8-inch zucchini
½  cup matzo meal
¼  cup minced fresh parsley
¼  cup grated sapsago cheese
¾  cup skinned and diced fresh tomato
½  cup finely chopped onion
¼  cup finely chopped green pepper
1  cup cooked rice
1  tablespoon diced pimiento (optional)
¼  teaspoon celery seed
¼  teaspoon dried mint
¼  teaspoon garlic powder

Slice the zucchini in half lengthwise. Scrape out the pulp from the centers and set it aside. Place the zucchini in a pan in a little boiling water and simmer gently for a few minutes until it's partially cooked. (The zucchini should be firm enough to withstand stuffing.) Combine the pulp and the other ingredients in a bowl. Drop whole tomatoes in boiling water for a couple of minutes to facilitate removing the skin. Skin and dice tomatoes and add them to the other ingredients. Stuff the zucchini and lay them in a nonstick baking pan or casserole dish. Cover and bake in a preheated 350 degree oven for 45 minutes. Then uncover and brown.

Serve plain or with spaghetti sauce (see Index for Our Favorite Spaghetti Sauce), or substitute canned tomato sauce.

*Serves 4 to 6*

## "LITTLE BEEF" PATTIES

½ cup roasted whole buckwheat groats
6 ounces fat-trimmed flank steak, ground
2 tablespoons beet juice from cooked or canned beets
1 tablespoon dry wine
1 teaspoon soy sauce
1½ cups chopped onions
⅔ cup chopped mushrooms
2 tablespoons minced shallots (optional)
1 teaspoon finely minced garlic
¼ teaspoon garlic powder
¼ teaspoon ground black pepper
½ cup whole wheat pastry flour
2 egg whites
"Little Beef" Patty Sauce (recipe follows)

Bring 1 cup water to a boil. Add the buckwheat and cook covered about 10 minutes. Turn off heat and let buckwheat steam, covered, another 10 minutes or longer. Fluff buckwheat with a fork and place 1 measured cupful into a large mixing bowl. (Freeze the extra cooked buckwheat for use the next time you make this recipe.)

In a nonstick skillet, brown the meat over moderate heat until the pinkness is gone. Pour off rendered fat, if any. Add beet juice, wine and soy sauce and heat until liquid simmers. Add onions, mushrooms, shallots, garlic and spices to the skillet. Sauté until the liquid evaporates and the vegetable-meat mixture is brown. Stir the sautéed mixture into the cooked buckwheat. Sprinkle in the flour and mix well. Beat the egg whites to soft peaks and fold them into the mixture. Shape into 6 patties and lay them on a nonstick baking sheet. Bake in a preheated 400 degree oven for 20 minutes, lightly covered with aluminum foil. Remove foil and bake another 10 minutes to brown tops. Serve hot with "Little Beef" Patty Sauce.

*Makes 6 3-ounce patties.*

## "LITTLE BEEF" PATTY SAUCE

1 15-ounce can tomato sauce
½ can (5 ounces) enchilada sauce (Rosarita brand recommended)
⅛ cup prepared mustard
¼ teaspoon ginger
¼ teaspoon garlic powder
¼ teaspoon onion powder

Combine all ingredients in saucepan; heat to blend flavors. Serve hot over patties.

*Makes about 3 cups*

## BREADED EGGPLANT

2 eggplants, thinly sliced
2 15-ounce cans tomato sauce
1½ teaspoons basil or 1 teaspoon oregano
¼ cup grated sapsago cheese (optional)
1 cup cornmeal
½ cup matzo meal or unprocessed bran
½ cup whole-wheat pastry flour, or brown-rice flour

Slice the eggplant. Combine the tomato sauce, spices, and cheese in a bowl. In another bowl, combine the dry ingredients for breading. Using tongs, dip the eggplant in the tomato-sauce mixture. Then bread the eggplant by holding each eggplant slice above the breading bowl and spooning the breading mixture carefully over both sides. (This breading method avoids getting the breading mixture lumpy with tomato sauce.) Lay the eggplant slices on a nonstick baking sheet. Bake in a preheated 400 degree oven for 20 minutes, or until the top looks dry. Spoon any remaining sauce over the eggplant and continue baking it until it's tender and browned.

*Serves 8*

## VEGETABLE CASSEROLE

⅓  cup dried pinto beans
⅓  cup dried navy beans
¾  cup frozen green beans
¾  cup frozen limas
½  cup sliced carrots
½  cup chopped onions
¼  cup canned salsa
½  cup tomato juice
 1  minced shallot (optional)
½  cup unsweetened apple juice
½  teaspoon curry powder
¼  teaspoon garlic powder
1¼  cups sliced zucchini
1¼  cups sliced crookneck squash
 1  cup chopped cabbage
¾  cup frozen peas
1½  cups cauliflower florets
½  cup sliced water chestnuts
1⅓  cups nonfat milk
 1  tablespoon cornstarch

Soak the pinto and navy beans overnight in a cooking pot, in plenty of water. Discard water, add fresh water, and begin cooking beans. When the beans are half-done, add the frozen green beans, corn, lima beans, carrots, onions, salsa, and tomato juice. Season. When these vegetables are half-done, add the squash, cabbage, peas, and cauliflower. Just before serving, add the water chestnuts. Then add the cold milk, which has been mixed with the cornstarch. Stir until mixture thickens.
*Serves 8*

## SALSA I

*Use this tasty recipe as a sauce or salad dressing.*

1 15-ounce can whole-packed tomatoes, undrained and
   chopped
1 ripe tomato, peeled, if desired, then chopped
½ onion, finely chopped
1 tablespoon diced canned green chilies (use more or
   less, according to taste)
½ tablespoon vinegar (use more or less, according to
   taste)
   Pinch of oregano and/or basil

Combine all the ingredients, stirring well. Chill.
Serve over green salad, baked potato, rice, or cooked
vegetables.
*Note:* To peel the tomato, drop it into boiling water
for a few seconds; puncture and slip off the skin.
*Makes 2 cups*


## SALSA II

*Another version of this favorite Mexican accompa-
niment.*

1 cup canned green chilies, finely diced
2 cups chopped green onion
2 cups canned salsa
¼ cup canned diced tomatoes
¼ cup lemon juice
1 teaspoon garlic powder

Combine all the ingredients, stirring well. Chill.
Serve over green salad, baked potato, rice, or cooked
vegetables.
*Makes 7¼ cups*

## ENCHILADA SAUCE

2½ cups canned tomato sauce
1¼ cups water
½ tablespoon undiluted frozen apple juice concentrate, thawed
1 tablespoon cornstarch
1 teaspoon chili powder
1 teaspoon paprika
1 teaspoon oregano
1 teaspoon basil
1 teaspoon cumin

Begin heating the tomato sauce. Add 1 cup water. Mix the cornstarch with ¼ cup water and add to the pot. Add the apple juice and season.
*Makes 3¾ cups*

# FIVE

The
Pritikin
Kitchen

# 20

## Kitchen Equipment

In the world of fats and sugars and chemical additives, your Pritikin kitchen will be your fortress. With your refrigerator and cabinet shelves stocked with the ingredients for the delicious recipes in this book, it will be hard indeed for you to return to your old eating ways.

At the supermarket you'll need to pay careful attention to labels. Stock up on interesting spices and seasonings and learn to use them creatively. For cooking, most of what you need is probably already at hand. Your favorite recipes often can be adapted easily to the diet with substitutions—and in many cases, the final result will be more delicious than before!

No special cooking equipment is needed, but you should invest in a blender and some nonstick pans if you don't own them already. Overall, you'll be pleased to find your grocery bills going down. Expect savings from about 25 percent upward.

### EQUIPMENT

Here's the equipment you'll want to have on hand:
- A blender with a powerful motor.
- Nonstick (Teflon) baking pans. We suggest a muffin pan for corn or bran muffins, two loaf pans for breads, two round pizza pans, and two square or oblong pans for casseroles.
- A T-Fal or other nonstick skillet.
- Nonstick spatulas and spoons (regular and slotted)— a must with nonstick equipment.
- Stainless steel or enamelware pots and pans. A variety

161

of saucepans, skillets, and large boiler pots (for soup and beans).

- Good chopping knives and a cutting board.
- A colander

Those are the essentials. In addition, you'll find these optional items handy:

- Canisters—glass or plastic see-through are better for keeping bugs out of grains; tall ones are nice for long, whole-wheat spaghetti.
- Plastic with seal-tops.
- Ice-cube trays for freezing stocks and sauces.
- A bulb baster to remove unwanted grease.
- Cake-cooling racks for cooling breads and draining cheese.
- Cheesecloth.
- A pastry brush with natural fibers.
- Ramekins—individual casserole dishes.
- A vegetable-steaming basket.
- Large and small tea strainers.
- Wire whisks for blending batters, sauces, and egg whites.
- An egg separater—a more reliable way to separate egg whites from the yolk than the haphazard hand method.
- A garlic press.
- A grater.
- Mashers.
- A melon baller.
- A scoop—traditionally for ice cream, but nice to scoop other foods.
- A sifter.
- A soup ladle. Also good for chili, vegetable stews, fruit sauces, etc.
- A strawberry huller.
- A pie spatula and server.
- Tongs.
- Vegetable brushes—for vegetable scrubbing.
- Vegetable peelers.
- Spin drier for lettuce.
- Popsicle forms for fruit-juice popsicles.

- Sherbet glasses for serving fruit cups or other appropriate desserts.
- Thermometer for making cheese. (Make sure the thermometer goes down to 70° F.)
- A Weight Watcher's scale, or a similar scale, for weighing meats and portions.

### *Appliances or Large Gadgetry*

- An electric mixer for making bread.
- A portable electric mixer (hand model) for beating egg whites, making whipped toppings of nonfat dry milk and juices, etc.
- A food processor. This is a major investment but well worth it. You'll use it to slice, chop, shred, blend, grate, purée, and grind vegetables.
- A rotary slicer for extra-fine slicing of potatoes, cabbages, beets, carrots, or any other food.
- A pressure cooker.
- A crockpot—a convenient, slow electric cooker.
- A toaster oven—especially useful for making open-faced toasted hoop cheese sandwiches, baking potatoes, heating small leftovers, warming or toasting large pita breads, bagels, etc., heating corn tortillas, making pita pizzas.
- A nonstick waffle iron.
- A yogurt maker.
- A juicer.
- An ice-cream maker—you just make the batter with your own ingredients and put it into the machine, then fit the machine into the freezer and wait. No messing with hand-cranking or rock salt.

### *Pots and Pans*

- Aluminum tins and pie pans—regular size and individual pot-pie size. Both are useful for heating leftovers in oven.
- Nonstick or quality stainless-finish baking pans with nonstick properties—square, rectangular, and large deep-dish for lasagne, manicotti, chili rellenos, crêpes, etc.
- A nonstick cake-roll pan, 15½-by-10½-by-1. Essen-

tially a cookie sheet with a raised rim and so more
versatile.
- Nonstick cake pans, round.
- Nonstick cookie sheets for baking oven-fried potatoes
  or chicken, heating several tortillas or pitas, etc.
- A nonstick crepe pan—terrific for making crepes and
  pseudo-omelets.
- A double boiler—desirable for making white sauces
  (as in a "creamed" turkey, chicken, tuna, salmon, or
  vegetable dish), cereal cooked with milk, etc.
- A nonstick or stainless steel wok—owners swear by it
  for cooking Chinese food and vegetables. Because of
  the wok's design compared to a regular pot, the heat
  distribution is superior and produces a unique, crisp-
  tender result.
- Nonstick muffin pans.

## THE SPICE SHELF

You'll want to learn all about seasonings and spices
and lay in a good stock of them. A spice chart like the
one published by Celestial Seasonings will be helpful. The
best way to learn is to experiment, and the best guide is
your own palate. You will become intuitive about your
spices in time.

If you like food well seasoned, experiment with a variety: garlic and onion powder, bay leaves, oregano, basil,
chives, parsley, sage, marjoram, rosemary, thyme, dillweed, cumin, black pepper, mustard. To emphasize the
sweetness of a dish, use allspice, ginger, coriander, cinnamon, nutmeg, curry, mace, cloves, mint, cardamom.

Here's a list of these and other spices to use:

Allspice                        whole
Anise seeds                     Chervil
Basil                           Chili powder
Caraway seeds                     (avoid salted brands)
Cardamom, ground                Chives
Cayenne pepper                  Cinnamon
Celery seeds, ground and        Cloves, ground and whole

Coriander
Curry powder
Cumin
Dillweed
Fennel
Garlic powder
Ginger, ground
Herb seasonings
Horseradish (powdered)
Italian seasoning
Mace, ground
Marjoram
Mint
Mustard (dry)
Nutmeg

Onion powder and flakes
Paprika
Parsley
Pepper (black and white),
   ground
Peppercorns (black)
Rosemary
Saffron
Sage, ground
Savory
Tarragon
Thyme
Turmeric
Vanilla extract
Vegetable flakes

Now that your kitchen has the essentials, it's time for a trip to the supermarket. The next chapter will tell you what foods to buy.

# 21

## Stocking Up

### MEAT, FISH, AND POULTRY

I like to consider this category as a source of flavoring for the more nutritious vegetable and grain dishes, rather than as main dishes in themselves.

In stocking your freezer, the emphasis should be on the leanest cuts. You may wish to keep lean beef, cut up as desired or ground, fish fillets, chicken and turkey breasts. Meat in good or standard grades, rather than choice or prime, is preferable for lower fat content. Avoid cholesterol-rich organ meats and inordinately fat meats such as bacon, hot dogs, and sausage. Shellfish are restricted (see Table of Foods to Use and to Avoid, Chapter 1). No duck or goose. Use *lean* fish, such as halibut, sole, sea bass, snapper.

Canned tuna is a good choice for your pantry shelf, but buy the water-packed variety.

To make it easier to stick to allowed portions of meat, fish, and fowl, you may wish to cut up your purchases, weigh them, then wrap them separately for freezer storage.

You'll find you can cook lean cuts of meat with as much flavor and tenderness as the fat ones you used to eat. The secret is to cook them slowly, seasoned with herbs and spices, and possibly some cooking wine or broth. You can add flavor by cooking with vegetables in the same pan—onions, parsley, carrots, mushrooms, celery, tomatoes, or whatever strikes your fancy.

If you cook with nonstick pans, you'll have no need for fats. Use water for sautéeing, flavoring the water occasionally with a little broth or tomato juice, stirring from time to time. With ground meat liquid is rarely required. As the meat sticks, you can loosen it with a spatula.

# VEGETABLES

By serving interesting vegetable dishes and soups combined with or alongside different grains, you'll shift the emphasis of the meal from the meat, fish, and fowl dishes that once held center stage. Include a couple of cooked vegetables or a vegetable medley in each meal, and as a change of pace, substitute a vegetarian entree for meat. If you like a richer flavor, try cooking vegetables in a bit of fat-free chicken stock.

Stock the refrigerator with a supply of basic vegetables like several kinds of lettuce, celery, tomatoes, green onions, green peppers, cucumbers, carrots, mushrooms, parsley, and radishes, plus an array of seasonal vegetables. (Some folks prefer to refrigerate onions and potatoes as well.) In the pantry, store canned vegetables such as beets, artichoke hearts, asparagus spears, green or wax beans, water chestnuts, pimientos, and green chilies. Canned tomato products in various forms are indispensable: tomato juice, sauce, paste, pureé, and diced or whole tomatoes, as well as specialties such as green chili salsa. In the freezer, keep bags and cartons of frozen out-of-season vegetables, but avoid those packed in sauces. Your best bet for beans is to purchase them dried, in bulk. Buy garbanzos, pintos, kidney and navy beans, etc., along with a supply of lentils and split peas. You may want to keep canned beans on hand as well, but check to find brands free of sugar and preservatives.

You may be used to sautéeing vegetables rapidly in a bit of fat. You'll find they're actually more flavorsome sautéed with water or a fat-free stock. Use a bit of water at the bottom of your skillet instead of oil, bring it to a boil, then add the vegetables and stir while the liquid evaporates until they're brown. Or sauté your vegetables directly on a dry skillet, making sure you don't use too high a heat and that you watch the cooking process closely to avoid scorching.

You can save the leftover liquid from cooking vegetables, store it in plastic containers in the freezer, and use it to make stocks that will enhance the flavor of soups, casseroles, and sauces.

You'll find a food processor helpful for chopping quantities of potatoes, carrots, and onions. With a change of blades it will shred cabbage, carrots, radishes, and potatoes. It will also grind beans and slice mushrooms, bell peppers, radishes, and onions.

You'll very likely want to get a pressure cooker and one of the new long-cooking electric pots. The first is a great time-saver for beans, stews, and vegetables; the second acts as a flavor-enhancer.

When using a pressure cooker, be sure to fill it only half full to prevent overpressurizing. When you take the lid off and check food, place the cooker under the faucet and run cold water over it. When the hissing stops, it's safe to remove the lid.

Garbanzo beans, which would normally have to soak overnight and simmer for at least two hours, take only forty-five minutes in a pressure cooker. Soft vegetables take only three to five minutes, harder ones up to ten minutes.

## SALADS

A green salad with lots of raw vegetables will enhance any meal. And who says you can't concoct a great dressing without fatty ingredients?

Hoop cheese, a versatile food you can use with a number of other foods, will mix with nonfat buttermilk to make a mock sour cream with a thick, creamy-smooth texture. It makes a good "mayonnaise" base in all kinds of salads—fish, chicken, potato, cole slaw, macaroni, and fruit. Season the "mayonnaise" appropriately for the dish. You can add whatever seasonings and condiments you like. You'll probably find you like this new dressing *better* than the somewhat heavier, more pungent flavor of mayonnaise. It also works as a sandwich spread. If you can't find hoop cheese, another form of uncreamed cottage cheese can generally be used.

You'll find that Tillie Lewis brand Italian salad dressing is an acceptable substitute for oil and vinegar, though quite salty. You may want to dilute its brininess with equal parts of vinegar and water and add extra spices, capers, grated sapsago cheese, or chunks of fresh hoop cheese. It's also useful for marinades.

You can make a delicious buttermilk dressing from acceptable dressing mixes by substituting nonfat buttermilk or nonfat yogurt, or mock sour cream (see Index) for the mayonnaise in the package directions.

Homemade croutons—cubed, seasoned bread chunks slow-toasted in the oven—will dress up your salads. You'll want to keep lots of condiments, too—dill pickles, pickled vegetables like cauliflower and red peppers, vinegar, mustard, horseradish, and hot sauce.

Bean and seed sprouts are delightful additions to any salad. It takes only three days to sprout mung, lentil, wheat, or alfalfa seeds, if you want to grow your own.

## SAUCES

In any creamed food, like creamed chicken or vegetables, a white sauce is as tasty as ever when nonfat milk is substituted for whole milk or cream. Normally, white sauce is a combination of butter, flour, and whole milk. Just omit the butter and substitute nonfat milk for the milk. (Use two tablespoons flour per cup of nonfat milk.) Then put the ingredients into your blender, blend until smooth, transfer to a saucepan to heat, and stir until thickened. Use your seasonings to flavor it.

You can create delicious sauces and gravies using fat-free stocks (vegetable, meat, poultry, or fish) or leftover liquid from cooking vegetables as a base. To de-fat meat or poultry stock, chill the liquid until the fat congeals. Then skim off the fat with a spoon. To remove any remaining fat, pour the stock through several thicknesses of cheesecloth. To your de-fatted stock, add any desired liquid. You can use fluid (or dried) nonfat milk or evaporated skim milk when you want a creamy appearance (by increasing the proportion of milk to stock, you can make an excellent white sauce). Throw in a few sliced mushrooms or onions to make it even zippier, then season to your taste.

Thicken your sauce with one scant tablespoon of cornstarch (if you prefer arrowroot*, use a little more) per cup of liquid, making a paste by mixing the thickener with a little cold liquid before adding it to the pot. Heat contents of pot until simmering, add paste, and stir while simmering until thickened.

Use these basic techniques to thicken, expand, de-fat and flavor the gravy from any dish you are preparing. The addition of cooking wines in permitted small quantities will add a nice gourmet touch to some recipes. Try a splash of burgundy in tomato sauce or some sherry in a fish dish.

For convenience, keep a supply of fat-free stocks in the freezer in small plastic containers, baggies, or ice-cube trays.


## DAIRY PRODUCTS

You'll now be using nonfat milk as a substitute for whole milk in recipes. In addition to regular (fluid) nonfat milk, keep on hand for occasional use a box of nonfat dry milk and some cans of evaporated skim milk.*

You'll also want nonfat buttermilk, nonfat yogurt, and 100 percent uncreamed cottage cheese, such as hoop cheese or dry curd cottage cheese.

The buttermilk you may frequently find in the store is partly unhomogenized with added particles of butter. If you strained these fat particles out, the buttermilk would then be about comparable in fat to lowfat milk. If you are unable to find a nonfat buttermilk or one up to 1 percent fat by weight, you can make your own using our recipe.

*If an arrowroot paste is used, the saucepan should be removed from heat while stirring in paste.

* Evaporated skim milk has the advantage of a heavier texture than nonfat milk, making it a good substitute for whole milk in some recipes. However, a given amount contains much more protein than nonfat milk—thus requiring limited use. It also contains questionable additives.

In the case of yogurt, we have found that the lowfat plain variety is the closest you can come to nonfat yogurt in the market. However, making your own is quite simple (especially with a yogurt maker) and economical, too.

One hundred percent uncreamed cottage cheese is now widely distributed in different forms; hoop cheese can be found in some areas in pressed brick form, others resemble cottage cheese. If you don't see one of these cheeses in the dairy case (or if you want to investigate the possibility of obtaining other nonfat dairy products), talk to the deli supervisor or phone local commercial dairies. They may be very accommodating. Whatever the outcome, you can make delicious homemade cheese with the recipes in this book.

For extra flavor, try sapsago (green) cheese, a hard cheese from Switzerland which can be grated in place of parmesan. While sapsago is low in fat for a hard cheese, it is not a 100 percent skim milk cheese, so is restricted accordingly. Eggs are a staple, though you'll only use the whites. When recipes call for whole eggs, use the whites of two eggs or substitute liquid for the missing yolk.

The labeling of dairy products is confusing, as fat content given by weight can mislead you into thinking you are purchasing a product low in fat. When fat is calculated as percent of total calories—the criterion of major importance on the Pritikin Diet—almost all but 100 percent skim milk products are unacceptable. The accompanying table illustrates this point with various dairy products:

| Food Item | Fat Percent by Weight | Fat Percent as Percent of Total Calories |
|---|---|---|
| Whole milk | 3.5 | 48.4 |
| Lowfat milk | 2.0 | 30.5 |
| Nonfat (skim) milk | 0.1 | 2.4 |
| Creamed cottage cheese | 4.0 | 36.7 |
| Lowfat cottage cheese | 2.0 | 17.6 |
| Uncreamed cottage cheese | 0.3 | 3.1 |
| New York deluxe pot cheese | 5.0 | 44.0 |

## CEREALS

Cereals will be a breakfast mainstay now, but you
needn't get bored with them—try a variety. Basic grains
like cracked wheat, rolled and steel-cut oats, whole
ground cornmeal, and whole grain combinations are
highly recommended because they are the least refined.
Whole wheat, rye, and oat flakes are also good. Erewhon,
El Molino, and Stone-buhr are distributors of fine quality whole grain cereals; you will probably discover others
in your area. Preferred popular cereal brands include
Wheatena, Zoom, Wheat Hearts, and Cream of Rye.
More refined cereals such as Cream of Wheat and Cream
of Rice are less desirable, though still acceptable. You
might also purchase unprocessed bran flakes, providing
extra dietary fiber, to add to your cereals.

Of the well-known dry cereals, only Grape Nuts and
Shredded Wheat are acceptable, though the wholesome-
ness of Shredded Wheat is marred by a preservative. You
will find Grape Nuts to be much more than just a cereal;
its versatility extends to use in breading, crumb pie crusts,
crumb toppings and layers in casseroles, puddings, and
dessert specialties. A superior cereal would be your own
whole grain dry cereal, made by toasting rolled oats
and/or wheat, rye, or oat flakes. (See recipes for Homemade Dry Cereal.) Eat it plain for munching, or with milk
and fruit as a cold cereal.

For a change from cereals, try pancakes from a whole-
wheat mix, or make your own batter. Use the batter for
waffles, too. For an unconventional but tasty breakfast or
snack, have hot or cold brown rice with sliced bananas,
cinnamon, and nonfat buttermilk or milk.

## BREADS

Read labels of breads at the supermarket to avoid additives. Sourdough breads, rolls, and biscuits are usually
best. You should also check out whole-grain breads or
rolls (wheat, rye, and pumpernickel). Specialty breads
are a good buy, too. Use corn tortillas for Mexican

entrees and for making corn chips, pita, and other breads for interesting sandwiches.

Most store-bought breads contain fats, sugars, and salt. Your best bet is to arrange with a local baker to bake up twenty loaves from one of the recipes in this book and store them in your freezer. You can also buy pita bread in packages of six and store several packages (sometimes you can get a discount on large quantities from a Middle Eastern bakery) in the refrigerator or freezer.

For baking, keep fresh cornmeal, flour, double-acting baking powder, and baking soda on hand. Check to make sure the baking powder doesn't contain aluminum.

Keep a variety of crackers around—they'll be particularly welcome at snack time and with soups. Types to try are Finn Crisp, unseasoned Rye-Krisp, all the Scandinavian flatbreads, matzo, rice cakes, whole-wheat or rice wafers, and cold-water crackers. You can also find (but you may have to search a bit) dietetic pretzels that don't contain salt or shortening—even the big, thick, twisted ones come that way.

## PASTA AND GRAINS

Keep (whole-wheat, preferably) macaroni, spaghetti, manicotti, grandini, and lasagne. When you buy noodles, make sure they don't contain egg. For a gourmet change, try Oriental pasta or coiled vermicelli instead of regular spaghetti. Keep brown rice, wild rice, barley, toasted or untoasted buckwheat (kasha), bulgur wheat (a fast-cooking par boiled wheat), cracked wheat, millet, whole ground cornmeal, triticale (a cross between wheat and rye), whole-wheat, flour and whole-wheat pastry flour among your staples. Rye flour, buckwheat flour, and brown rice flour (for those with wheat allergies) are useful additions when making your own bread.

## FRUITS

Take advantage of year-round and seasonal fresh fruits—don't skimp on quality or variety. You'll find bananas to be an indispensable fruit for breakfasts, snacks, and baking. Citrus fruits and apples are also reliable stand-bys. Try several varieties of apples (pippin, golden and red delicious, Granny Smith from New Zealand, and Rome beauty for baking). Sliced melon is a nice eye-opener in the morning, an attractive garnish with a luncheon or dinner plate, and a refreshing dessert. And, of course, melon balls are great in a fruit cup. In addition to the usual cantaloupe and watermelon, try crenshaw and honeydew.

When the fresh summer fruits are out, load up on nectarines, apricots, peaches, plums, grapes, and berries of all kinds. Try the exotic fruits, too, like mangoes, papaya, pineapple, and kiwi fruit.

You'll also want to look for frozen and canned fruits with no sweeteners added. Dietetic brands of canned fruit often carry fruit packed in water or juice, and it's easy to find major brands of pineapple canned in its own juice. A good selection of unsweetened fruit juices awaits you at a health- or natural-food store—often better than at the regular supermarket. There, you may also find fruit "preserves" without added sugar or honey. Dried fruits like raisins, currants, and dates are acceptable in small amounts and are particularly useful in sweetening your own baked goods.

*However*, even though these fruit products are unsweetened, the processing they undergo makes their natural fruit sugars more concentrated. Fruits processed by cooking (canned fruit is cooked), freezing, drying, or even by extracting the juice from the pulp—mechanically damaging the pulp—have a higher concentration of free sugars, which may raise the blood triglycerides markedly if eaten in excess; hence, we restrict their use. Gorging on fresh fruit might have a similar effect, though fresh fruit's abundance of complex carbohydrates are digested at a very manageable rate.

## DRINKS

Sample a wide variety of fruit juices and keep your favorites chilled in the refrigerator. For some, the hardest time of day to stick to the diet is cocktail hour. Try having mineral water or club soda with a twist of lemon or lime or a little frozen apple juice concentrate mixed in, or a spiced, tomato juice "Virgin Mary" if you're used to an afternoon drink.

A satisfying hot drink can be made with hot milk mixed with a bit of carob powder, vanilla, and a hint of cinnamon. In the blender, you can concoct creamy shakes with fruit juice and buttermilk along with a banana or berries. Or mix up plain milk with fruit, carob powder, or vanilla. Frozen berries or just ice cubes will add a nice, icy froth.

You will find, though, that you will be less thirsty on your new diet owing to the reduced salt intake and the large quantity of high-water content vegetables you will be eating.

## SWEETS AND SNACKS

The ideal sweet or snack is fresh fruit. You would do well to become a connoisseur of juicy, ripe fresh fruit! Of course, when the variety of fresh fruit drops in off-season months, you will rely more on frozen and canned fruit (unsweetened). You can keep dried fruits around, too. (Don't forget restrictions on all fruit categories.)

A favorite quick treat in our family is sliced banana (and other fruit, if you want) over cold brown rice, topped with non-fat buttermilk and a sprinkling of cinnamon. Or try a dish of fruit topped with Grape Nuts, raisins, or non-fat milk or buttermilk, and cinnamon. A fruit milkshake is another easy and very refreshing snack. Or whip up some orange juice, or any other juice, in the blender with lots of ice for a delicious "freeze."

If you feel a bit more industrious, try some of the tempting dessert recipes in the book to satisfy your sweet tooth. Puddings, pies, cakes, cookies, jams: all can be made without fats and are sweetened with fruit and fruit products.

Snacking on simple fare can be most satisfying. Crackers, a warm sourdough roll, a juicy orange, home-crisped corn chips with salsa, a sliced hoop cheese and banana sandwich, or raw vegetable sticks might just hit the spot. Popcorn without oil is not much more trouble to make, especially if you have kidpower to help. You can use the kind of popper for open fire use, an enclosed mesh "cage" with a long handle that you shake (and shake and shake!) over a heat source until the corn is popped, though any covered pan that conducts heat well will also work. Or treat yourself to one of the new electric hot-air poppers, which does not require added fat.

If you plan ahead, you can have snack foods on hand which require more prep time, such as garbanzo "nuts" and garbanzo "nut" butter, granola, cheese and bean dips (see Index). Prepared in larger quantity, they can be stored in extra containers in the refrigerator or freezer.

Feel free to snack on leftovers like spaghetti or soup. Remember, this kind of snacking, as opposed to conventional snacking, provides you with the most healthful of foods. So don't worry if you spoil your appetite a little.

## STORAGE

If you cook food in large quantities and store the excess, you'll save time. When you cook soup, for instance, make a big potful and put the rest in the freezer.

Store cooked foods in meal-sized plastic containers, Pyrex ware, or in plastic bags with labels. You can store cooked beans, bean entrees, breads, crêpes, pancakes, homemade cheese, lasagne, spaghetti sauces, salad dressings, and pizza this way.

Here's a quick checklist of foods your kitchen might now contain:

### Refrigerator

*Dairy products:* Nonfat milk, nonfat buttermilk,* nonfat yogurt,* 100 percent uncreamed cottage cheese,* e.g., hoop cheese or dry curd cottage cheese, sapsago (green cheese).

* Make at home if unavailable in stores.

*Vegetables:* Lettuce, tomatoes, green peppers, cucumber, celery, carrots, parsley, radishes, green onion, onions and potatoes,** other vegetables in season. Cooked beans, leftover cooked vegetables, soups.

*Beverages:* Fruit and vegetable juices, mineral water or club soda, iced linden tea.

*Grain foods:* Cooked grains—brown rice (seasoned), kasha, and/or bulgur wheat; brown rice (plain) for snacks, dessert recipes, and fillers (such as extending meat). Leftover pancakes, waffles, French toast, corn tortillas. Breads,** such as whole wheat, sourdough, pumpernickel or rye, pita, and sprouted wheat berry.

*Fruits:* All fruits of choice, such as citrus fruits, apples, melon, and seasonal fruits.

*Condiments and Miscellaneous:* Capers, vinegar, pimientos, dill pickles, peppers, and other vegetables packed in wine vinegar, mustard, horseradish (not creamed), Kikkoman mild low-salt soy sauce, hot sauce, Pace Picante Sauce, Tillie Lewis Italian salad dressing, cooking wines.

## Cupboard

*Spices:* Your old favorites, plus those you want to experiment with.

*Canned goods:* Tomato sauce, tomato purée, whole tomatoes, tomato paste, whole green chilies, green chili salsa, enchilada sauce, canned juices (vegetable and fruit), canned fruits, evaporated skim milk, canned vegetables and beans, canned soup (e.g., Anderson's Split Pea).

*Crackers:* Scandinavian flatbreads, matzo crackers, Finn Crisp, Rye-Crisp, dietetic pretzels.

*Pasta:* Spaghetti, lasagne, manicotti, coiled vermicelli, macaroni, noodles, etc.

Cereals: An assortment of whole grains including cracked wheat, whole rolled and steel-cut oats, whole ground cornmeal, and grain combinations (try Erewhon, Stonebuhr, and other superior brands). Packaged hot and cold

** These items do not require refrigeration, but they will last longer if refrigerated. Refrigerator space will pobably be a consideration here.

cereals, such as Wheatena, Zoom, Cream of Rye, Cream of Wheat, Grape Nuts. Whole wheat, rye, oat flakes.
*Other grains:* Brown rice, wild rice, bulgur wheat, buckwheat (kasha), barley, rye, millet, triticale, etc.
*Dry staples:* Flours, baking powder, baking soda, cornstarch, arrowroot, matzo meal, pearl tapioca, unflavored gelatin, dry yeast, non-fat dry milk, carob powder or pure carob, pectin, rennet tablets (Junket), potato pancake mix (acceptable ingredients), homemade croutons.

### Freezer

*Meats, Poultry and Fish:* Lean beef cut up or ground, chicken and turkey breasts, fish fillets or steaks, packaged for individual or family servings.
*Vegetables and Fruits:* Cartons and bags of frozen vegetables and unsweetened berries, concentrated unsweetened fruit juices.
*Breads:* Miscellaneous fat- and sugar-free breads, corn tortillas, pita bread (whole-grain breads preferred).
*Prepared Foods:* Homemade vegetable or defatted stocks from beef, chicken, and fish; sauces, including spaghetti sauce and enchilada sauce; Mock Sour Cream (stir vigorously before using); soups, casseroles, and entrees.

The next chapter gives many helpful hints on how to reduce fat intake, substitute acceptable items for unacceptable ones, and ends with a final, summary shopping list.

# 22

## Hints and Substitutions

### REDUCING FAT INTAKE

The following are practical ways of getting the fat out of your cooking—and your life.

- Chill all soups and stews with a beef or poultry base, and all potted meat and poultry dishes, to remove congealed fat that rises to the top of the container. Then pour stock through several thicknesses of cheesecloth to collect any remaining fat.
- When there is no time to chill cooked foods to remove fat, drop several ice cubes in the pot and remove the cubes and the fat that congeals on them. Or you can try removing surface fat with a turkey baster, then strain through several layers of cheesecloth.
- Use only the leanest cuts of meat and keep portions small.
- Always remove skin of poultry before serving, and preferably before cooking.
- If 100 percent uncreamed cottage cheese is unavailable, look for cottage cheese up to 1 percent fat by weight, or rinse creamed cottage cheese in colander until water runs clear.
- Use only egg yolk-free pasta products.
- Make your own nonfat yogurt or nonfat buttermilk with a lowfat commercial starter. Afterwards, always save some homemade yogurt or buttermilk to serve as a starter for the next batch.
- Experiment with hamburger patties to stretch them with vegetables and rice.

The accompanying table shows what foods to use in place of foods not allowed on the diet.

## TABLE OF SUBSTITUTIONS

| *Unacceptable Item* | *Acceptable Substitute* |
| --- | --- |
| Butter, oil, other fats | • Substitute depends on function of fat; see section on Other Substitution Hints, page 183. |
| Sugar, honey, molasses | • Fruit juice, natural strength or frozen concentrate<br>• Fresh fruit, frozen or canned fruit (unsweetened, grated, mashed or liquidized in blender)<br>• Raisins or other dried fruits (may be soaked in water or juice to plump fruit and obtain sweeter liquid) |
| Egg yolks | • Egg whites (2 whites per yolk)<br>• 1 or 2 tbsp. permissible liquid for each missing yolk |
| Cream, whole milk | • Nonfat milk<br>• Evaporated skim milk (more comparable in heaviness to cream or whole milk, but contains much more protein than nonfat milk as well as questionable additives; restrict use)<br>• Nonfat buttermilk (in some recipes)<br>• Other permissible liquid |
| Sour cream | • 100 percent uncreamed cottage cheese (e.g., hoop cheese or dry curd) blended with nonfat milk or buttermilk to sour cream consistency (see *Mock Sour Cream*)<br>• Nonfat yogurt, homemade; see recipe or use yogurt maker |
| Yogurt | • Nonfat yogurt, homemade; see recipe or use yogurt maker |
| Creamed cottage cheese, ricotta | • 100 percent uncreamed cottage cheese (e.g., hoop cheese or dry |

| *Unacceptable Item* | *Acceptable Substitute* |
| --- | --- |
| cheese | curd) mashed with acceptable milk or water to desired consistency<br>● *Easy Ricotta Cheese*<br>● *Creamy Nonfat Cheese* |
| Mozarella, other part-skim cheeses | ● Hoop cheese (pressed brick form) crumbled or sliced thin (in some recipes) |
| Parmesan cheese, grated, romano cheese, grated | ● Sapsago cheese (also called green cheese), grated |
| Cream cheese | ● Hoop cheese (pressed brick form), or any other kind of 100 percent uncreamed cottage cheese<br>● *Easy Ricotta Cheese*<br>● *Creamy Nonfat Cheese* |
| Ice cream | ● Use home ice-cream maker to create your own |
| Nuts | ● *Garbanzo "Nuts"*<br>● Roasted chestnuts<br>● Diced water chestnuts<br>● Grape Nuts cereal |
| Peanut Butter | ● *Garbanzo "Nut" Butter* |
| Seeds | ● Uncooked rolled oats, oven-toasted until crunchy |
| Egg noodles | ● Vegetable (eggless) noodles<br>● Yolk-free noodles<br>● Spaghetti, broken up<br>● Macaroni |
| Mayonnaise | ● *Mock Sour Cream*, with seasoning<br>● Nonfat yogurt, homemade, with seasoning; see recipe or use yogurt maker<br>● Combination of *Mock Sour Cream* and nonfat yogurt, with seasoning |
| Tartar sauce | ● To basic mayonnaise substitute, add: capers, mustard, finely chopped |

*Unacceptable Item*          *Acceptable Substitute*

|  | onion, garlic, dillweed, herbs, optional dash lemon juice |
|---|---|
| Catsup | • Combine to catsup consistency: tomato paste, vinegar, small amount of apple juice concentrate, garlic powder, onion powder |
| Soy sauce | • Low-salt soy sauce<br>• Regular soy sauce, diluted |
| Bouillon cubes | • Fat-free stock, equivalent to volume each cube flavors |
| Chocolate | • Carob powder, unsweetened (suitable in many recipes where chocolate is used) |
| Jam, jelly, fruit butter | • Unsweetened fruit, with added fruit juice if desired, cooked and then thickened with cornstarch, arrowroot, gelatin, or pectin (with optional added vanilla and spices). *Note:* Fruit may cook down to sufficient thickness without using thickening agent<br>• Mashed banana, persimmon, other fruits |
| Salt | • Other spices of choice |
| Soft drinks | • Mineral or carbonated water with added fruit juice |
| Coffee | • Carob powder, unsweetened—not as substitute for beverage but to simulate coffee flavor in some recipes<br>• Coffee substitutes (roasted barley, chicory, etc., combinations) still under study—but neither recommended nor prohibited. |

## OTHER SUBSTITUTION HINTS

Here's what to use instead of butter or oil in different cooking techniques:

*Sautéing vegetables:* Use a little liquid such as water or vegetable or chicken broth in the bottom of a skillet. Bring liquid to a boil, then add vegetables and stir until browned, allowing most of the liquid to evaporate. While sautéing, add extra liquid if vegetables look too dry.

You can also brown vegetables directly in a dry nonstick skillet, making sure you do not use too high a heat and that you watch the cooking process carefully to avoid scorched vegetables. This can also be applied to sautéing rice for a pilaf; or use a nonstick pan and oven-toast, watching carefully so as not to burn.

*Browning:* Lean ground beef is easily browned in a nonstick skillet over moderate heat with no added fat or liquid. Loosen meat with a spatula as it sticks, and stir to obtain even browning. Other meats require a little liquid to sauté. Start with a cold nonstick skillet and add meat with a tablespoon or two of water, broth, or tomato juice. Using moderate flame, cook meat until nicely browned, stirring occasionally. Vegetables may be added at this time for browning.

Another technique especially good for foods such as pot roasts, stew meat, chicken, and fish involves quick-browning under the broiler, after which the cooking proceeds on top of the stove or in the oven. While browning the foods, be sure to baste them in rendered juices to avoid dryness, or use an additional basting liquid. If chicken is used, remove the skin first and baste generously during browning.

*Frying:* On stove top, use nonstick skillet without fat to "fry" patties, potato pancakes, French toast, pancakes, etc. Use a nonstick baking sheet without fat to oven-"fry" breaded chicken, potatoes, eggplant, patties, etc. Some foods lend themselves well to both methods; others do better with one method or the other.

*Marinades:* Replace oil or fat with compatible liquids, like lemon juice, vinegar, vegetable broth or fat-free stock, tomato juice, fruit juice, nonfat milk, low-salt soy sauce, cooking wines.

*Basting:* Use acceptable liquids such as those suggested under Marinades, as well as rendered juices from food being cooked.

Sweetening tips: Fruits and fruit juices are most often required for sweetening. However, there are more subtle ways to sweeten foods. Cooking with carrots is one good way. They can impart a sweet flavor to soups and entrees that normally call for a tablespoon or two of sugar, such as a spaghetti sauce. If a little sugar is called for in a recipe, try adding a diced or chopped carrot. Or put in a large whole carrot to simmer with the sauce, then remove before serving. If you want to make it even sweeter, add a swig of apple or pineapple juice. You can use carrots to sweeten a navy bean casserole, rather than the usual molasses and brown sugar. Cook the carrots and some apple juice in the bean liquid.

Naturally sweet vegetables like sweet potatoes, squash, and yams make great pies and hot casseroles, and when chilled are gooey-sweet snacks. Sweet corn is another vegetable that lends a natural sweetness.

For some cooking and baking, to complement the sweetness you are trying to achieve, the flavor of vanilla will help. Use vanilla extract or whole vanilla beans. For chocolate you can substitute carob powder, but beware of the carob bars sold in health food stores, which generally have sugar and fat additives comparable to a chocolate bar.

Also, use spices to best advantage. Certain spices, such as oregano or peppers, impart a slightly bitter quality, as opposed to sweet basil, for example. Spices such as coriander, cinnamon, nutmeg, allspice, curry, cardamom, ginger, and mace tend to complement a sweet flavor. The omission of salt from recipes, moreover, will automatically sweeten a dish.

To make gravy from fat-free stock: Remove all traces of fat from meat, fish, or fowl stock by refrigerating or freezing the stock until fat is congealed. Remove fat with a large spoon and pour stock through several thicknesses of cheesecloth to remove remaining fat. You may want to freeze the defatted stock in premeasured amounts or in ice-cube trays.

Add to the fat-free stock desired seasoning and other

liquids of choice, such as vegetable broth, nonfat milk, a dash of soy sauce. Then thicken according to the following methods.

Thickening hints: For sauces, stews, and many soups (cream-type and others), cornstarch or arrowroot can be used for thickening. Arrowroot clears completely, so it should be used where greater transparency is desirable. While it makes a delicate sauce, it does not reheat well. Cornstarch may leave a little cloudiness but is preferable for some uses, such as thickening a white sauce, as it gives desirable color. (Arrowroot may be purchased at health- or natural-food stores.)

To use cornstarch or arrowroot, follow these suggestions: Make a thin paste of the cornstarch or arrowroot in a little cold liquid (water or other acceptable liquid). One level tablespoon of arrowroot will thicken one cup of liquid. Cornstarch has slightly more thickening capacity, so a little less will be needed to thicken the same amount of liquid.

Bring liquid to be thickened to a boil. If using cornstarch, simmer liquid gently as you slowly pour in the paste, stirring as you pour. With arrowroot, remove saucepan from heat as you do this step, then return to heat and again bring to a boil. Stir while liquid thickens.

Flours, such as wheat and potato, are also good thickening agents and can be used instead of cornstarch or arrowroot for some recipes.

For some foods, a thickening agent such as those described is not required to achieve good results. For example, a spaghetti sauce is preferably thickened by reduction; that is, reducing it to the proper thickness. The sauce is slowly simmered, uncovered, until enough liquid evaporates to produce the desired consistency. This method also works well with soups. Also, a very handy way to thicken soups like split pea, minestrone, bean, or vegetable is to purée a portion of it in the blender, and then return it to the soup pot. With this method, the blended soup vegetables act as a thickener.

The shopping list that follows sums up everything we've talked about in the last few chapters, plus some items we may not have mentioned. You'll want to refer to

it whenever you go shopping for your Pritikin Kitchen.
But remember, some of these items are high in salt content, or are to be restricted for other reasons as discussed elsewhere in this book.

## SUMMARY SHOPPING LIST

### DAIRY FOODS
Nonfat (skim) milk
100 percent uncreamed cottage cheese (e.g., hoop cheese or dry curd cottage cheese; should not be more than 1 percent fat by weight), or large-curd cottage cheese you can rinse.
Sapsago (green) cheese
Buttermilk, up to 1 percent fat by weight
Eggs (use whites only); no egg substitutes

### CEREALS AND GRAINS
Unprocessed miller's bran (to add to cereals, soups, etc., as needed)
Cracked wheat
Whole rolled oats
Rice (long or short grain)—brown preferred, wild or white OK
Buckwheat (kasha)
Bulgur wheat (parboiled wheat; Ala, Jolly Joan, other brands)
Other grains (millet, barley, triticale, etc.)
Blends of grains (without added wheat germ, sweeteners, nuts, etc.)
Hot cereals (Wheatena, Zoom, Roman Meal, Cream of Wheat, Cream of Rice, etc.)
Grape Nuts cereal
Wheat, oat, rye flakes

### CRACKERS, BREADS
Whole-grain crackers without fats or sugar (e.g., Hol-Grain Rice or Wheat Waferets, unsalted; whole rye crackers, as Rye-Krisp; Scandinavian flatbread; Ryvita; Finn Crisp)

Matzo (whole-wheat available; avoid matzo with egg or
     shortening)
Rice cakes (puffed rice pressed into round cakes)
Corn tortillas, not fried (*no* flour tortillas)
Pita bread, whole-wheat variety preferred
Sprouted wheat berry bread (Wayfarer's or Essene
     brands)
Sourdough bread, rolls, loaves
Any whole-grain bread without fats, sugars

## PASTA PRODUCTS

Spaghetti, lasagne, macaroni, manicotti, noodles (includ-
     ing artichoke noodles), etc. (Avoid kinds with soy
     flour or egg solids, whole-wheat preferred)
Oriental pasta

## DRY STAPLES

Whole-grain flours (whole-wheat, brown rice, whole
     ground cornmeal, etc.) and unbleached white flour
Thickeners: cornstarch, arrowroot, potato flour
Dry yeast, for bread making
Rennet tablets (Junket), for cheese making
Pectin, if desired
Plain gelatin (unflavored)
Nonfat dry milk, as Carnation (not recommended for use
     as beverage)
Tapioca, pearl (raw)
Baking powder (Rumford, Royal, Cellu—no additives
     containing aluminum)
Baking soda
Carob powder, unsweetened or pure carob
Matzo meal
Pancake mix, acceptable ingredients (e.g., Stone-Buhr
     brand)
Potato pancake mix, acceptable ingredients

## DRIED LEGUMES

All dried peas and beans except soybeans

## FRESH PRODUCE

All fruits and vegetables except avocados
Chestnuts (but no other nuts)

Fruit juice, fresh
Raisins
Currants

## FROZEN FOODS
Plain (no sauces) frozen vegetables
Frozen berries and other fruits, unsweetened
Frozen apple, orange, and pineapple juice, unsweetened

## CANNED FOODS
Tomato products, including tomato and V-8 juice
Assorted vegetables and beans (avoid kinds with sugar,
   like corn or stewed tomatoes, or with undesirable addi-
   tives like EDTA); no olives
Green chili salsa (Ortega)
Enchilada sauce (Rosarita)
Tuna, water-packed
Evaporated skim milk
Anderson's Split Pea soup
Applesauce, unsweetened
Water- or juice-packed fruit

## CONDIMENTS AND COOKING LIQUIDS
Capers
Vinegars, e.g., rice, wine, cider
Mustard
Hot sauce (acceptable brand)
Pace Picante sauce
Dill pickles
Peppers or other vegetables packed in wine vinegar
Salt-reduced soy sauce (Kikkoman)
Horseradish, uncreamed
Lemon and lime juice
Wines for cooking

## MEAT, FISH, POULTRY
Lean meat (including *leanest* ground meat)
Chicken, turkey, Cornish game hens (white meat pre-
   ferred)
Fish and acceptable shellfish

## BEVERAGES AND MISCELLANEOUS

Linden flower tea *(Tilea europea)*

Perrier or other mineral or spring water

Club soda

Powdered (dry) salad dressing mix (check ingredients), to be mixed with wine vinegar or acceptable buttermilk

Tillie Lewis Italian salad dressing (dilute with vinegar or water, adding more spices if desired)

Dried chopped vegetables (onion, green pepper, red pepper, etc.)

Vanilla extract, pure (Lester or Iris brand)

Assorted herbs and spices

# 23

## How to Cheat

You can, er, cheat on this diet. It's allowed. But only honest cheating is allowed. If you cheat dishonestly or carelessly, you'll blow the whole thing.

Cheating is not obligatory, however—let's get that straight. Anyone who is seriously ill would be crazy to cheat. To know how much you can cheat without getting into trouble, you'll have to do some computing.

There are four categories in which you may cheat. There is also a suggested cheating advisability order, indicating the likelihood of getting away with it safely. The descending cheating advisability order (cholesterol cheating being the least advisable) is: (1) *sugar;* (2) *protein;* (3) *fat;* and (4) *cholesterol.*

The guide that follows will tell you exactly how much of each item you may safely chisel on. If you use up the cheating ration for one of the four categories by cheating on a particular food, you have completely expended the ration for that category. Thus, you can do no other cheating in that category for that time limit without breaking the rules.

For instance, by eating one six-ounce avocado, you would deplete your entire fat-cheating ration for the week. Or if you split your weekly fat-cheating ration, you could have half the avocado on one day and three ounces of olives on another day. Either way, you would have exhausted your entire weekly fat-cheating ration, leaving only sugar, protein, and cholesterol to sin with.

Your normal Pritikin Diet keeps your fat intake to 8 percent, your protein to 13 percent, sugar to 0 percent. The daily cholesterol limit is 70 milligrams. The cheating scheme expands these to the maximum safe limit. Thus,

| Cheating Item | Fat | Cholesterol | Sugar | Protein | Maximum Weekly Allotment |
|---|---|---|---|---|---|
| Fats | | | | | |
| Butter | X | X | | | 2 oz. |
| Oil | X | | | | 1½ oz. |
| Sugars | | | | | |
| Sugar (including honey) | | | X | | 12 level tsp. |
| Meat and Fish | | | | | |
| *Lowfat meats, poultry, fish | | X | | ½ | 8 oz. |
| Fatty meats, poultry, fish | X | X | | ½ | 8 oz. |
| Liver, beef | | X | | | 2 oz. |
| Eggs | | | | | |
| *Egg whites, cooked | | | | X | 24 |
| Egg yolks | | X | | | 1 |
| Dairy | | | | | |
| *Nonfat (skim) milk | | | | X | 2 qts. |
| *Buttermilk, nonfat or up to 1% fat by weight | | | | X | 2 qts. |

| Cheating Item | Fat | Cholesterol | Sugar | Protein | Maximum Weekly Allotment |
|---|---|---|---|---|---|
| Lowfat milk | x | x | | x | 2 qts. |
| Whole milk | x | x | | ½ | 1 qt. |
| Cream | x | x | | x | 8 oz. |
| *100% skim milk cheeses | | | | x | 1 lb. |
| *Cottage cheese, up to 1% fat | | | | | 1 lb. |
| Lowfat cottage cheese | ½ | ½ | | x | 1 lb. |
| Creamed cottage cheese | x | | | x | 1 lb. |
| *Sapsago (green) cheese | | | | ½ | 4 oz. |
| Hard cheeses, e.g., cheddar, mozzarella | x | x | | ½ | 4–6 oz. |
| *Nonfat yogurt | | | | ½ | 2 qts. |
| Lowfat yogurt | x | ½ | | x | 2 qts. |
| Whole milk yogurt | x | ½ | | x | 1 qt. |
| Ice cream | x | x | ½ | | 2 qts. |
| Ice milk | x | x | ½ | ½ | 1 qt. |
| **Beans, Peas, Nuts, Seeds** | | | | | |
| *Beans and peas | | | | x | 2 lbs. |
| Nuts and seeds | x | | | | 2 oz. |
| **Vegetables** | | | | | |
| Avocados, olives | x | | | | ½ lb. |

| Cheating Item | Fat | Cholesterol | Sugar | Protein | Maximum Weekly Allotment |
|---|---|---|---|---|---|
| Fruit | | | | | |
| *Whole fruits | | | | | unlimited if triglycerides stay below 100 |
| *Canned, frozen, cooked fruit, unsweetened | | | x | | 12 oz. |
| *Fruit juices, unsweetened | | | x | | 12 oz. |
| *Dried fruits | | | x | | 2 oz. |
| Miscellaneous | | | | | |
| *Liquor for cooking use | | | x | | 2 oz. |
| *Wines for cooking use | | | x | | 4½ oz. |
| *Plain gelatin, unsweetened | | | | x | 3 oz. |
| Mayonnaise | x | | | | 1½ oz. |

x  Weekly ration for that particular cheating category used up with the given weekly allotment of a specific food item.

½ Half of weekly ration of that particular cheating category used up with the given weekly allotment for the food item.

* All food items considered approved foods on the Pritikin Diet. (Cheating occurs when the restrictions on these foods are exceeded.)

fat is stretched to 11 percent, protein to 16 percent, sugar to 1½ percent, and daily cholesterol intake to 100 milligrams.

Frankly, cheating is something that horrifies our veteran dieters. It strikes them as a netless high-wire balancing act. We, however, regard this as an optional outlet for beginners in transit from their old diet to the new.

However you cheat, we believe that you should do it openly, even publicly, and without pangs of conscience. The worst thing that could happen would be for the Pritikin Diet to be a source of guilt feelings. This would just make it likelier that you'll toss out the whole diet one day out of frustration. We'd hate to see that happen.

The accompanying tables gives maximum weekly cheating allotments for sugar, protein, fat, and cholesterol. Foods shown on the table are taboo foods you are most likely to cheat with, as well as approved foods you may be tempted to eat in excess or permitted limits. Notice that some foods, such as ice cream, use up more than one allotment (in this case fat, sugar, *and* protein).

*Remember:* While cheating is permitted, breaking the rules will be regarded as a serious infraction of dietary discipline, punishable by all the horrors we've described elsewhere in this book.

For those who are confused by paperwork and are likely to break the rules when they cheat, here are some helpful pointers:

1. Less animal protein may satisfy you if you "dilute" it with rice or other grains, pasta, or potatoes, in casserole-type preparations.

2. If you have access to range-fed animals, so much the better. They have lower fat levels than feed-lot animals.

3. It could take *two weeks* of regulation breakfasts to overcome the bad effects of one conventional breakfast of hotcakes, syrup, butter, sausages, eggs, salt, toast and butter, coffee with cream and sugar.

4. No cheating is permitted on tobacco. It spoils everything. If you are faithful to the Pritikin Diet and

smoke, it's the same as bringing your food quality
down to the level of the regular American diet.
5.  The degree of fidelity to your diet will tell you the
    degree of health potential you are creating for your-
    self.

# 24

## Hanging In
## While Dining Out

Dietary sabotage away from home is impossible to avoid,
but it can be countered successfully. Confronted with this
kind of terrorism, many people simply give up. Of course,
with surrender you forfeit some of your benefits.

When the waitress brandishes her ball-point over the
order pad and chants, "French, Roquefort, or Thousand
Island?" do you meekly pick one of the unholy trio?

As you board the Red-Eye Special for a coast-to-coast
flight, do you kiss your diet goodbye, settle down with an
anesthetizing double Scotch, and stuff yourself with those
warmed-over unspeakables?

Do you ever even *consider* a countersuggestion when
the neighbors invite you over for a cheese soufflé or
baked Alaska?

These are the challenges we meet every day. It's entirely up to *you* how much you want to improve your
health and whether you want to eat for yourself or to suit
the convenience of restaurant owners, airline steward-
esses, and the neighbors.

I am here to tell you that you do not have to sneak out
of the house waving a white flag, announcing to one and
all your defeat. You *can* hang in while dining out. All it
takes is some planning.

The main problems are restaurants, travel, and guestmanship. In this chapter you will find suggestions from
Pritikin Program dieters who have solved these problems
for themselves, and tell you how you can solve them.

## RESTAURANTS

In all likelihood, there's a meal for you *somewhere* in that kitchen. You will have to take care that it gets to you unspoiled by butter, oil and sauces. As a rule of thumb, the better the restaurant, the better your chances of cooperation from the management.

### Restaurant selection

*Vegetarian* restaurants are a good bet; so are *health-food* restaurants. You may, of course, already have a convert in the owner and then your problems will be minimal.

Among *American* restaurants, one featuring a salad bar can be a lifesaver. It's almost always possible to be served vinegar or lemon wedges, and thus avoid oily dressings.

*Cafeterias* have the advantage of showing you exactly what you're getting before surprises are delivered to your table. The problem is, almost everything they serve is swimming in fats and sugars, leaving you with slim pickings.

Restaurants featuring *Weight Watcher* meals are usually acceptable, offering food that can easily be adapted to your regimen.

*Chinese* restaurants are good because their food is customarily cooked to order. You can often get the chef to prepare a wok of steamed vegetables with a diced breast of chicken worked into it. Be sure to ask them to hold the MSG, sugar, oil, and salt. A little dash of soy sauce goes a long way toward flavoring your food. You may order your vegetables cooked in a clear chicken broth; with mounds of hot rice it constitutes an excellent meal.

*Italian* restaurants' pasta isn't as good as the whole-wheat variety you've stocked in your kitchen, but it'll do. Order unbuttered spaghetti with a marinara sauce (oil-free), a cup of minestrone if it's not the fatty kind, and a dry salad dressed with lemon juice or vinegar. Remembering to avoid parmesan, and consign those olives and anchovies to the ashtray.

*Seafood* restaurants are OK, too. Stay away from the high-cholesterol shellfish and butter and tartar sauce.

Have your seafood choice prepared without fats—broiled, baked, or poached (*not fried*).

Smorgasbord or buffet tables usually contain acceptable dishes. Just don't get boggled by the attractive displays of the shrimp, liver pâté, and oily stuff.

### Things to remember before leaving home

- Don't get into the habit of eating out too often. It can get wearying to make a production of ordering *your* foods in the enemy camp.
- Eat something to take the edge off your appetite *before* you leave home. This will minimize the seductive power of an unfriendly menu.
- Restaurants appreciate being called *in advance* for special requests. This courtesy improves your chances of getting what you want.
- When it comes right down to the nitty-gritty, it's your *strength of character* that will determine whether the restaurateur is going to serve you—or you're sheepishly going to take what is served everybody else.
- Remember that a *good restaurateur* enjoys making you happy. He survives on repeat business.
- Steer clear of *cheap restaurants*. Usually the prices aren't that much lower—but the food is. Cheap restaurants pack their dishes with fats and sweets to compensate for the lack of real food.
- Beware or *hospital restaurants*. Paradoxically, they are among the worst for fatty, cholesterol-laden, sugary foods.
- If you're too easily corrupted by gastronomic allurements, join your friends at the restaurant *after dinner* for socializing.

### Things to remember when ordering

- Don't nod "yes" when you're asked if you want sour cream with your baked potato. Try it just *with chives*.
- You can spice the blandness of your hardy *baked potato* with a nonoil *salsa*. West Coast restaurants are more likely to have salsa on hand than others.
- Ask for *sourdough rolls or bread* immediately. If they don't have them, eat the rolls they do have. The slight

amount of vegetable shortening in them won't hurt you as an occasional substitute for your good whole-grain breads at home.

• Don't be afraid to ask for half orders or to split an order with a friend. Two can get by with a *single* serving of fish, an extra baked potato, and an extra salad. Ask for an extra plate, then split the fish entree.

• Tote along a small bag of *your own hors d'oeuvres* to munch on before your salad or entree comes. (Chances are only one in five that you'll raise the waiter's eyebrow.)

• If there are only one or two dishes that won't throw you off your diet, don't hesitate to load up on them and forget the rest. You may feel cheated eating nothing but salad and soup and (occasionally) having to pay for a noneaten entree as well. Just remember that *less is more!*

• Sometimes the only acceptable vegetable is a baked potato—since most restaurants smother vegetables in butter or margarine. In that case, *eat two baked potatoes.*

• If you eat at one restaurant regularly, *let the owner look over your diet* and favorite recipes. If he wants to keep your business, usually he'll manage to include several of them among his repertoire.

• Try talking *your favorite Chinese restaurateur* into preparing a chicken and tomato dish (instead of the usual beef and tomatoes) with a sweet-sour flavor (sans sugar) and a won-ton soup with soft (not fried) noodles.

• In *vegetarian restaurants,* don't forget to *defend yourself* against their oils, cheeses, nuts, avocado, honey, etc.

• In *seafood restaurants,* it's all right to order fish prepared with wine, lemon juice, spices, or mustard. Just make sure it isn't fried.

• In *salad bars,* stay away from marinated vegetables (too much oil). Load up on red onions, bamboo shoots, garbanzo beans (chickpeas), raw cauliflower, broccoli, celery, radishes, etc. Avoid croutons, cheese toppings, cole slaw, grated eggs, and the like.

• You can survive in a *Mexican restaurant* by ordering

a pile of warmed corn tortillas (careful that you're not getting an omelette!) and getting the chef to custom-blend a taco or enchilada without cheese. Chicken or bean enchiladas, with an enchilada sauce, may have some oil, but not much. You can complement these with a lettuce and tomato salad—possibly on top of your enchilada or inside your taco.

* Let the waiter know that you are not kidding. Warn him that you're going to *send the food back* if it has a trace of oil or butter. This is particularly important at the beginning of a stay in a resort where you will be at the chef's mercy for days on end. *Conditioning the chef* should start with Meal One.
* If the menu is a disaster, don't be afraid to pack up friends or family and *try another restaurant.*
* Make your baked-potato order a restaurant habit. If you don't, three guesses what you're going to find alongside your entree.

### Breakfast ideas

* Hot oatmeal or Cream of Wheat, Shredded Wheat or Grape Nuts.
* Ask for nonfat milk (or carry along your own nonfat dry milk).
* Order a grapefruit half, a sliced orange, melon, berries, or sliced banana.
* Ask for dry toast or rolls and a pot of hot water with lemon slice.

### Lunch and dinner ideas

* Don't fret over occasional deviations in a restaurant. But if you visit a restaurant regularly, be very strict—and supplement whatever is available with permissible foods from home.
* A great standby: a large green salad without dressing (lemon juice or vinegar only).
* Standby dessert: any fresh fruit.
* Standby appetizers: split pea, navy bean, lentil, or vegetable soups (if made without fat).
* Fresh vegetables—without butter—are ideal. Try arti-

chokes, mushrooms, zucchini, corn on the cob, green beans or peas, and baked potatoes.

*Items you may wish to include in your restaurant survival kit:*

A lemon

Linden tea bags

Bran (the co-author carries his in a tobacco pouch)

Mini bottle of salsa

Whole-wheat pita or sourdough bread

Plastic bag of raw vegetables (carrots, cauliflower, celery, etc.)

Cooked rice or bulgur wheat

Fresh fruit

A "doggy" bag for taking home leftovers and other items

# TRAVEL

## The airlines

Competition has brought courtesy to the airlines. I'm amazed by the considerate treatment I receive while traveling. Indeed, the airlines are giants of graciousness compared to railways and bus lines.

Did you know that you can stick to your Pritikin Diet on most long-distance flights of most airlines? All you have to do is order ahead. Eight hours' advance notice is usually enough, but twenty-four hours is better still.

Best procedure is to call the company and specify the foods you want as well as what you *can't* eat. If you order a baked potato, specify without butter. Tell them you don't eat salad dressings with oil. Etc.

Their computers are programmed for several diets, but you run a risk with any one or combination of them. They're all too high in fat, including the Low Calorie, Vegetarian, Low Sodium, Low Cholesterol, Low Fat, Diabetic, and Kosher. For instance, the vegetarian offerings tend to swim in butter, and eggs pop up on the breakfast menu. It's better to figure out what you want to eat and specify each dish.

You can be 100 percent sure if you pack your own flight bag with emergency rations, in case the "diet" menu provided by the stewardess contains surprises. Here are some of the staples:

Coffee substitute or linden tea bag

Uncreamed cottage cheese in plastic container

Sourdough or other acceptable rolls or bread, crackers

Fresh fruit

A thermos of nonfat milk

Plastic baggies of *Homemade Dry Cereal* (see Index) or a small box of Grape Nuts

A thermos of hot soup

Plastic containers of cooked rice, salad, and raw vegetable sticks

### *Travel-safe tips*

- Eat before boarding the plane, and carry backup foods.
- If you order merely a "dietetic meal," you may wind up being served eggs.
- If you can avoid staying overnight on your trip—i.e., return the same day—your risk of going off the diet will be minimized.
- Your travel success, in the air or by any other transportation, will depend much on how well you operate at home. Do you have a supply of good bread in the freezer? Soups? Snacks and crackers? Raw vegetables in the refrigerator? If so, all you have to do is pack a flight bag—or brown paper bag—with enough for your flight.
- Remember that you should eat *less* if you travel, since your walking may be restricted. You'll feel better, too.

### *Campers and cars*

A camper is a diet saver. With your traveling kitchen, you are no longer at the mercy of "greasy spoon" eateries en route and can carry your staples with you. It's the best guarantee I know of not to break your diet while traveling.

Your car can also be outfitted with hot and cold storage facilities. An ice chest can keep your salads, cheese, fruit, frozen soups, and other perishables. Thermoses will keep hot water for your oatmeal, linden tea, dried soups, heated vegetables, and the like.

If you stay in a motel, try to find one with a kitchenette. Prepare to do your own cooking by bringing along an electric pot, nonstick frying pan, and a small supply of

brown rice, oatmeal and other cereals, fresh fruit and vegetables. You may also want to bring some cold chicken,
uncreamed cottage cheese, oven-roasted *Garbanzo "Nuts"*
(see Index), and sourdough or other acceptable bread.

## Other ideas

- Be sure to take at least enough food for your first
  day—all meals. Then you can shop at leisure to fill in
  for the rest of the trip.
- Bread and tortillas keep well in refrigeration.
- If you avoid thinking in terms of rigid breakfast,
  lunch, and dinner categories, you can eat whenever
  you're hungry. That way you'll be less likely to stop
  off at restaurants, where the chances of departing
  from the diet are high.
- Be strict in limiting your time away from home.
- Plan your trip so that you can choose to stop over in
  places that allow you to rent apartments, or provide
  kitchenettes.
- *Garbanzo "Nuts," Homemade Dry Cereal,* or *Granola*
  (see Index) are great diet savers!
- If you travel with nondieters, keep separate food storage facilities.
- Remember that bulgur wheat is the fastest-cooking
  grain.
- Use a wide-mouthed thermos for hot soups, steamed
  vegetable combinations, or hot baked beans.
- Sealed plastic containers are excellent for plain rice,
  rice salad, *tabouli,* cole slaw, tomatoes and other raw
  vegetables, as well as for marinated bean salad, tossed
  green salad, potato salad, fish salad, chicken salad,
  etc.

## Breakfasts

- Carry oranges and bananas (for eating whole or slicing up for cereal toppings).
- If you pack a wide-mouthed thermos with boiling
  water and uncooked cereal in the proper proportions,
  the cereal will absorb the water overnight and be
  ready to eat in the morning.

- Hot pots with a two- or three-cup capacity are ideal for preparing morning cereals; immersion heaters are second best, but also useful.
- If you've repacked your oatmeal and have lost the directions, remember it's one part oats to two parts boiling water. Just stir until thick and eat.
- Rolled oats is the one natural cereal you can eat without cooking.
- Don't forget nonfat dry milk powder.

## Lunches and dinners

- Don't go hungry, whatever you do. It's vital to eat every few hours. If you're desperate, buy some fruit and acceptable crackers or bread.
- Styrofoam picnic ice chests are good for carrying frozen food and other perishables.
- Thermoses for soup and plastic containers for rice, beans, or vegetable combinations are handy take-alongs. Supplement with acceptable whole-grain or sourdough bread, crackers, and fruit.
- Earthwonder of Springfield, Missouri, puts out a line of dehydrated foods that require only water and heating. Many are acceptable. Check camping or sporting goods stores for other brands. Read ingredients on the packages carefully.
- For short excursions, you can make excellent picnic lunches based around whole-wheat pita or other acceptable sandwich breads filled with: lettuce, tomato and cucumber, and: 1) Bean Dip or other bean preparations; 2) "Little Beef" Burgers or other patties made from fish, rice or potatoes; 3) thin slab of hoop cheese, or other kind of uncreamed cottage cheese spread on bread; or 4) thin slice of chicken or turkey breast, or salads made with chopped chicken, turkey or fish, and a dressing using *Mock Sour Cream* seasoned with prepared mustard and herbs.
- Consider, too, a "sweet" sandwich, using *Garbanzo "Nut Butter"* and thin slices of banana, or thin slices of banana with a thin slab of hoop cheese, or other kind of uncreamed cottage cheese spread on bread.

- Lunches can be nicely rounded out with fruit and crackers or oven-roasted *Garbanzo "Nuts."*

See Index for all recipes mentioned above.

## OVERSEAS TRAVEL

You should not find travel abroad any more of an impediment to your diet than anywhere in the United States. In fact, it may be loads easier. For one thing, other countries have not committed the chemical mayhem on their foodstuffs that we have. European countries rigorously control preservatives and additives of many foods.

European marketplaces abound with delicious, robust fresh fruits and vegetables. If you've schlepped your hot pot, immersion heater, and wide- and narrow-mouthed thermoses with you (and haven't forgotten your electric current converters), you'll eat better than you can here.

Our former patients John and Virginia Morse, of Scottsdale, Arizona, have brought to our attention the following facts:

- Vegetarian restaurants abound throughout Europe; so do health-food stores.
- You can usually find acceptable—or darned near acceptable (and divine-tasting!)—breads throughout Europe.
- Finding nonfat milk was no problem anywhere.
- The overseas airlines cooperated in providing acceptable meals—to the letter. On TWA, vegetarian and low-cholesterol meals came close to the Pritikin Diet.
- The best way to see Europe is to settle in a large city by renting a flat for a couple of weeks, then make daily excursions. It'll cut your costs—as well as the risk of going off the diet.

## GUESTMANSHIP

Your halo will get heavy the first time that you, with your new resolve to stick to the diet, dine with friends.

Do you tell them you're on a diet? Do you instruct

them as to which foods you can and cannot eat? Do you ask them to set aside some undressed salad for you?

And, if the lobster's already in the pot, did you remember to bring some emergency rations with you?

If you want to preserve your new good feelings, all of your answers ought to be YES! Let's face it: Your "When-in-Rome . . ." days are over.

Once you've resolved to winnow out the poisons from your food, you've won half the battle. The other half is yours with a few simple tactics.

The challenge facing you is very simple: How much more good health do you want? All you can get? Half of what you can get? Ten percent?

If you want the highest quality of life you can get with the Pritikin Program, then it's incumbent on you not to fall apart in the tender loving care of your friends. We've already shown you how to avoid the traps of restaurants and travel. The traps our best friends place for us can be the worst.

In creating a strategy to preserve your diet, here are a few principles to guide you:

- Perhaps for the first time in your life, start saying "No, thank you." And say it whenever you're offered a taboo.
- People respect those who respect themselves.
- Don't turn off your friends by proselytizing. Everyone will be very curious about your new diet—as people are about all diets. In fact, you'll get tired answering their questions.
- Be thoughtful of your hosts. Warn them long enough in advance that you can't eat their roast suckling pig so that they can steam up a few vegetables for you.
- Most people enjoy helping friends stick to their diets—particularly when the extra food preparation is so simple, as it is for the Pritikin Diet basics.
- Those who fail to honor your wish to stay healthy may not really be your friends after all.
- If you spend more time with compatible people who are also on the diet, you'll find that mealtimes with them are extremely pleasant occasions for sharing recipes, hiking experiences, and other joys of the world's healthiest diet program.

- If you are wishy-washy or inconsistent about your diet with friends, there is a strong tendency for them to regard you as a hypocrite.

And here are some tried-and-proven suggestions from the pioneers:

- If you're paranoid enough to think that your host (or anyone else, for that matter) *really* gives a damn what you're drinking, here's a trick you can use. Sneak into the kitchen and put a couple drops of coffee or decaffeinated coffee into your water or soda water. Anyone who can tell the difference between that and whisky by merely looking is a genius.
- If your hosts are reluctant to prepare anything suitable for you, join them *after* dinner. Or find new friends.
- The simplest way to present your dietary needs to your host is by asking them to steam any vegetables they happen to have on hand.
- The more candid you are about the importance of your diet, the easier it is for others to help you.
- Once you're at the table and discover that the food has been smothered in butter, oil, and/or salt, take just a bite or two if you must—and then rearrange the food on your plate. (This is a technique perfected by travel writers Temple and Nancy Fielding when reviewing several restaurants a night for their guidebooks.)
- Perhaps the most useful bit of advice is to eat substantially from *your* food before leaving home—so you won't be at the mercy of your hunger and your host's fatty foods.
- Eat at home more often.

## PLAYING HOST

Hostmanship is less of a problem than guestmanship because your friends are playing on your home court. You call the shots. How do you stick to your diet without offending them?

Here are some answers Pritikin Center veterans have come up with for themselves and share with you:

- When you've explained why you're on your diet, most people are enthusiastic about *trying* it—even if they don't opt to *live* with it.
- Courtesy goes a long way. Tell your friends what your menu is. Don't be afraid to try some of the gourmet recipes in this book. That's the best way to show that a good diet need not be bland or tasteless.
- Give your friends a choice of menus.
- Keep a stick of butter, some olive oil, and some salt on hand for those who can't make do without them. After a few weeks on the diet, you'll probably find that you're no longer tempted by them—even when they're right under your nose. (Sweets, potato chips, peanut butter, and ice cream are another story. They are the most common diet busters.)
- You can always serve two entrees, one for the dieters and experimenters, the other for the meat lovers. Again, however, you run the risk of being accused of hypocrisy by making a health-menacing, fat-rich menu for those who know how dangerous you consider it to be.
- Potluck dinners are a simple way of solving the problem. If you provide an entree, bread, and salad dressing for yourself, each guest can bring whatever he or she regards as a turn-on. (Similarly, as a guest you can always suggest that you bring along an entree for your hosts and other guests to sample.)
- Bear in mind that your diet may be the most valuable gift you can give your guests.

I shall shortly unveil all of those mouth-watering recipes I've been promising you. Consider them your reward for not knuckling under to temptation while dining away from home.

But first, read the next chapter carefully. It's your key to getting the most out of this exquisite selection of menus.

# 25

## Computing Food Values

You may wonder how a Pritikin Diet follower knows whether his or her food intake actually falls within the recommended caloric ratio of 7 to 10 percent fat, 10 to 13 percent protein, and 80 percent carbohydrates (of the proper kind).

*The simplest way to check to ensure diet compliance is to follow carefully the dietary guidelines outlined in this book, including the table of food restrictions in Chapter 1.*

A much more difficult method would be to analyze a typical day's food intake. You could have a laboratory make a chemical assay, or you could do this by computation. To make the computations, it would be necessary to:

1. Weigh each separate ingredient consumed during the day and compute the day's total.
2. Use handbook data to determine percent by weight of fat, protein, and carbohydrate in 100 grams of each separate ingredient.
3. Again using handbook data, convert the gram data from step 2 into calories of fat, protein, and carbohydrate.
4. Obtain separate totals for calories of fat, protein, and carbohydrate consumed during the day by adding figures for calories of fat, protein, and carbohydrate from all ingredients in the day's diet. Add the three totals together to get a grand total.
5. Divide each separate total by the grand total to obtain percentages of fat, protein, and carbohydrates consumed.

Not many people will want to bother with that kind of bookkeeping. Just think of the work involved in weighing the separate ingredients that go into making a cup of vegetable soup, for instance!

Nevertheless, knowing how to make some of these calculations may be of practical value from time to time. You may want to know how many of the calories are fat in a canned product that you think falls within the parameters of the Pritikin Diet. Our recommendation for a top limit of fat content for any food is *about 15 percent* (except for your limited intake of meat, fish, or fowl, all of which exceed this percentage). If you follow the general rule of avoiding foods with a fat content exceeding 15 percent, your foods will tend to average a maximum fat content of 10 percent, since so many of the grains and other foods you will be consuming will be lower than 10 percent.

Let's get back to that can of food you were looking at longingly. You've checked the label and are full of anticipation because it seems to be free of no-nos. To find whether the fat content is acceptable, check the label for this information: calories per 100 grams (or the equivalent, 3½ ounces) and grams of fat per 100 grams. You can then make an on-the-spot determination of fat calories. Simply multiply the number of fat grams by 9, since there are about 9 calories in an average gram of fat. Now that you know the number of fat calories per 100 grams, you need only divide that figure by the total number of calories in 100 grams. The answer, converted to a percentage figure by moving the decimal point two places to the right, tells you the fat content in percent of total calories. Hope it was below 15 percent!

Just for practice, let's try out the procedure with a can of tuna packed in spring water picked up from a supermarket shelf. The label information gives data on calories per 3½ ounces, or 100 grams: calories per 3½ ounces— 120; fat content by gram weight for 3½ ounces—2 grams. (Note that gram weights on cans are always rounded out.) Now we're ready to go:

*Computing fat calorie information from label data:*
Label data: 120 calories per 3½ ounces (100 grams)
2 grams fat per 3½ ounces (100 grams)

$$2 \times 9 = 18 \text{ calories} \qquad \frac{18}{120} = .15 = 15 \text{ percent fat}$$

Suppose you wanted to calculate the protein content of that same can of tuna. Protein content by weight for 3½ ounces, or 100 grams, is given as 25 grams. Follow the same procedure as used for the fat calculations, but use 4 instead of 9, because there are about 4 calories in an average gram of protein.

*Computing protein calorie information from label data:*
Label data:  120 calories per 3½ ounces (100 grams)
            25 grams protein per 3½ ounces (100 grams)

$$25 \times 4 = 100 \text{ calories} \quad \frac{100}{120} = .83 = 83 \text{ percent protein}$$

To obtain information about carbohydrate calories from gram data, the same number, 4, is used that you use for protein. That's because there are also about 4 calories in an average gram of carbohydrate. (Actually, the figures 9 for fat and 4 for protein or carbohydrate are a bit of an oversimplification, as we'll see later. But they are good enough for our purposes.)

If nutritional data on the label of a food product is given in terms of serving or portion size, rather than on the basis of 100 grams, the identical procedures are followed, except that to determine percentage of fat (protein or carbohydrate) of total calories, divide the calories of fat (protein or carbohydrate) in a serving or portion by total calories per serving or portion.

Incidentally, if you fixed that 3½ ounces of tuna into salad for your lunch, you would have used up a good part of your protein budget for the day. Let's say you consume about 2,000 calories daily. The upper recommended limit for protein intake—13 percent—of 2,000 calories is 260 protein calories. Since you ate 100 protein calories in your tuna salad made with 3½ ounces of tuna, you would then have left a maximum of 160 protein calories for the day to be obtained from all other food sources.

The most authoritative handbook for computing food values is *Composition of Foods,* Handbook No. 8, issued by the United States Department of Agriculture and obtainable from the Superintendent of Documents, U.S. Government Printing Office, Washington, D.C. 20402.

Tables of interest in the handbook include one on cholesterol content of animal foods (Table 4) and another
which gives more accurate factor values for conversion of
gram data to calorie data (Table 6). While the rough figures of 9 for fat and 4 for protein and carbohydrate suf-
fice for our purposes, it is interesting to note variations in
factor values based upon averages within each food
group, as shown in the table.

|              |        | Nuts/   |            |        |      | Meat/     |
|--------------|--------|---------|------------|--------|------|-----------|
|              | Grains | Legumes | Vegetables | Fruits | Milk | Fish      |
| Protein      | 3.3    | 3.5     | 2.6        | 3.4    | 4.3  | 4.3       |
| Fat          | 8.4    | 8.4     | 8.4        | 8.4    | 8.8  | 9.0       |
| Carbohydrate | 3.9    | 4.1     | 3.7        | 3.6    | 3.9  | Approx. 4 |

Table 1 of the handbook gives food composition by
gram weight for 100 grams, edible portion, of some 2,500
food items, raw, processed, and prepared. To convert the
fat, protein, and carbohydrate gram data for any food
item to percent of total calories, you would have to make
your own computations. The procedure used is exactly
the same as that used in the canned tuna calculations
above, though you could use the more accurate conversion factors shown above instead of the rounded-out numbers 9 and 4.

The table at the end of this chapter, Caloric Ratios of
Common Foods, is a ready reference providing data on
percent of total calories of fat, protein, and carbohydrate
for most foods you will be using. You will find the table
handy in several ways. A quick glance at the column
headed Fat Percent will tell you whether a particular food
exceeds the recommended maximum figure of 15 percent.
Also, to determine the number of fat calories in 100
grams or 3½ ounces, you need merely multiply the percentage figure given under the column headed Fat Percent
by the figure in the left-hand column headed Calories Per
100 Grams. Calculations for protein or carbohydrate
would be done similarly, using the percentage figures from
the appropriate column.

If you are not the kind of person who is comfortable
with calculations, don't worry. You will do just as well
with the Pritikin Diet by simply following the dietary
guidelines set out in this book!

## CALORIC RATIOS OF COMMON FOODS*

### I. FOOD FROM ANIMALS

| | CALORIES PER 100 GRAMS | % FAT | % PROTEIN | % CARBO-HYDRATE |
|---|---|---|---|---|
| **MEAT** | | | | |
| BEEF | | | | |
| Flank Steak: | | | | |
|   Total edible, choice grade, cooked | 196 | 33 | 66 | — |
|   Total edible, good grade, cooked | 191 | 31 | 69 | — |
| Hamburger (ground beef), lean, cooked | 219 | 46 | 53 | — |
| Rib, entire (6th–12th ribs): | | | | |
|   Total edible, choice grade, cooked | 440 | 81 | 19 | — |
|   Separable lean, choice grade, cooked | 241 | 50 | 50 | — |
| Rump: | | | | |
|   Total edible, choice grade, cooked | 347 | 71 | 29 | — |
|   Total edible, good grade, cooked | 317 | 67 | 33 | — |
|   Separable lean, choice grade, cooked | 208 | 40 | 60 | — |
|   Separable lean, good grade, cooked | 190 | 34 | 66 | — |
| Sirloin steak, double-bone: | | | | |
|   Total edible, choice grade, cooked | 408 | 77 | 23 | — |
|   Total edible, good grade, cooked | 365 | 72 | 28 | — |

* Values based on data from U.S. Department of Agriculture Handbook No. 8, *Composition of Foods*, Table 1, "Composition of foods, 100 grams, edible portion." (100 grams = approximately 3½ ounces.) Total percentages may not equal 100 primarily due to rounding of values. In addition, factors for converting the gram data from Table 1 to calorie equivalents are based on averages for that food group, as shown in Table 6 of *Composition of Foods*. As deemed useful, values for cooked food have been given wherever possible.

|  |  |  |  |  |
|---|---|---|---|---|
| Separable lean, choice grade, cooked | **216** | 40 | 60 | — |
| Separable lean, good grade, cooked | **190** | 29 | 71 | — |

**VEAL**

| | | | | |
|---|---|---|---|---|
| Loin, total edible, medium-fat class, cooked | **234** | 52 | 48 | — |
| Rib, total edible, medium-fat class, cooked | **269** | 57 | 43 | — |
| Round with rump, total edible, medium-fat class, cooked | **216** | 46 | 54 | — |

**LAMB**
Leg of lamb:

| | | | | |
|---|---|---|---|---|
| Total edible, choice grade, cooked | **279** | 61 | 39 | — |
| Total edible, good grade, cooked | **266** | 59 | 41 | — |
| Separable lean, choice grade, cooked | **186** | 34 | 66 | — |
| Separable lean, good grade, cooked | **183** | 33 | 67 | — |

Rib:

| | | | | |
|---|---|---|---|---|
| Total edible, choice grade, cooked | **407** | 79 | 21 | — |
| Total edible, good grade, cooked | **378** | 76 | 24 | — |
| Separable lean, choice grade, cooked | **211** | 45 | 55 | — |
| Separable lean, good grade, cooked | **206** | 43 | 57 | — |

**MEAT**
**PORK**
Composite of trimmed lean cuts (ham, shoulder, loin and spare ribs):

| | | | | |
|---|---|---|---|---|
| Total edible, medium-fat class, cooked | **373** | 74 | 26 | — |
| Total edible, thin class, cooked | **341** | 70 | 30 | — |
| Separable lean, medium-fat class, cooked | **236** | 49 | 51 | — |
| Separable lean, thin class, cooked | **228** | 46 | 54 | — |

Loin:

| | | | | |
|---|---|---|---|---|
| Total edible, medium-fat class, cooked | **391** | 73 | 27 | — |
| Total edible, thin class, cooked | **333** | 67 | 33 | — |

| | | | |
|---|---|---|---|
| Separable lean, medium-fat class, cooked | **254** | 50 | 49 | — |
| Separable lean, thin class, cooked | **254** | 50 | 49 | — |

**POULTRY**
**CHICKEN**
All classes:

| | | | |
|---|---|---|---|
| Light meat without skin, raw | **117** | 15 | 85 | — |
| Light meat without skin, cooked | **166** | 18 | 81 | — |
| Dark meat without skin, raw | **130** | 33 | 68 | — |
| Dark meat without skin, cooked | **176** | 32 | 68 | — |

Roasters:

| | | | |
|---|---|---|---|
| Light meat without skin, cooked | **182** | 24 | 76 | — |
| Dark meat without skin, cooked | **184** | 32 | 68 | — |

Hens and cocks:

| | | | |
|---|---|---|---|
| Light meat without skin, cooked | **180** | 24 | 76 | — |
| Dark meat without skin, cooked | **207** | 41 | 59 | — |

Fryers:

| | | | |
|---|---|---|---|
| Light meat without skin, raw | **101** | 13 | 87 | — |
| Breast, raw | **110** | 20 | 81 | — |
| Thigh, raw | **128** | 39 | 60 | — |

**TURKEY**

| | | | |
|---|---|---|---|
| Flesh only, all classes, cooked | **190** | 29 | 71 | — |
| Light meat, all classes, cooked | **176** | 20 | 80 | — |
| Dark meat, all classes, cooked | **203** | 37 | 63 | — |

**DUCK**

| | | | |
|---|---|---|---|
| Domesticated, flesh only, raw | **165** | 55 | 49 | — |
| Wild, flesh only, raw | **138** | 66 | 34 | — |

**SQUAB**

| | | | |
|---|---|---|---|
| Light meat without skin, raw | **125** | 30 | 70 | — |

**FISH AND SHELLFISH**
**FISH**

| | | | |
|---|---|---|---|
| Barracuda, Pacific, raw | **113** | 21 | 79 | — |

Bass:

| | | | |
|---|---|---|---|
| Black sea, raw | **93** | 12 | 88 | — |
| Striped, raw | **105** | 23 | 77 | — |
| White, raw | **98** | 21 | 78 | — |
| Carp, raw | **115** | 33 | 67 | — |
| Catfish, raw | **103** | 27 | 73 | — |

Cod:

| | | | |
|---|---|---|---|
| raw | **78** | 3 | 96 | — |
| canned | **85** | 3 | 96 | — |
| Flatfishes (flounders, soles, sanddabs), raw | **79** | 9 | 90 | — |

| | | | | |
|---|---|---|---|---|
| Haddock, raw | **79** | 1 | 99 | — |
| Halibut: | | | | |
| Atlantic and Pacific, raw | **100** | 11 | 89 | — |
| California, raw | **97** | 13 | 87 | — |
| Herring: | | | | |
| Atlantic, raw | **176** | 58 | 42 | — |
| Pacific, raw | **98** | 24 | 76 | — |
| Mackerel: | | | | |
| Atlantic, raw | **191** | 58 | 42 | — |
| Pacific, raw | **159** | 59 | 41 | — |
| Ocean perch: | | | | |
| Atlantic, raw | **88** | 12 | 87 | — |
| Pacific, raw | **95** | 14 | 85 | — |
| Perch: | | | | |
| White, raw | **118** | 31 | 70 | — |
| Yellow, raw | **91** | 9 | 91 | — |
| Pike: | | | | |
| Blue, raw | **90** | 9 | 91 | — |
| Northern, raw | **88** | 11 | 89 | — |
| Walleye, raw | **93** | 12 | 89 | — |
| Pompano, raw | **166** | 52 | 48 | — |
| Salmon: | | | | |
| Atlantic, raw | **217** | 56 | 44 | — |
| Chinook, raw | **222** | 63 | 37 | — |
| Atlantic, canned, solids and liquids | **203** | 54 | 46 | — |
| Chinook, canned, solids and liquids | **210** | 60 | 40 | — |
| Sockeye, canned, solids and liquids | **171** | 49 | 51 | — |
| Seabass, white, raw | **96** | 5 | 95 | — |
| Snapper, red and gray, raw | **93** | 9 | 91 | — |
| Sturgeon: | | | | |
| Raw | **94** | 18 | 82 | — |
| Cooked, steamed | **160** | 32 | 68 | — |
| Swordfish, raw | **118** | 31 | 69 | — |
| Trout: | | | | |
| Brook, raw | **101** | 19 | 81 | — |
| Rainbow (steelhead), raw | **195** | 53 | 47 | — |
| Tuna: | | | | |
| Bluefin, raw | **145** | 26 | 74 | — |
| Yellowfin, raw | **133** | 20 | 79 | — |
| Canned in water, solids and liquids | **127** | 6 | 94 | — |
| Whitefish, lake, raw | **155** | 48 | 52 | — |
| Yellowtail (Pacific coast), raw | **138** | 35 | 65 | — |
| | | | | |
| SHELLFISH | | | | |
| Abalone, raw | **98** | 5 | 81 | 14 |

| | | | | |
|---|---|---|---|---|
| Clams: | | | | |
| Soft, meat only, raw | **82** | 21 | 73 | 6 |
| Hard, meat only, raw | **80** | 10 | 59 | 30 |
| Mixed, canned, drained solids | **98** | 23 | 69 | 8 |
| Mixed, canned, liquor | **19** | 5 | 52 | 45 |
| Crab: | | | | |
| Steamed | **93** | 18 | 79 | 2 |
| Canned | **101** | 22 | 74 | 4 |
| Lobster, northern: | | | | |
| Whole, raw | **91** | 19 | 79 | 2 |
| Canned or cooked | **95** | 14 | 84 | 1 |
| Mussels, Atlantic and Pacific, meat only, raw | **95** | 21 | 65 | 14 |
| Oysters: | | | | |
| Eastern, meat only, raw | **66** | 25 | 54 | 21 |
| Pacific and western, meat only, raw | **91** | 22 | 50 | 29 |
| Canned, solids and liquids | **76** | 26 | 48 | 26 |
| Scallops | | | | |
| Raw | **81** | 2 | 81 | 17 |
| Cooked, steamed | **112** | 11 | 88 | — |
| Shrimp: | | | | |
| Raw | **91** | 8 | 85 | 7 |
| Canned, drained solids | **116** | 9 | 89 | 2 |

## EGGS AND DAIRY PRODUCTS
### EGGS

| | | | | |
|---|---|---|---|---|
| Whites, raw | **51** | *trace* | 93 | 6 |
| Yolks, raw | **348** | 79 | 20 | 1 |
| Whole eggs, poached | **163** | 64 | 34 | 2 |

### MILK
Fluid milk:

| | | | | |
|---|---|---|---|---|
| Whole (3.5% fat by weight) | **65** | 47 | 23 | 29 |
| Lowfat (2% fat by weight) | **59** | 30 | 30 | 39 |
| Skim (.1% fat by weight) | **36** | 2 | 43 | 55 |
| Dry: | | | | |
| Skim (nonfat solids), regular | **363** | 2 | 42 | 56 |
| Skim (nonfat solids), instant | **359** | 2 | 43 | 56 |

### CHEESE
Cottage, large or small curd:

| | | | | |
|---|---|---|---|---|
| Creamed | **106** | 35 | 55 | 11 |
| Uncreamed (e.g., hoop, dry curds) | **86** | 3 | 84 | 12 |
| Cheddar | **398** | 71 | 27 | 2 |
| Swiss | **370** | 67 | 32 | 2 |
| Blue or Roquefort | **368** | 73 | 25 | 2 |
| Parmesan | **393** | 58 | 39 | 3 |

YOGURT

| | | | |
|---|---|---|---|
| Made from partially skimmed milk | 50 | 30 | 29 | 40 |
| Made from whole milk | 62 | 48 | 21 | 31 |

| | | | |
|---|---|---|---|
| BUTTER | 716 | 99 | <.5 | <.5 |

## II. FOOD FROM PLANTS

| | CALORIES PER 100 GRAMS | % FAT | % PROTEIN | % CARBO-HYDRATE |
|---|---|---|---|---|
| **OILS, MARGARINE** | | | | |
| Oils, salad or cooking | 884 | 100 | 0 | 0 |
| Margarine | 720 | 99 | <.5 | <.5 |
| **GRAINS** | | | | |
| Barley, pearled (light), raw | 349 | 2 | 8 | 89 |
| Buckwheat: | | | | |
| Whole-grain (kasha), raw | 335 | 6 | 12 | 82 |
| Flour, dark | 333 | 6 | 12 | 82 |
| Cornmeal, white or yellow: | | | | |
| Whole ground, unbolted | 355 | 9 | 7 | 84 |
| Oatmeal (rolled oats): | | | | |
| Dry | 390 | 16 | 13 | 72 |
| Cooked | 55 | 15 | 13 | 73 |
| Popcorn: | | | | |
| Unpopped | 362 | 11 | 9 | 80 |
| Popped, plain | 386 | 11 | 9 | 80 |
| Rice: | | | | |
| Brown, raw | 360 | 4 | 7 | 89 |
| Brown, cooked | 119 | 4 | 7 | 88 |
| White, raw | 363 | 1 | 7 | 92 |
| White, cooked | 109 | 1 | 7 | 92 |
| Rye: | | | | |
| Whole-grain, raw | 334 | 4 | 11 | 85 |
| Flour, medium | 350 | 4 | 11 | 85 |
| Wheat: | | | | |
| Bulgur (parboiled whole wheat), variety average, dry | 356 | 3 | 10 | 82 |
| Whole-grain, variety average, raw | 330 | 5 | 13 | 81 |
| Flour, whole (from hard wheats) | 333 | 5 | 14 | 81 |
| Flour, white all-purpose (patent) | 364 | 2 | 12 | 86 |

DRIED LEGUMES

| | | | |
|---|---|---|---|
| Black, brown, Bayo beans, raw | 339 | 4 | 23 | 74 |
| Chickpeas or garbanzos, raw | 360 | 11 | 20 | 69 |
| Lentils: | | | | |
|   Whole, raw | 340 | 3 | 25 | 72 |
|   Whole, cooked | 106 | trace | 26 | 74 |
|   Split without seed coat, raw | 345 | 2 | 25 | 74 |
| Lima beans: | | | | |
|   Raw | 345 | 4 | 20 | 75 |
|   Cooked | 138 | 4 | 20 | 75 |
| Peanuts | | | | |
|   Raw, with skins | 564 | 70 | 16 | 13 |
|   Roasted, with skins | 582 | 70 | 16 | 14 |
| Peanut butter (without sweetener) | 581 | 71 | 17 | 12 |
| Peas, split: | | | | |
|   Raw | 348 | 2 | 24 | 73 |
|   Cooked | 115 | 2 | 24 | 74 |
| Pinto, calico, red Mexican beans, raw | 349 | 3 | 23 | 74 |
| Soybeans: | | | | |
|   Raw | 403 | 37 | 29 | 34 |
|   Cooked | 130 | 37 | 29 | 34 |

NUTS, SEEDS

| | | | |
|---|---|---|---|
| Almonds | 598 | 76 | 11 | 13 |
| Brazil nuts | 654 | 86 | 7 | 7 |
| Cashews | 561 | 68 | 11 | 21 |
| Chestnuts: | | | | |
|   Fresh | 194 | 6 | 5 | 88 |
|   Dried | 377 | 9 | 6 | 85 |
| Coconut: | | | | |
|   Meat, fresh | 346 | 85 | 3 | 11 |
|   Meat, dried, unsweetened | 662 | 82 | 4 | 14 |
| Filberts (hazelnuts) | 634 | 82 | 7 | 11 |
| Macadamias | 691 | 87 | 4 | 9 |
| Peanuts, see Dried Legumes | | | | |
| Pecans | 687 | 87 | 5 | 9 |
| Sesame seeds, dried | 582 | 77 | 11 | 12 |
| Sunflower seed kernels, dried | 560 | 71 | 15 | 14 |
| Walnuts, English or Persian | 651 | 82 | 8 | 10 |

VEGETABLES

| | | | |
|---|---|---|---|
| Artichokes, globe or French, cooked | 44* | 4 | 15 | 80 |
| Asparagus, cooked | 20 | 8 | 27 | 64 |
| Avocados, raw | 167 | 82 | 4 | 13 |
| Bamboo shoots, raw | 27 | 9 | 23 | 69 |

* Calories range from 8–44; they are lowest in freshly harvested artichokes.

Beans:

| | | | | |
|---|---|---|---|---|
| limas, cooked | 111 | 4 | 24 | 72 |
| snap green, cooked | 25 | 7 | 16 | 77 |
| yellow or wax, cooked | 22 | 8 | 16 | 76 |
| Bean sprouts (mung beans), raw | 35 | 5 | 27 | 68 |
| Beets, red, cooked | 32 | 3 | 10 | 86 |
| Broccoli, raw | 32 | 8 | 27 | 66 |
| Brussels sprouts, cooked | 36 | 9 | 28 | 63 |
| Cabbage, raw | 24 | 7 | 13 | 80 |
| Carrots, raw | 42 | 4 | 7 | 89 |
| Cauliflower, raw | 27 | 6 | 24 | 69 |
| Celery, raw | 17 | 5 | 13 | 82 |
| Chives, raw | 28 | 9 | 16 | 74 |
| Collards, cooked | 29 | 17 | 23 | 60 |
| Corn kernels, sweet, cooked (approximate values) | 83* | 9 | 9 | 81 |
| Cucumbers: | | | | |
| pared, raw | 14 | 6 | 10 | 83 |
| unpared, raw | 15 | 5 | 14 | 80 |
| Eggplant, cooked | 19 | 9 | 13 | 78 |
| Endive, curly and escarole, raw | 20 | 4 | 21 | 74 |
| Garlic cloves, raw | 137 | 1 | 12 | 86 |
| Kale, cooked | 28 | 21 | 28 | 51 |
| Leeks, raw | 52 | 5 | 12 | 83 |
| Lettuce: | | | | |
| Butterhead varieties, e.g., Bibb, raw | 14 | 12 | 22 | 66 |
| Crisphead varieties, e.g., iceberg, raw | 13 | 6 | 16 | 78 |
| Romaine, or cos, raw | 18 | 14 | 18 | 69 |
| Mushrooms, raw | 28 | 9 | 25 | 55 |
| Mustard greens, cooked | 23 | 14 | 23 | 62 |
| Okra, cooked | 29 | 9 | 17 | 74 |
| Olives, ripe, canned | 129 | 90 | 3 | 7 |
| Onions, mature, raw | 38 | 2 | 11 | 88 |
| Onions, green, raw | 36 | 5 | 10 | 84 |
| Parsley, raw | 44 | 11 | 20 | 69 |
| Parsnips, cooked | 66 | 6 | 6 | 87 |
| Peas, edible-podded, raw | 53 | 3 | 16 | 81 |
| Peas, green, cooked | 71 | 5 | 26 | 69 |
| Peppers, bell, raw | 22 | 8 | 13 | 78 |
| Potatoes, baked in skin | 93 | 1 | 8 | 91 |
| Potatoes, boiled in skin | 76 | 1 | 8 | 91 |
| Pumpkin, canned | 33 | 7 | 7 | 85 |
| Radishes, raw | 17 | 5 | 16 | 80 |
| Rutabagas, cooked | 35 | 2 | 7 | 90 |

* Two variables markedly affect carbohydrate content of corn: corn variety and edible stage. Differences can be as great as 40 calories per 100 grams of kernel.

| | | | |
|---|---|---|---|
| Spinach, cooked | 23 | 11 | 32 | 56 |
| Squash, summer, cooked | 14 | 6 | 16 | 78 |
| Squash, winter, cooked, baked | 63 | 5 | 7 | 88 |
| Sweet potatoes, cooked, baked in skim milk | 141 | 3 | 4 | 93 |
| Swisschard, cooked | 18 | 9 | 25 | 66 |
| Tapioca, dry | 352 | <.5 | <.5 | 99 |
| Tomatoes, ripe, raw | 22 | 8 | 12 | 76 |
| Tomato juice, canned or bottled | 19 | 4 | 12 | 81 |
| Turnips, cooked | 23 | 7 | 10 | 83 |
| Water chestnut, raw | 79 | 2 | 5 | 94 |
| Watercress, raw | 19 | 13 | 29 | 57 |
| Zucchini, *see* Squash, summer | | | | |
| | | | | |
| **FRUITS** | | | | |
| Apples, raw | 58 | 9 | 1 | 90 |
| Apple juice, canned or bottled | 47 | *trace* | 1 | 99 |
| Apricots, raw | 51 | 3 | 7 | 90 |
| Bananas, raw | 85 | 2 | 4 | 94 |
| Blackberries (incl. boysenberries), raw | 58 | 13 | 7 | 80 |
| Blueberries, raw | 62 | 7 | 4 | 89 |
| Breadfruit, raw | 103 | 2 | 6 | 92 |
| Cantaloupe, *see* Muskmelons | | | | |
| Casaba melon, *see* Muskmelons | | | | |
| Cherries: | | | | |
|   Sour red, raw | 58 | 4 | 7 | 88 |
|   Sweet, raw | 70 | 4 | 6 | 90 |
| Cranberries, raw | 46 | 13 | 3 | 84 |
| Dates, dried | 274 | 1 | 3 | 96 |
| Figs: | | | | |
|   Raw | 80 | 3 | 5 | 92 |
|   Dried | 274 | 4 | 5 | 91 |
| Gooseberries, raw | 39 | 4 | 7 | 89 |
| Grapefruit, raw | 41 | 2 | 4 | 93 |
| Granadilla, raw | 90 | 6 | 8 | 85 |
| Grapes: | | | | |
|   Slip skin (incl. Concord), raw | 69 | 12 | 6 | 82 |
|   Adherent skin (incl. Thompson seedless, muscat), raw | 67 | 4 | 3 | 93 |
| Guava, raw | 62 | 8 | 4 | 87 |
| Kumquats, raw | 65 | 1 | 5 | 94 |
| Lemon juice | 25 | 7 | 7 | 86 |
| Loganberries, raw | 62 | 8 | 5 | 87 |
| Loquats, raw | 48 | 3 | 3 | 94 |
| Lychees, raw | 64 | 4 | 5 | 92 |
| Mangos, raw | 66 | 5 | 4 | 92 |
| Muskmelons: | | | | |
|   Cantaloupe, raw | 30 | 3 | 8 | 90 |
|   Casaba, raw | 27 | *trace* | 15 | 87 |

| | | | |
|---|---|---|---|
| Honeydew, raw | 33 | 8 | 8 | 84 |
| Nectarines, raw | 64 | trace | 3 | 96 |
| Oranges, raw | 49 | 3 | 7 | 90 |
| Orange juice | 45 | 4 | 5 | 91 |
| Papayas, raw | 39 | 2 | 5 | 92 |
| Peaches, raw | 38 | 2 | 5 | 92 |
| Pears, raw | 61 | 5 | 4 | 90 |
| Persimmons, raw | 127 | 3 | 2 | 95 |
| Pineapple, raw | 52 | 3 | 3 | 95 |
| Plums, raw | 66 | trace | 2 | 97 |
| Pomegranates, raw | 63 | 4 | 3 | 94 |
| Quinces, raw | 57 | 1 | 2 | 97 |
| Raisins, natural, uncooked | 289 | 1 | 3 | 96 |
| Raspberries, red, raw | 57 | 7 | 7 | 86 |
| Strawberries, raw | 37 | 11 | 6 | 82 |
| Tangerines, raw | 46 | 4 | 6 | 91 |
| Watermelon, raw | 26 | 6 | 6 | 87 |

# SIX

## Selected Pritikin Program Recipes

# 26

# Introduction
# to the Recipes

Now that you understand the diet, how do you make it work?

Theory is one thing, three-meals-plus-snacks-a-day is another. Are these foods tasty? Is the diet practical? Or will it make you a slave to your kitchen? Is it expensive?

Let's discuss palatability. Be assured that in time your diet will taste better than your old way of eating. It may not at first, though. And you will launch yourself only with plenty of will power. You may miss the old sugar, the salt, the meat, the butter. But not for long.

If you stick to the diet, within a week or two you will not notice the missing salt. In fact, you'll begin to relish the flavors of natural food, including natural salt.

Curiously, many people adapt effortlessly to meatless meals. Butter and margarine are usually sacrificed with some gnashing of teeth during the first week or so, and thereafter nary a whimper is heard.

Some of the nonfat dairy food substitutions, like nonfat buttermilk, are almost undetectable. Others, like uncreamed cottage cheese in its various forms, may taste as good or better than their creamed or partially creamed equivalents. Both nonfat buttermilk and uncreamed cottage cheese are called for in various recipes. If the uncreamed cottage cheese you purchase is in pressed brick ("hoop cheese") form, you may need to mash it with a little skim milk to cottage cheese-consistency for recipes calling for uncreamed cottage cheese.

If no uncreamed cottage cheese or other skim milk dairy products such as nonfat buttermilk or nonfat yogurt are available where you live, make your own from simple recipes we have provided or, in a pinch, you can use products with up to 1 percent fat by weight. Unfortunately, unlike cottage cheese, hard cheeses have no skim milk counterparts, as they depend upon butterfat for flavor. The Pritikin Diet offers no gastronomical solace to hard-cheese lovers—but time will dull this craving, especially when you discover the exciting dishes provided here.

The recipe section that follows was created by award-winning cookbook author and nationally syndicated food columnist June Roth to provide a solid foundation for your new lifestyle. June Roth, with assistance from members of the Pritikin Longevity Center staff, explores the culinary possibilities of the Pritikin Diet with great flair and resourcefulness—and illuminates by example the sort of creativity that you can bring to bear on meal preparation in your own home. The recipes are divided into three categories: for the gourmet cook, for the family cook, and for the single cook. Each category boasts delicious breakfast, lunch, and dinner selections. Do not feel that you have to limit yourself to any one section. The recipes are categorized roughly according to complexity and number of mouths to feed.

Look through the recipes in the Maximum Weight Loss chapter, too. It includes many basic recipes that you may want to incorporate into your repertory of recipes, even if you are not trying to lose weight.

As for practicality and efficiency of food preparation, these will improve with habituation to the diet. You may despair at first. *Don't.* In a few days you will adjust to the new shopping and storage techniques that will expedite meal preparation.

Economy is one of the diet's major triumphs. The elimination of expensive meat and prepared food purchases alone should cut your food budget by a quarter to a third.

## MEAL PLANNING

Many of the recipes may be served as often as you like—their ingredients being at optimal levels of recommended fat, protein, cholesterol, and fruit-sugar limits. Others, particularly those for the gourmet cook, some

lessert selections, and those requiring meat, fish, fowl, or
other high protein foods such as cheese, beans, and egg
whites, must be used less often, so as not to violate Pritikin Diet guidelines. Some gourmet recipes ought to be
saved for special occasions and not be considered daily
fare.

To conform to your new health guidelines, try to down-
play the old meat, fish, or fowl entree as the basis of your
meals. Play director and build up the bit parts of the vegetables and grains to compensate for the dimming of the
old stars.

For instance, serve a salad as your first dinner course.
Make it a large salad, adding interesting raw (or cooked)
vegetables and serve it with an imaginative dressing.
Make the next course a hearty soup. Then move on to a
Pritikin-style entree, served with some vegetable side
dishes and a choice of grain, pasta, or potatoes. And don't
stint on the bread.

Diplomates of the Pritikin Centers do not seem to miss
the old conventional slab of beef or pork when Pritikin
meals are creatively prepared.

It may be hard for you to shuck some venerable, but
tired and false, notions of good nutrition. At the Pritikin
Center we often have to reassure people that a meal with
cooked dried beans, rice, and corn is not "too much
starch." Where once upon a time we were supposed to
"stay away from starches," good dieting now requires
planning meals around complex carbohydrate foods with
their high starch content. This means raising the priority
of grains, preferably unrefined, in the form of such foods
as rice, pasta, cereals, and bread, along with potatoes and
other vegetable foods.

Meat generally should be regarded as a flavoring condiment, a kind of spice. A small amount of flesh foods can
flavor an entire casserole or stew. In many of the recipes
in this book you can cut down on the amount of meat
without diminishing taste. This, by the way, would not be
an idle experiment. If you can cut down on animal protein, you can effectively stretch your meat ration over
more meals. One way of reducing the percentage of animal protein in these recipes is merely to augment the

quantity of grains and vegetables. First try the recipe as described, so that on a second go-round you know how much modification you can attempt. You'll have a better feel that way of what will work and what won't work.

This stretching technique can be demonstrated with specific recipes from the family cook section:

*Stuffed Cabbage.* Increase the quantity of rice (or add another grain for interest) and decrease the amount of meat by the same amount. You might also reduce the amount of meat and add a comparable amount of chopped cooked vegetables, such as celery, mushrooms, carrots, onion.

*Baked Haddock and Vegetables.* Add more vegetables, using ones already called for and adding others, such as celery and mushrooms. Some zucchini and broccoli, if partially precooked, would also be nice additions.

*Chicken in the Pot.* Extend further with more vegetables. More onion, possibly cabbage wedges, or whatever the cook fancies.

In some cases, you could eliminate the meat altogether, thus converting a meat entree to a vegetarian one, without any problems. In the Eggplant Parmigiana recipe, you could just as well use a marinara-type sauce. Or you could compromise and cut the meat to a quarter-pound. At the Pritikin Centers, a favorite dish is salmon loaf with curry sauce—one ounce of canned salmon in each serving. Ordinarily, salmon, a high-fat content fish, should be avoided. But when sufficiently diluted with other ingredients, even that small amount—especially of canned salmon with its potent flavor—can make a very good salmon dish.

To hold down your overall protein intake, you can employ this same "stretching" technique with other high protein foods besides meat, fish, or fowl. You could add a variety of vegetables to the topping of the Pita Pizza (Single Cook Recipes) and proportionately decrease the cheese. Chopped onion, celery, mushrooms, green pepper, etc.—all partially precooked—are standard pizza adornments that work well with this recipe.

You can also profitably stretch fruit juice ingredients of dessert recipes. Since your appetite for sugary tastes will drop in time, this touch of miserliness will not be as painful as you may think. Simply dilute the juice called for with water. You may wish to dilute those you drink, too, by adding water or sparkling mineral water. In that way, the minuscule four ounces per day fruit juice allotment goes farther.

One last and very important suggestion: substitute whole grains for refined grains wherever possible. Your taste buds will soon grow to prefer the more robust flavor and interesting texture of whole grain foods over the relatively pallid refined grain foods—and you will benefit enormously from the enhanced nutritional value and increased dietary fiber of the unrefined products. In most cases, substitution presents no problem: instead of white rice, or white pasta, use brown rice and whole wheat pasta.

When substituting whole wheat flour for white flour in baking, if the flour is coarsely ground, simply lower the amount of whole wheat flour to ⅞ cup for every cup of white flour called for. With all of the recipes in this book calling for unbleached white flour, you'll be boosting the nutritional value by substituting whole wheat flour. Even in certain cake recipes where you feel you must have some white flour to achieve a light enough texture, you can mix together whole wheat pastry flour with some unbleached white flour.

Tinkering with recipes carries some risks. In most recipes, however, the tolerances are not too fine. When using recipes from ordinary sources, your adapting skills must be versatile. Once you master them, you will be amazed at how broad the culinary opportunities are. You may even wish to pattern new recipes on old favorites.

Your meal plans may be as simple or as fussy as you wish, depending upon the occasion, the amount of time you have for food preparation, and your food preferences—*except that intake of fat, cholesterol, protein and fruit sugars must never exceed allowed maximums.*

A stipped-down (but nutritionally superb) model of the Pritikin Diet could consist of such simply prepared foods as follows:

*Breakfast*

Whole orange or a half grapefruit
Bowl of steaming hot whole-grain cereal
Skim milk

*Lunch*

A hearty bean and vegetable soup
Large, mixed raw-vegetables salad with acceptable dressing
Piece of fresh fruit for dessert

*Dinner*

Steamed vegetables (with a little lean meat, chicken or
fish, if desired) over a mound of brown rice
Piece of fresh fruit for dessert

The meals above could include acceptable bread or
crackers and beverages, if desired. Snacks for the day
could consist of more bread or crackers, fresh vegetables
for munching, and perhaps another piece of fruit.

On the other hand, on many days, or on special occasions, you may require or desire more elaborate, festive,
or gourmet meal preparations. To show you just how
glamorous a Pritikin Diet meal can be, let's look at some
special-occasion menus and recipes.

*Sunday Breakfast Menu*

Broiled Grapefruit
Belgian Waffles with Strawberries
Beverage

*Holiday Luncheon Menu*

Onion Soup in Individual Crocks
Manicotti Florentine
Bibb and Red Pepper Salad
Fruit Salad Alaska
Beverage

*Special Occasion Dinner Menu*

Vichyssoise
Tournedos Chasseur
Stuffed Mushrooms
Braised Endive
Carrots with Apple Glaze
Romaine Salad with Lemon-Mustard Dressing
Pumpkin Mousse Pie
Beverage

# 27

## Recipes for the Gourmet Cook

### *BREAKFAST RECIPES*

#### NOVA LOX AND ONION OMELET

1 small Nova Scotia smoked salmon fin
1 medium onion, sliced
¼ teaspoon dried dillweed
4 egg whites

Place the fin (including the skin) in a large nonstick skillet. Add the sliced onion and the dillweed. Cover and cook the salmon under low heat for 10 minutes, or until the fish can be easily separated from the skin and bones. Remove the fin and cut the cooked salmon into small shreds, discarding the skin and bones. Beat the egg whites until soft peaks form. Gently fold in the shredded salmon and the onions. Return the salmon mixture to the skillet and cook it over medium heat for 1 minute, then cover and cook it until the top is solidified. Loosen edges with a spatula and flip the omelet over. Cover the pan and brown the other side. Turn the omelet out on a round platter and cut it into pie-shaped wedges. Serve with chilled sliced tomatoes, if desired.

*Note:* Do not use regular smoked salmon, known as "lox," as it is very salty compared to the Nova Scotia type. Use smoked fish on rare occasions because smoked products have some suspected carcinogens.

*Serves 4*

## DEVILED EGGS

6 hard-boiled eggs
¼ cup uncreamed cottage cheese
¼ teaspoon dry mustard
¼ teaspoon curry powder
1 teaspoon lemon juice
   Paprika, to taste

Peel the eggs and cut them in half lengthwise. Scoop out the yolks and discard. Mash the cottage cheese with a fork or press it through a sieve. Add the mustard, curry, and lemon juice; mix well. Spoon the mixture into the cavities of the hard-boiled egg whites and swirl the filling into decorative peaks. Dust the filling with paprika. Chill the eggs until they are ready to serve.

*Serves 6*

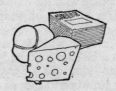

## CHEESE DANISH

1 cup uncreamed cottage cheese
4 slices sourdough bread
¼ cup undiluted frozen apple juice concentrate, thawed
1 teaspoon ground cinnamon
¼ teaspoon ground ginger

Spread the cottage cheese generously on each slice of bread. Drizzle the apple juice over the cheese. Sprinkle on the cinnamon and the ginger. Put the bread slices under the broiler until they are lightly browned. Serve at once.

*Serves 4*

## BELGIAN WAFFLES WITH STRAWBERRIES

    4 egg whites
    1 cup unbleached flour
1¼ cups skim milk
    1 teaspoon vanilla extract
    2 cups sliced fresh strawberries
    2 teaspoons undiluted frozen apple juice concentrate,
        thawed

Beat egg whites until stiff peaks form. In another bowl, combine the flour, milk, and vanilla until smooth; then fold the mixture through the beaten egg whites, taking care not to break down the air bubbles. Spoon the batter into a hot nonstick waffle iron and bake. Meanwhile, combine ½ cup each of the sliced strawberries and the apple juice in an electric blender and process the two into a smooth sauce; pour it over the remaining sliced strawberries and serve as a topping with the waffles.

*Note:* If you prefer a layer of whipped topping between the waffles and the strawberries, process 1 cup uncreamed cottage cheese with 4 teaspoons undiluted frozen apple juice in a blender until fluffy. (If more liquid is required, add some skim milk.) Serve with plain fresh strawberries, or with strawberry sauce as directed above.

*Note:* If waffles stick to Teflon iron, use a light coating of vegetable spray for the first waffle only.

*Serves 4*


## BLUEBERRY COTTAGE CHEESE PANCAKES

    1 cup uncreamed cottage cheese
¼ cup skim milk
¾ cup unbleached all-purpose flour
    4 egg whites
1½ teaspoons lemon juice
    1 cup whole fresh blueberries
        Mock Sour Cream, optional (see Index)

Combine the cheese, milk, and flour. Beat the egg whites with a fork until just frothy; add to cheese mixture.

Add the lemon juice and stir. Add the blueberries. Spoon the batter onto a nonstick griddle; turn when the tops begin to bubble and the bottoms are lightly browned.

Serve at once with Mock Sour Cream, if desired.
*Serves 4*

### BAKED APPLE PUDDING

1½ cups unbleached all-purpose flour
2 cups skim milk
¼ cup undiluted frozen apple juice concentrate, thawed
2 teaspoons vanilla extract
4 egg whites
4 apples
¼ cup orange juice
1 teaspoon ground cinnamon
¼ teaspoon ground ginger

Combine the flour, milk, apple juice, and vanilla. Beat the egg whites lightly with a fork until they are foamy; add them to the batter and mix well. Set the batter aside. Peel and slice the apples; spread them in a neat layer over the bottom of an 8-by-12-inch nonstick baking pan. Sprinkle the orange juice evenly over the apples. Add half the cinnamon and the ginger to the batter and sprinkle the other half over the apples. Pour the batter over the apples. Bake in a preheated 400 degree oven for 30 minutes, or until they are lightly browned and well set. Cut the pudding into squares and serve with Mock Sour Cream, if desired (see Index).

*Serves 6*

## *SOUPS*

### ONION SOUP GRATINÉE

 5  large onions, thinly sliced
 6  cups water
 2  beef bones, precooked and defatted
 1  bay leaf
¼  teaspoon ground pepper
 2  tablespoons unbleached all-purpose flour
 4  slices sourdough toast
 4  tablespoons grated fresh sapsago cheese

Place 1 sliced onion in a small baking pan and set aside. Place the remaining onions in a large saucepan with the water, prepared beef bones, bay leaf, and pepper. Cover and cook this until the onions are tender. Remove the bay leaf and the bones. Sprinkle the flour over the onion slices in a baking pan; put it under the broiler until the flour has browned and some of the onions have burned. Add a little water and stir until smooth. Add a small amount of the soup, stirring until smooth, then return all to the soup. Heat the soup, stirring constantly until boiling and slightly thickened. Pour the soup into 4 individual crocks, and trim the toast to fit on top of each. Sprinkle the toast with grated cheese. Put it under the broiler until the cheese melts. Serve at once.
*Serves 4*

### MINESTRONE

¼  cup uncooked brown rice
 1  medium onion, chopped
 1  clove garlic, minced
 1  leek, diced and then washed (optional)
 3  stalks celery, chopped
 2  medium carrots, diced
 2  cups shredded cabbage
 1  zucchini, chopped
1½  quarts liquid (water or a combination of water and tomato juice) or more, if a thinner soup is desired

1 28-ounce can whole pack tomatoes, chopped, or
diced tomatoes, with juice
3 tablespoons tomato paste (or more, if a stronger tomato flavor is desired)
2 tablespoons minced parsley
½ teaspoon thyme
½ teaspoon oregano
3 cups cooked dried beans (red, navy, lentil, kidney,
garbanzo, or combinations)

Slowly add the rice to boiling liquid containing all the
other ingredients except the beans. Reduce the heat and
simmer 1 hour, stirring occasionally. Add the cooked
beans. Put about ⅓ of the contents of the soup pot in a
blender to blend. Return the blended mixture to the soup
pot and stir well. Heat through and serve.

*Note:* For a variation, omit the rice and add uncooked
whole-wheat pasta (shells, elbow macaroni, or broken
spaghetti) to the simmering soup about 10 minutes before
the end of the cooking period.

*Serves 8*

## SWEDISH YELLOW PEA SOUP

2 cups dried yellow peas
2 quarts water
1 onion, thinly sliced
½ teaspoon dried marjoram
⅛ teaspoon ground ginger
⅛ teaspoon ground pepper
2 beef bones

Soak the peas in water overnight; bring them to a boil
and skim off the residue. Add the onion, marjoram,
ginger, pepper, and beef bones. Cover and simmer the
soup for several hours, or until the peas disintegrate. Remove the bones.

To serve, it's best to chill the soup and remove the top
layer of the solidified fat before reheating the soup.

*Serves 6 to 8*

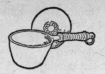

## CIOPPINO

2 large onions, diced
2 cloves garlic, minced
1 green pepper, chopped
2 cups tomato juice
½ cup red burgundy wine
1 28-ounce can tomatoes
1 teaspoon dried oregano
1 teaspoon dried parsley
½ teaspoon dried basil
¼ teaspoon ground pepper
1 pound halibut, cut in chunks
2 potatoes, peeled and diced

Put the onions, garlic, green pepper, and tomato juice into a large saucepan; cook the vegetables until they are tender. Add the wine, tomatoes, oregano, parsley, basil, and pepper. Cover the pot and cook for 10 minutes. Add the fish and the potatoes; cover and cook for 15 minutes more or until the potatoes are tender. Uncover and cook for an additional 5 minutes.
*Serves 6*

## VICHYSSOISE

4 large potatoes, peeled and cut up
1 large white of leek, sliced
2 cups water
1 tablespoon chopped fresh parsley
¼ teaspoon white pepper
2 cups skim milk
2 tablespoons cornstarch
¼ cup chopped fresh chives

Place the potatoes, leek, water, parsley, and pepper in
saucepan. Cover the pan and cook over a low heat until
ne potatoes are very tender. Mash the potatoes and the
ooked leek with the soup water, or process them in an
lectric blender. Combine the milk and the cornstarch
ito a smooth paste; stir it into the potato mixture. Heat
nd stir constantly until the soup has thickened. Chill.

Serve the soup in chilled bowls with a garnish of
hopped chives.

*Serves 4 to 6*


## BROCCOLI BISQUE

1  10-ounce package frozen chopped broccoli
1  small onion, sliced
1  whole clove garlic
⅛  teaspoon ground pepper
1  cup water
2  cups skim milk
1  tablespoon cornstarch

Place the broccoli, onion, clove, pepper, and water in a
aucepan. Cover the pan and cook the broccoli until it is
ery soft. Remove the clove. Process the broccoli and the
quid in an electric blender; then return it to the sauce-
an. Combine the skim milk and the cornstarch into a
mooth paste; stir it into the broccoli mixture. Heat, stir-
ng constantly, until the bisque has thickened slightly.
erve at once.

*Serves 4 to 6*


## ESCAROLE LENTIL SOUP

2  cups dried lentils
1  quart water
1  onion, diced
1  bay leaf
¼  teaspoon ground pepper
1  teaspoon paprika
1  head escarole

Pick over and wash the lentils. Soak them in water for several hours. Drain. Bring the water to a boil; add the lentils, onion, bay leaf, pepper, and paprika. Cook the lentil mixture over a very low heat, stirring occasionally, until the lentils are soft, about 1½ to 2 hours. Meanwhile, wash the escarole and trim off all of the white parts, using only the green leaves. Place the escarole in a saucepan, cover with water, and cook until soft. Drain. Add the escarole to the lentil soup just before it is ready to serve. The lentils should be soft but about half will retain their shape.

*Serves 6*

## GAZPACHO

4 large tomatoes, cut up
1 clove garlic, peeled
2 tablespoons wine vinegar
¼ teaspoon ground pepper
1 cup tomato juice
1 cucumber, peeled and diced
1 green pepper, seeded and diced
3 scallions, finely sliced

Process the tomatoes in an electric blender or food processor until smooth. Add the garlic, vinegar, and pepper; process again. Pour the purée into a container; add the tomato juice and stir well. Chill.

Serve the gazpacho in small chilled bowls. Pass bowls of diced cucumber, green pepper, and scallions for garnish.

*Serves 4 to 6*

## MEAT, POULTRY, AND FISH

### BRAISED SADDLE OF VENISON

    1  saddle of young venison
    1  clove garlic, mashed
  ¼  teaspoon dried thyme
  ¼  teaspoon ground pepper
    1  onion, sliced
    2  carrots, scraped and sliced
    2  stalks celery, sliced
  ¼  wedge cabbage, shredded
    1  cup red wine
    2  tablespoons tomato paste
    1  tablespoon lemon juice
    1  cup water
  10  medium potatoes, peeled

Rub the venison with the garlic, thyme, and pepper. Combine the onion, carrots, celery, and cabbage and place in the bottom of a roasting pan. Place the venison on top of the vegetables. Pour the mixture of wine, tomato paste, lemon juice, and water over all. Arrange the potatoes around the roast. Cover tightly and place in a 350 degree oven for 1 hour, or until fork tender and done to desired degree of rareness.

*Note:* A saddle of veal may be substituted for the venison.

*Serves 8 to 10*

### POACHED SALMON WITH CUCUMBER SAUCE

    2  pounds fresh salmon steaks
  ¼  cup lemon juice
    1  carrot, sliced
    1  onion, thinly sliced
    2  cloves
    1  bay leaf
    1  black peppercorn
  ½  cucumber, peeled and chopped
  ½  small onion
    1  cup thin Mock Sour Cream (see Index)

Arrange the salmon steaks in a large skillet. Pour the lemon juice over the salmon. Fill the skillet with 1 inch of water. Add the sliced carrot, onion, cloves, bay leaf, and peppercorn. Bring to a boil, then reduce the heat and cover. Simmer the fish and the aromatics gently for 20 minutes, or until it flakes easily when tested with a fork. Remove the fish to a platter and serve with the carrots, if desired. Mix the cucumber, onion, and Mock Sour Cream together and serve as a sauce.

*Serves 8*

## WHITEFISH QUENELLES

 4  pounds whitefish
 4  onions
 2  carrots, scraped
 3  sprigs fresh parsley
 2  sprigs fresh dill
 4  egg whites
 ¼  cup fine matzo meal or unbleached all-purpose flour
 1  teaspoon ground white pepper

Have your fish man fillet the fish and give you the head, bones, and skin. (If possible, have him grind the fish fillets for you.) Place the head, bones, skin, 2 of the onions, carrots, parsley, and dill into a deep pot. Add about 1 quart of water and bring it to a boil. Reduce the heat. Meanwhile, grind the fish and the remaining 2 onions together. Beat the egg whites with a fork until they are frothy; add egg white to the fish. Add the matzo meal and the pepper. Form the fish mixture into round balls, using about ½ cup of fish for each ball. Drop each quenelle carefully into the simmering fish stock. Cover and simmer for 2 hours. Cool. Remove the quenelles from the broth with a slotted spoon. Serve hot or chilled.

*Note:* Do not discard the broth. Use it as fish stock, as the base of a chowder, or reduce the volume by boiling it, uncovered, then strain and chill it to be served as a jellied soup. Carrots may be cut up and served with the fish, if desired.

*Serves 10*

## CHICKEN WITH MUSHROOMS

    4 boneless and skinless chicken breast halves
    ¼ pound fresh mushrooms, sliced
    ½ cup white wine
    1 teaspoon lemon juice
    ½ teaspoon dried dillweed
    ½ cup evaporated skim milk
    ½ cup permissible bread crumbs

With a meat mallet, pound the chicken breasts flat between two sheets of waxed paper. Set them aside. Simmer the mushrooms in the white wine, lemon juice, and dillweed; cook the mushroom mixture until the wine is almost evaporated. Lift the thin layer of chicken found on the underside of the breast and stuff it with a portion of the mushrooms. Pat the protective layer of chicken back in place, and fold both sides of the breast under to enclose. Roll the breasts in the evaporated skim milk and then in bread crumbs, covering well. Arrange the stuffed breasts in a baking pan. Bake in a 350 degree oven for 35 minutes, or until the chicken is tender.
*Serves 4*


## CORNISH HENS WITH APPLE GLAZE

    4 Cornish hens, about 1 pound each
    1 cup undiluted frozen apple juice concentrate, thawed
    ½ teaspoon ground cinnamon
    1 tablespoon cornstarch
    3 lemon slices

Wash the hens and arrange them in a small roasting pan. In a saucepan, combine the apple juice, cinnamon, and cornstarch. Mix until smooth. Add the lemon slices. Cook and stir the apple-juice mixture over a medium heat until the mixture thickens. Brush this glaze over the hens. Roast the hens in a 375 degree oven for 1 hour, or until they are fork tender, basting with additional sauce several times during cooking.
Cut the hens in half and serve.
*Serves 8*

## OSSO BUCO

4 pounds veal shanks, cut into 2-inch chunks and
    trimmed of fat
2 onions, diced
1 clove garlic, minced
2 bay leaves
1 teaspoon dried rosemary
½ teaspoon ground pepper
1 cup dry white wine
1 carrot, grated
1 celery stalk, minced
¼ cup chopped fresh parsley
2 cups chopped fresh tomatoes
2 tablespoons tomato paste
½ cup water

Using a heavy nonstick skillet, sear the cut sides of
the veal shanks. Add the onions, garlic, bay leaves, rosemary, pepper, and white wine; cover and simmer over low
heat for 5 minutes. Add the carrot, celery, parsley, and
tomatoes. Stir the tomato paste into the water and add to
the veal. Mix well. Simmer the veal, covered, for 35
minutes or until it is tender. Remove the veal to a platter
and discard the bay leaves from the skillet. Cook the remaining sauce over a high heat for several minutes to
reduce the volume and to thicken. Pour the sauce over
the shanks and serve.

*Note:* It's best to cook this dish in advance, so as to be
able to chill it and remove any fat that solidifies; then reheat and serve.

*Serves 8*

## TOURNEDOS CHASSEUR

4 tournedos (4 ounces each) cut from the tail of a beef
    tenderloin
2 shallots, minced
¼ pound mushrooms, minced
1 cup dry white wine
1 cup beef consommé, defatted

1 tablespoon tomato paste
2 teaspoons cornstarch
¼ cup chopped fresh parsley
  Freshly ground pepper

Using a heavy skillet, sear the tournedos on both sides; remove them to a warming platter. Add the shallots, mushrooms, and white wine to the skillet; cook until the wine is reduced in half. Add the consommé and the tomato paste; cover and simmer for several minutes. Mix the cornstarch with just enough water to make a thin paste; spoon some of the consommé mixture into the cornstarch paste and then return all to the skillet, stirring constantly as the sauce thickens. Return the tournedos to the skillet, cover and simmer the meat for several minutes or until they are done to your taste.

Serve with the sauce, topped with a sprinkling of fresh parsley and freshly ground pepper.

*Serves 4*

## MOUSSAKA

1½ pounds very lean ground beef
 2 onions, diced
 1 6-ounce can tomato paste
 1 cup water
 1 cup dry white wine
 3 tablespoons chopped parsley
 ½ teaspoon cinnamon
 ½ teaspoon ground nutmeg
 ¼ teaspoon ground pepper
 ½ cup toasted sourdough bread crumbs
 1 large eggplant

Brown the meat in a large nonstick skillet, breaking apart the meat into bits. Skim off most of the rendered fat, if any. Add the onions, tomato paste, water, wine, parsley, cinnamon, nutmeg, and pepper. Cover and simmer for 1 hour. Stir in the bread crumbs. Meanwhile, peel and slice the eggplant into thin slices. Cover the bottom of an 8-by-12-inch baking pan with the sauce. Arrange a layer of the eggplant slices, side by side, over the sauce. Continue to fill the pan with layers of the sauce and the eggplant, ending with the sauce. Sprinkle the top with additional bread crumbs and nutmeg. Bake in a 350 degree oven for 1 hour.

*Serves 6*

## *MEATLESS MAIN DISHES*

### WILD RICE AND MUSHROOM RING

1 cup raw wild rice
4 cups water
1 pound fresh mushrooms, sliced
½ cup dry white wine
⅛ teaspoon ground nutmeg
⅛ teaspoon ground pepper

Wash the raw rice thoroughly. Bring water to a boil; add rice, reduce heat to low, and cover saucepan. Simmer the rice for 40 minutes, fluffing it occasionally with a fork. Meanwhile, simmer the mushrooms in a skillet with the white wine, nutmeg, and pepper, until the wine has almost evaporated. Combine the cooked rice and the mushrooms. Pack the rice mixture into a 1-quart nonstick ring mold. Set the mold into a pan of water and place it on the middle rack of the oven. Bake at 350 degrees for 30 minutes. Unmold the ring on a large round platter. Fill the center with steamed green peas, if desired.

*Serves 4 to 6*

## ALMOST PAELLA

6 tablespoons vegetable stock or water
2 large onions, thinly sliced
2 cloves garlic, crushed
1 large green pepper, de-seeded and sliced
2 sticks celery, finely chopped
1 cup mushrooms, sliced
1 cup long-grain brown rice
1½ cups vegetable stock or water
Pepper
½ cup fresh peas, shelled
½ cup green beans
¼ teaspoon saffron threads, crushed
4 large tomatoes, skinned and sliced

Heat the vegetable stock or water in a saucepan. Meanwhile, in a large skillet, sauté the onions, garlic, pepper, celery, and mushrooms in the additional 6 tablespoons of stock or water. After 5 minutes, add the rice and stir over the heat for 3 to 4 minutes, until the rice is glossy and slightly opaque. Add the stock, some pepper, and bring up to the boil, then add the peas and the beans. Mix the saffron with a couple of tablespoons of water and add to the pan with the tomatoes. Taste the liquid to check the seasoning, because the paella must not be stirred again. Cover the skillet and simmer gently, in the oven or on the burner, for about 40 minutes, or until the rice is cooked and all the liquid is absorbed.

*Serves 6 to 8*

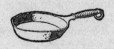

## CRÊPES

1 cup whole-wheat pastry flour
1¼ cups skim milk
4 egg whites, stiffly beaten

Blend the milk with the flour until smooth, then carefully fold in the stiffly beaten egg whites. Heat a medium-sized nonstick skillet until very hot. Then pour in a scant ¼ cup batter, rotating the pan to cover the bottom and to distribute the batter evenly. Brown the crêpe on both sides until golden.

*Note:* Crêpes are a versatile dish for any meal, with fillings ranging from cheese to Chinese vegetables, fruits, meat, and fish. Experiment!

# RATATOUILLE CRÊPES

  1 onion, sliced
  3 medium zucchini, sliced
  2 medium crookneck squash, sliced
 10 mushrooms, sliced
  1 green pepper, cut into strips
  1 clove garlic, minced
  1 6-ounce can tomato paste
  2 tablespoons chopped pimientos
  1 teaspoon Italian herb seasoning
 ¼ teaspoon pepper
 14 to 16 premade crêpes
    Chopped parsley, to garnish

In a heated nonstick skillet, add the onions to brown. Stir constantly over a medium flame to prevent scorching. Then add a few tablespoons of water, bring to a boil, and add the other vegetables, cooking until the vegetables are almost limp. Stir in the tomato paste, 1 can of water, pimiento, and seasoning. Simmer for 10 to 15 minutes.

Place about 3 tablespoons of vegetable mixture on each crêpe; fold the sides to overlap. Place the crêpes on serving plates, allowing 2 per person. Spoon the remaining mixture over the folded crêpes. Garnish with chopped parsley.

*Serves 8*

## POTATO STUFFED CABBAGE

1 large head cabbage
5 pounds potatoes, peeled
2 onions
½ cup raw rice
1 teaspoon dried dillweed
¼ teaspoon pepper
2 egg whites
1 28-ounce can tomatoes
1 apple, peeled and sliced
¼ teaspoon ground ginger

Parboil the cabbage and separate the leaves. Level the knife against outer side of each leaf and remove the excess of the heavy center without cutting into the leaf. Set aside several large outer leaves. Grate the potatoes and the small cabbage leaves near the core. Grate one of the onions over the potatoes and the cabbage. Add the rice, dillweed, and pepper. Beat the egg whites with a fork until they are frothy; add this to the potato mixture. Fill each cabbage leaf with 2 tablespoons of the filling. Fold the bottom over the filling, fold sides in, and roll up. Secure with toothpicks, if necessary. Line the bottom of a Dutch oven with the larger outer cabbage leaves sliced up. Slice the second onion and add it to the pot. Add the tomatoes, apple, and ginger. Place the rolled stuffed cabbage leaves into the pot. Add water if the sauce becomes too thick. Cook the cabbage rolls over very low heat for 4 to 5 hours.
*Serves 8*

## STUFFED ARTICHOKES

4 whole fresh artichokes
¼ cup lemon juice
1 bay leaf
2 peppercorns
4 whole cloves
2 slices toatsed sourdough bread
1 cup chopped fresh mushrooms

 1 onion, diced
 2 tablespoons chopped parsley
½ teaspoon garlic powder

Trim the points from the artichoke leaves and cut the
stem so that the artichoke can be placed upright. In a
skillet roll the artichokes in lemon juice, then arrange
them upright. Add an inch of water. Place the bay leaf,
peppercorns, and cloves in the water. Crumble the toast
as fine as possible. Add the chopped mushrooms, onion,
parsley, and garlic powder. With a spoon, scatter this
mixture among the leaves of the artichokes, using very
small amounts in each place. Cover and cook the artichokes over a low heat for 30 minutes, or until a lower
leaf pulls off easily. Serve with wedges of lemon, if
desired.

*Note:* To eat the artichoke, scrape the fleshy part of
each leaf across the teeth and pile the leaves neatly on the
plate. When you reach the central thistle, remove it with a
fork and eat the soft heart of the artichoke below.

*Serves 4*

## MANICOTTI FLORENTINE

12 whole-wheat manicotti pasta shells
 1 10-ounce package frozen chopped spinach
 1 tablespoon chopped scallions
¼ teaspoon ground nutmeg
 1 cup crumbled hoop cheese (or other uncreamed cot-
     tage cheese)
¼ cup skim milk
 2 teaspoons chopped parsley
 1 egg white
 2 cups tomato juice
¼ cup tomato paste
½ teaspoon garlic powder
½ teaspoon dried oregano
¼ teaspoon dried basil

Cook the manicotti shells in boiling water until *al
dente;* drain. Meanwhile, cook the spinach, scallions, and

nutmeg in a small amount of water and drain well. Mash
the cheese with the skim milk and the parsley; add this to
the drained cooked spinach. Beat the egg white with a
fork until it is frothy; add it to the spinach mixture. Combine the tomato juice, tomato paste, garlic powder, oregano, and basil; cover and cook the liquid mixture over a
low heat for several minutes. Meanwhile, stuff the spinach
mixture into the cooked manicotti shells. Spoon a layer of
tomato sauce over the bottom of a baking dish. Arrange
the stuffed shells side by side. Top with the tomato sauce.
Bake in a 350 degree oven for 30 minutes.

*Serves 6*

## EGGPLANT CANNELLONI

   1 large eggplant, sliced very thin
   2 cups lemon juice plus enough water to cover
       eggplant

### SAUCE
3⅓ cups premade Our Favorite Spaghetti Sauce (see In-
       dex) or 1⅔ cups canned tomatoes, blended in
       blender
  ¾ cup tomato purée
  ¾ cup tomato sauce
1½ cups sliced mushrooms (optional)
1½ cups chopped onion
  ¼ teaspoon garlic powder
   1 teaspoon oregano
   1 teaspoon Italian seasoning

### FILLING
1¾ cups hoop cheese (or other uncreamed cottage
       cheese)
  ½ cup skim milk
   2 egg whites, stiffly beaten
  ½ cup finely chopped Bermuda onion
  ½ cup finely chopped celery
  ½ cup finely chopped green pepper
  ¼ teaspoon garlic powder
  ¼ cup grated sapsago cheese

BATTER

- 3 egg whites
- 2 cups skim milk
- 3 tablespoons brown-rice flour (or use an additional 3 tablespoons whole-wheat pastry flour)
- 1 cup whole-wheat pastry flour

Peel the eggplant carefully. Using a sharp knife, cut the eggplant lengthwise into thin slices. Cover the eggplant slices in the lemon-water mixture and refrigerate until ready to use. Combine the canned tomatoes, tomato purée, tomato sauce, and seasonings. Add the mushrooms and onions. Simmer gently for 20 to 30 minutes.

*Filling:* Mash the hoop cheese and the skim milk with a potato masher. Add the stiffly beaten egg whites and the remaining filling ingredients.

*Batter:* Beat the egg whites until stiff and add the skim milk and the flour. Stir to combine.

Dip the eggplant in the batter and brown on both sides in a crêpe pan. While the eggplant is still warm, spoon enough filling on to be able to roll it up like a crêpe. Place seam-side down in a rectangular nonstick baking pan. Just before baking, spoon the tops with the sauce. Bake at 375 degrees for 20 minutes. If desired, sprinkle with some more sapsago cheese when serving.

This dish is a great hit at cocktail parties. Instead of serving each person a whole cannelloni, allow the cannelloni to cool sufficiently and cut each one into 4 or 5 hors d'oeuvres. This dish can be prepared in advance and refrigerated overnight. But be sure to increase the baking time to about 30 minutes if placed in the oven chilled.

*Serves 6*

## STUFFED ACORN SQUASH

- 2 acorn squash
- 2 scraped carrots, grated
- 1 8-ounce can water-packed crushed pineapple
- 2 tablespoons dried white raisins
- ¼ teaspoon ground ginger

Cut the squash in half; scoop out the seeds, and place the squash in a baking pan. Combine the grated carrots, pineapple, raisins, and ginger. Spoon this mixture into the squash cavities. Bake in a 350 degree oven for 30 minutes, or until the squash are tender.

*Note:* If available, use crushed pineapple that has been packed in its own unsweetened juice instead of the water-packed variety.

*Serves 4*

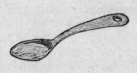

## STUFFED ZUCCHINI

3 large zucchini
1 onion, thinly sliced
1 green pepper, diced
1 clove garlic, minced
½ cup chopped fresh tomatoes
1 cup tomato juice
1 teaspoon dried oregano
1 slice sourdough toast

Cut the zucchini in half lengthwise. Scoop out the pulp, leaving ¼-inch-thick shells. Save the zucchini shells for stuffing. Dice the scooped-out zucchini; place them in a large nonstick skillet with the onion, green pepper, garlic, chopped tomatoes, ¼ cup of the tomato juice, and oregano. Cook until the vegetables are limp. Fill the reserved zucchini shells with the cooked mixture and arrange in a baking dish. Pour the remaining tomato juice around the stuffed zucchini. Crumble the toast and sprinkle it on the tops of the stuffing. Bake in a 350 degree oven for 30 minutes, or until the shells are tender.

Serve with the tomato juice gravy spooned over the shells.

*Serves 6*

## *MAIN DISH VEGETABLES*

### FRENCH PEAS AND LETTUCE

2 10-ounce packages frozen peas, or 2 pounds fresh
    peas, shelled
1 onion, diced
¼ teaspoon dried tarragon
¼ head lettuce, shredded
1 cup water

Place the peas, onion, and tarragon in a saucepan. Top
with the shredded lettuce. Add water and cover. Simmer
over low heat for 10 minutes.
*Serves 6*

### CAULIFLOWER POLONAISE

1 head cauliflower
2 hard-boiled egg whites, chopped
3 tablespoons fresh chopped parsley
3 tablespoons toasted permissible bread crumbs

Boil or steam the whole head of cauliflower until it is
tender. Remove the cauliflower to a serving platter. Combine the egg whites with the parsley and the bread
crumbs; sprinkle the topping over the cooked cauliflower
and serve.
*Serves 6*

## STUFFED MUSHROOMS

12 large mushrooms
1 tablespoon chopped parsley
¼ teaspoon garlic powder
¼ teaspoon onion powder
2 tablespoons permissible bread crumbs
1 egg white

Remove the stems from the mushrooms; trim the ends and chop stems fine. Add the parsley, garlic powder, onion powder, and bread crumbs. Beat the egg white with a fork until it is frothy and mix with the chopped mushrooms. Spoon the egg-white mixture into the mushroom caps. Place the mushrooms in a nonstick baking pan and bake in a 400-degree oven for 20 minutes.

*Serves 4*


## ASPARAGUS WITH LEMON-PARSLEY SAUCE

1 bunch fresh asparagus
¼ cup lemon juice
2 tablespoons chopped fresh parsley

Trim the scales and the woody ends from the asparagus. Wash well. Tie them loosely together in a bunch. Stand them upright in the bottom of a double boiler; add several inches of water and invert the top of the boiler to serve as a cover. (In this way the tender tops will steam while the bottoms boil.) Cook the asparagus just until they are tender. Remove them from the water, cut the string. Arrange on a platter. Stir the lemon juice and fresh parsley together; pour this over the asparagus and serve.

*Serves 4 to 6*

## HARVARD BEETS

1 bunch fresh beets
¼ cup lemon juice
1 tablespoon vinegar
2 tablespoons undiluted frozen apple juice concentrate, thawed
2 tablespoons cornstarch

Trim and peel the beets. Place them in a saucepan, cover with water, and cook, covered, until the beets are tender. Slice the beets. Measure 1½ cups of beet liquid and return that to a saucepan; add the lemon juice, vinegar, and apple juice mixed with the cornstarch. Heat and stir until the mixture thickens and becomes clear. Return the sliced beets to the sauce and heat through.

*Serves 4 to 6*

## GREEN BEANS AND TOMATOES OREGANO

1 pound fresh green beans, trimmed and sliced
2 fresh tomatoes, chopped
1 small onion, diced
½ teaspoon dried oregano
⅛ teaspoon ground pepper
1 cup water

Place the beans in a saucepan with the tomatoes, onion, oregano, pepper, and water. Cook the beans until they reach the tender-crisp stage, about 10 minutes. Drain and serve.

*Serves 6*

## BRAISED ENDIVE

4 head Belgian endive
½ cup dry white wine
1 tablespoon lemon juice
1 hard-boiled egg white, chopped
⅛ teaspoon ground nutmeg

Trim and wash the endives. If they are very thick, cut them in half lengthwise. Arrange them in a baking dish. Add the white wine. Drizzle the lemon juice over the endives. Cover the dish tightly and bake in a 350 degree oven for 20 to 30 minutes, depending on the size of the endives. Add the chopped egg white and nutmeg to garnish. Serve at once.

*Serves 4*

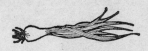

## STEAMED BROCCOLI RABE

1 pound broccoli rabe
¼ cup lemon juice
¼ teaspoon garlic powder
⅛ teaspoon dry mustard

Wash and trim the broccoli rabe. Place the broccoli in a steam unit over a saucepan of water. Steam for 10 to 15 minutes, or until tender. Remove to a serving dish. Combine the lemon juice, garlic powder, and mustard; pour this sauce over the hot vegetable. Serve at once.

*Note:* If it is difficult to find broccoli rabe, look for it in an Italian vegetable market.

*Serves 4*

## CARROTS WITH APPLE GLAZE

8 large carrots, scraped and thinly sliced
¼ cup undiluted frozen apple juice, thawed
1 tablespoon grated orange rind
1 teaspoon cornstarch
⅛ teaspoon ground ginger

Steam the carrots over boiling water for 15 minutes, or until they are tender. Combine the apple juice, orange rind, cornstarch, and ginger in a saucepan; mix until smooth, then cook and stir constantly until the mixture has thickened and cleared. Add the cooked carrots to the sauce. Serve hot.

*Serves 6 to 8*

## DILLED CROOKNECK SQUASH

2 yellow crookneck squash, sliced
1 cup orange juice
1 teaspoon dried dillweed
⅛ teaspoon ground pepper

Place all the ingredients in a saucepan; cook, covered, over a low heat for 15 minutes, or until they are tender.

*Serves 4*

## ZUCCHINI AND MUSHROOMS

2 zucchini, thinly sliced
½ pound fresh mushrooms, sliced
2 stalks celery, sliced
1 onion, sliced
1 cup water
½ teaspoon dried thyme
⅛ teaspoon ground pepper

Place the zucchini, mushrooms, celery, onion, and water in a saucepan. Add the thyme and the pepper. Simmer, covered, for 15 to 20 minutes, or until the vegetables are tender.

*Serves 4 to 6*

## RATATOUILLE

1 eggplant, peeled and diced
3 zucchini, sliced
2 green peppers, diced
1 onion, thinly sliced
1 clove garlic, minced
2 large tomatoes, halved, cut into ½-inch strips, and
   drained
½ teaspoon oregano
¼ teaspoon ground pepper

Combine all the ingredients in a large, heavy pot.
Cook, covered, over low heat for 20 minutes. Cook,
uncovered, 15 minutes more over moderate heat, stirring
with a wooden spoon to prevent scorching.

*Note:* An alternate cooking method is to place all the
ingredients in a covered casserole dish and bake in the
oven at 350 degrees until the vegetables are tender, about
1 hour.

*Serves 4*

## GRILLED HERBED TOMATOES

4 medium tomatoes
¼ teaspoon ground pepper
2 teaspoons dried dillweed
1 teaspoon grated sapsago cheese or hoop cheese

Arrange the tomatoes in a baking pan. Cut a cross into
the top of each tomato. Sprinkle the insides with pepper,
dillweed, and cheese. Place the tomatoes under the broiler
for 8 to 10 minutes, or until the tomatoes are heated
through. Do not, however, overcook them, otherwise they
will lose their shape.

*Serves 4*

## SCALLOPED POTATOES

5 large potatoes
1 onion, thinly sliced
¼ teaspoon ground nutmeg
⅛ teaspoon ground pepper
1 cup evaporated skim milk

Peel the potatoes and slice them paper thin. Layer the potatoes and the onions in a nonstick baking pan, sprinkling lightly with the nutmeg and the pepper as you layer. Pour the evaporated skim milk over them and bake the potatoes in a 350 degree oven for 45 minutes, or until they are tender; add extra skim milk if necessary.

*Serves 6*

## BAKED STUFFED POTATOES

3 whole potatoes
⅓ cup chopped onions, water-sautéed
1 egg white, stiffly beaten
1 cup nonfat buttermilk (see Index)
⅛–¼ teaspoon prepared mustard
½–1½ teaspoons dried or fresh parsley
⅛–¼ teaspoon dillweed
½ teaspoon onion powder
½ teaspoon garlic powder
¼ teaspoon horseradish (optional)
1 tablespoon grated sapsago cheese
¼–½ teaspoon paprika

Wash the potatoes thoroughly and bake them in a 350 degree oven for 1 to 1½ hours, or until tender. Cut the potatoes in half lengthwise and scoop out the insides with a spoon. Save the skins for stuffing. Whip the potatoes with the mustard, other seasonings, and buttermilk. Fold in the egg whites last. Using a cookie press or spoon, stuff the potato skins with the mashed potatoes and lay them out in nonstick baking pans. Sprinkle them with paprika and parsley and bake in a 350 degree oven until hot and browned.

*Serves 6*

## SWEET POTATO PUFF

2½  cups cooked, mashed sweet potatoes
 ¼  cup orange juice
 ¼  teaspoon ground ginger
 ⅛  teaspoon ground nutmeg
 2  egg whites

Add the orange juice, ginger, and nutmeg to the hot cooked and mashed sweet potatoes. Beat the egg whites until stiff peaks form and fold them through the sweet-potato mixture. Spoon the potatoes into a nonstick baking dish and bake in a 350 degree oven for 30 minutes.
*Serves 4 to 6*


# *SALADS AND DRESSINGS*


## ROMAINE SALAD WITH LEMON-MUSTARD DRESSING

 1  head crisp romaine lettuce
 1  small red onion, thinly sliced
 ¼  cup tarragon vinegar
 2  tablespoons lemon juice
 2  tablespoons water
 ¼  teaspoon dry mustard
    Dash of pepper

Tear the lettuce into pieces and place in a salad bowl. Add the sliced red onion. Combine the vinegar, lemon juice, water, mustard, and pepper; mix the dressing vigorously just before pouring it on the salad. Toss and serve.
*Serves 4 to 6*

## BIBB AND RED PEPPER SALAD

1 head Bibb lettuce
1 sweet red pepper
½ cup tomato juice
2 tablespoons nonfat yogurt (see Index for Yogurt)
1 tablespoon lemon juice
¼ teaspoon garlic powder

Wash, dry, and tear the lettuce into pieces and place in a salad bowl. Remove the seeds from the pepper and cut it into long strips. Pour the tomato juice, yogurt, lemon juice, and garlic into an electric blender and process until it is smooth. Use as a salad dressing.

*Serves 4 to 6*

## ARUGULA SALAD

1 head iceberg lettuce, torn up
1 bunch arugula, trimmed
½ cup cider vinegar
¼ cup water
¼ teaspoon garlic powder
⅛ teaspoon dry mustard
1 teaspoon undiluted frozen apple juice concentrate, thawed

Combine the lettuce and the arugula. Shake together the cider vinegar, water, garlic powder, mustard, and apple juice; pour the dressing over the salad and toss.

*Note:* If it is difficult to find arugula in your local store, look for it in an Italian vegetable market.

*Serves 6*

## ORANGE AND WATERCRESS SALAD

2 oranges, peeled and sliced in rounds
1 small bunch watercress, washed and trimmed
½ cup thin Mock Sour Cream (see Index)
2 teaspoons lemon juice
½ teaspoon dried dillweed

Arrange the orange slices and the watercress attractively on each of 4 plates. Combine the Mock Sour Cream, lemon juice, and dillweed; serve as a dressing for the salad.

*Serves 4*

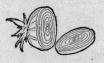

## DILLED TOMATOES AND ONIONS

2 large tomatoes, thickly sliced
1 large Bermuda onion, thinly sliced
2 tablespoons chopped fresh dill
  Wine vinegar, to taste

Arrange a platter of the sliced tomatoes and the onions. Sprinkle the fresh dill over the tomato slices.

Serve with a cruet of fine wine vinegar to be used sparingly.

*Serves 4*

## SPINACH AND MUSHROOM SALAD

1 pound fresh spinach
¼ pound fresh mushrooms
1 hard-boiled egg white
¼ cup tarragon vinegar
2 tablespoons water
⅛ teaspoon ground pepper
⅛ teaspoon ground paprika
1 tablespoon undiluted frozen orange juice concentrate, thawed

Trim and wash the spinach carefully and place in a salad bowl. Wash and slice the mushrooms; add them to the spinach. Discard the yolk of the egg, and chop the white; add it to the spinach. Combine the vinegar, water,

pepper, paprika, and orange juice; pour the dressing over
the salad. Toss and serve.
*Serves 4 to 6*

## CUCUMBER ONION SALAD

 1 large cucumber, peeled and thinly sliced
 1 large onion, thinly sliced
 ½ cup white vinegar
 ¼ cup water
 1 tablespoon chopped fresh dill
 1 tablespoon undiluted frozen apple juice concentrate,
      thawed
 ¼ teaspoon pepper

Combine the cucumber and the onion in a small, deep
bowl. Combine the vinegar, water, dill, apple juice, and
pepper; mix well and pour over the cucumbers. Cover
and store the salad in the refrigerator for at least 1 day,
stirring occasionally.
*Serves 4*

## BULGUR WHEAT SALAD (TABOULI)

 1 cup bulgur wheat
 1 cup finely chopped parsley
 ½ cup finely chopped green onions, or more, if desired
 1 pound tomatoes, coarsely chopped
 1 cup finely chopped fresh mint (optional, but very de-
      sirable)
 ⅓ cup lemon juice, or more, if desired
 ¼ teaspoon ground black pepper
   Lettuce (romaine preferred), for garnish

Cover bulgur wheat with boiling water and let soak for
2 hours. Drain well. Add remaining ingredients and mix
well. Let stand for several hours or overnight in refrigerator so that flavors blend.

Serve in a bowl surrounded with romaine lettuce leaves.
The romaine is used to scoop up the tabouli for eating.
*Serves 4*

# FRUITS AND DESSERTS

## ORANGE BASKETS

4 oranges
1 banana, sliced
1 apple, diced
½ cup seedless grapes

Cut the oranges in half. With a grapefruit knife, remove the fruit from the rind, leaving the rind intact. Slice ¼ inch from the cut side of the rind on each side toward the center without severing the portion in the center. Pull both ends of the slices toward the middle and tie with a small piece of ribbon, creating a basket. Cut the orange segments into a bowl. Add the banana, apple, and grapes; mix well. Fill the baskets with this mixture.

Garnish with a sprig of mint, if desired. Chill and serve.
*Serves 8*

## STRAWBERRY-FILLED MELON

2 small cantaloupes
1 pint fresh strawberries

Cut the melons into halves and remove the seeds. Scallop the edges by making zig-zag slices with a sharp knife. Scoop out melon balls. Wash and hull the strawberries and mix with the melon balls and return to the melon halves. Cut a small slice from the bottom of each melon if it does not stand upright. Chill and serve.
*Serves 4*

## PEARS IN APRICOT SAUCE

1 28-ounce can pear halves, water-packed
1 8-ounce can apricot halves, water-packed
1 tablespoon undiluted frozen apple juice concentrate, thawed
1 tablespoon Grape Nuts cereal

Drain the pears and arrange several halves, cut-side up, attractively in a shallow dessert bowl. Purée the apricot halves and the apple juice together in an electric blender. Pour the apricot sauce over the pear cavities. Top with a sprinkling of Grape Nuts cereal. Chill and serve.
*Serves 8*


## PINEAPPLE FRUIT BOATS

1 large ripe pineapple
1 cantaloupe melon

Cut the pineapple in half lengthwise, then cut each half in thirds lengthwise. Slide a knife between the rind and the pineapple flesh on all pieces, then cut the flesh into thick slices. Push every other slice half off the rind, creating a checkerboard effect. Scoop the melon into round balls, and place a melon ball in each of the open places on the rind. Chill and serve.
*Serves 6*


## KADOTA FIGS AND GRAPES

1 1-pound can kadota figs, water-packed
1 cup white seedless grapes

Combine the figs and the grapes in a small compote dish. Chill and serve.
*Serves 6*


## BROILED GRAPEFRUIT

1 grapefruit
2 tablespoons undiluted frozen apple juice concentrate, thawed
⅛ teaspoon cinnamon

Cut the grapefruit in half and use a grapefruit knife to loosen the segments. Spread the apple juice on the grapefruit and sprinkle lightly with the cinnamon. Broil the

grapefruit for several minutes, or until the top is lightly browned.
*Serves 2*

## ORANGE FLIP

1 cup unsweetened cranberry juice
1 quart fresh or frozen orange juice
2 cups unsweetened pineapple juice
¼ cup lemon juice
1 quart sparkling mineral water

Combine the juices and chill. Add mineral water and ice, if desired, just before serving.
*Serves 8-10*

## APRICOT COOLER

1 quart fresh or frozen orange juice
3 cups unsweetened apricot juice
1 quart sparkling mineral water

Combine the juices and chill. Add mineral water and ice, if desired, just before serving.
*Serves 8-12*

## CROSTATA di FRUTTA

1 cup Grape Nuts cereal
3 tablespoons frozen apple juice concentrate, thawed
¼ teaspoon ground cinnamon
1 tablespoon unflavored gelatin
½ cup pineapple juice
1½ cups plain nonfat yogurt (see Index for Yogurt)
½ teaspoon vanilla extract
1 pint fresh strawberries
1 1-pound can sliced peaches, water-packed, drained
1 tablespoon cornstarch
½ cup undiluted frozen apple juice concentrate, thawed
½ cup water

Moisten the cereal with 3 tablespoons apple juice concentrate (or a little more, if needed) and pat the cereal into a thin layer in a 10-inch nonstick pie pan. Sprinkle with cinnamon. Chill. Combine the gelatin and the pineapple juice; cook and stir over low heat until the gelatin is completely dissolved. Stir the gelatin mixture into the yogurt and the vanilla, mixing well. Spread this over the chilled crust and chill again until firm. Wash and hull the strawberries; dry well. Arrange a ring of strawberries around the rim of the pie pan over the filling. Arrange drained peaches like spokes in a wheel. Place a large strawberry in the center. (The entire surface of the filling should be covered by fruit, except for small gaps.) Combine the cornstarch, the remaining apple concentrate, and water in a saucepan; cook and stir until the mixture thickens and then clears. Spoon or brush this mixture over the fruit and the gaps. Chill.

*Serves 6 to 8*

## PUMPKIN MOUSSE PIE

 1 cup canned pumpkin
½ cup evaporated skim milk
½ teaspoon ground cinnamon
¼ teaspoon ground nutmeg
⅛ teaspoon ground ginger
 1 teaspoon vanilla extract
 1 envelope unflavored gelatin
½ cup boiling water
¼ cup undiluted frozen apple juice concentrate, thawed
 3 egg whites

Combine the pumpkin, skim milk, cinnamon, nutmeg, ginger, and vanilla. Stir the gelatin into boiling water until it is dissolved, then add the apple juice, stirring well. Pour this mixture into the pumpkin mixture and chill for 20 minutes. Beat the egg whites until stiff peaks form; fold them into the pumpkin mixture. Mound the filling into a pie pan and chill until it is firm.

*Serves 6 to 8*

## FRENCH APPLE TART

1 cup Grape Nuts cereal
3 tablespoons undiluted frozen apple juice concentrate, thawed
3 medium apples, peeled, cored, and thinly sliced
2 teaspoons lemon juice
  Cinnamon
1 tablespoon cornstarch
½ cup undiluted frozen apple juice concentrate, thawed
½ cup water

Moisten the cereal with 3 tablespoons apple juice concentrate (or a little more, if needed) and pat the cereal into a thin layer in a nonstick lined tart pan. Sprinkle with ¼ teaspoon cinnamon. Arrange the prepared apples in slightly overlapping circles, starting at the outside rim and working toward the center. Sprinkle them with lemon juice and ¼ teaspoon cinnamon. Cover with foil and bake in a 350 degree oven for 45 minutes, or until the apples are tender. Remove the tart from oven and cool it to room temperature. Combine the cornstarch, apple juice concentrate, and water in a saucepan; cook and stir until the mixture thickens and then clears. Spoon or brush this mixture over the apples. Chill.

*Serves 6 to 8*

## PEACH MELBA

1 pint nonfat yogurt (see Index for Yogurt)
1 teaspoon vanilla extract
1 cup fresh black or red raspberries, or frozen, without sugar
1 tablespoon undiluted frozen apple juice concentrate, thawed
6 canned peach halves, water-packed drained

Combine the yogurt and the vanilla. Purée the raspberries in an electric blender; add ¼ cup of the purée to the yogurt, mixing well. Freeze the yogurt mixture for several hours. Add the apple juice concentrate to the re-

maining purée and process it again until it is smooth.
Chill the peaches until they are ready to serve. When
chilled, place a peach half in each of 6 dessert compotes.
Top with a scoop of frozen yogurt. Spoon the raspberry
sauce over all.

*Serves 4*

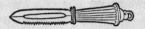

## APPLESAUCE SOUFFLÉ

```
    1  cup unsweetened pineapple juice
    2  envelopes unflavored gelatin
    1  cup skim milk
    1  tablespoon cornstarch
    1  teaspoon almond extract
 1½  cups applesauce, unsweetened
    2  egg whites
       Carob curls (optional)
```

Pour the pineapple juice into a small saucepan and stir
in the gelatin, mixing until dissolved. Heat this to the
boiling point, stirring constantly. Cool. Meanwhile, combine the milk, cornstarch, and almond extract in another
saucepan; cook and stir until the mixture comes to a boil
and is thickened. Stir the applesauce into the milk mixture. Add the gelatin mixture. Chill for 1 hour. Then beat
the egg whites until stiff peaks form; fold them carefully
into the applesauce mixture, taking care not to break the
bubbles of the whites. Spoon all into a soufflé dish that
has a 2-inch wax paper extension around the top of the
dish. Chill for several hours. Remove the wax paper. With
a vegetable parer, shave pure carob curls on top, if
desired.

*Serves 6 to 8*

## MANDARIN ORANGE PARFAITS

1 envelope unflavored gelatin
1 6-ounce can frozen orange juice, thawed
2 egg whites
1 teaspoon vanilla extract
½ cup nonfat dry milk
½ cup ice water
1 6-ounce can Mandarin oranges, water-packed, drained

In a saucepan, sprinkle the gelatin in ½ cup of cold water. Place over low heat; stir constantly, until the gelatin dissolves. Remove from heat. Add the undiluted orange juice and stir until it is melted. Chill, stirring occasionally, until the mixture thickens and mounds slightly when dropped from a spoon. Beat the egg whites until stiff peaks form; add the vanilla and beat in. Fold this into the orange mixture. Combine the dry-milk powder and ice water; beat them together until firm peaks form. Fold this into the orange mixture.

To serve, spoon the dessert into 8 parfait glasses. Top with drained Mandarin oranges and a sprig of fresh mint, if desired.

*Serves 8*

## FRUIT SALAD ALASKA

1 fresh apple, diced
1 16-ounce can pineapple chunks, water-packed or packed in its natural juice
1 orange, peeled and diced
4 tablespoons undiluted frozen pineapple juice concentrate, thawed
2 egg whites
⅛ teaspoon cream of tartar
½ teaspoon vanilla extract

Combine the apple, pineapple, orange, and pineapple juice; mix well to coat the fruits with the juice. Spoon the fruit into 4 individual soufflé baking dishes. Beat the egg whites until soft peaks form; add the cream of tartar and

continue beating until stiff peaks form. Add the vanilla.
Swirl the egg whites on top of the fruit salad, heaping it
thick and spreading it to the edge of the dishes. Place in a
preheated 450 degree oven for 4 to 5 minutes, or until the
meringue is lightly browned.

*Serves 4*

# 28

## Recipes for the Family Cook

*Holiday Dinner*

Barley Vegetable Soup
Fruited Turkey Roll
Sweet Potato-Squash Soufflé
Bean and Tomato Stew
Hearts of Lettuce Salad
Apple Bundt Cake

*Buffet Luncheon or Supper*

Curried Salmon-Rice Loaf
Broccoli-Noodle Casserole
Spicy Zucchini
Carrot Pudding
Tossed Salad with Yogurt Cheese Dressing
Lemon Pudding

*Saturday Breakfast*

Sliced Orange
Banana French Toast
Fruit Topping
Beverage

## BREAKFAST RECIPES

### HOMEMADE DRY CEREAL

2 cups "old-fashioned" rolled oats
1 cup rye flakes, available at health-food stores, or use an
    additional cup of oats
  Cinnamon, to taste
  Mace (optional)

Place the oats and the rye flakes in a colander. Pour water over them to dampen; drain well. Lay out in a thin layer in a shallow baking pan or on a cookie sheet. Place in a preheated 325 degree oven to toast, stirring from time to time to avoid overbrowning. Toast for about 20 to 30 minutes. Sprinkle lightly with cinnamon and mace, if desired, for the last 5 minutes of toasting. Cool and store covered in a dry place.

*Note:* The finished cereal may be put up in small plastic sandwich bags to be carried on trips, to the office, etc. The cereal may be eaten out of the bag (like peanuts) or served in a bowl with either hot or cold milk and a topping of sliced fruit.

*Serves 2 to 3*

### ONION CHEESE OMELET

1 small onion, sliced
4 egg whites
2 tablespoons grated sapsago cheese
½ teaspoon dried dillweed
  Dash of pepper

In a nonstick pan, sauté the onion in a small amount of water until tender. Beat the egg whites until soft peaks form. Add the cooked onions, sapsago cheese, and dillweed. Pour this into a large nonstick skillet and cook over low heat until the bottom has browned. Flip the omelet and cook, covered, over a low heat until it is firm.

*Serves 2*

## BUTTERMILK-CHEESE WAFFLES

5  egg whites
3  cups nonfat buttermilk, (see Index)
3  tablespoons Mock Sour Cream (see Index)
3  cups unbleached all-purpose flour
2  teaspoons baking powder
2  teaspoons vanilla

Beat the egg whites until they are thick and frothy; add the remaining ingredients and mix well. Pour the batter (about ¾ cup per waffle) into a hot nonstick waffle iron. Cook until the waffles are browned on both sides. Serve with a fruit topping (see Index) if desired.

*Note:* If waffles stick to Teflon iron, use a light coating of vegetable spray for the first waffle only.

*Serves 6 to 8*


## BANANA FRENCH TOAST

 2  bananas
½  cup evaporated skim milk
 5  egg whites
 1  teaspoon vanilla extract
⅛  teaspoon ground allspice
    Dash of nutmeg
10  slices of sourdough bread

Peel and slice the bananas and put them into an electric blender. Add the milk, egg whites, vanilla, and spices. Blend until smooth. Turn the batter into a shallow dish. Cut the bread into halves and dip them into the banana batter, then cook the bread over a low heat in a nonstick pan or griddle.

*Serves 6 to 8*

## OATMEAL HOTCAKES

2 cups "old-fashioned" rolled oats
1 cup water
1 cup skim milk
2 tablespoons evaporated skim milk
1 tablespoon nonfat dry milk
¼ teaspoon baking powder
2 egg whites

Stir together the oats, water, milks, and baking powder; mix well. Beat the egg whites until they are frothy and add to the mixture. Drop the batter by spoonfuls on a nonstick griddle and fry. When browned on one side, turn and brown the other side.

*Note:* Serve with a selection of fruit toppings (see Index).

*Serves 8*

## GRANOLA

2½ cups "old-fashioned" rolled oats
2 cups Grape Nuts cereal
½ cup rice flour
½ cup nonfat dry milk
1 teaspoon cinnamon
3 large apples, grated
2 to 3 tablespoons undiluted frozen apple juice concentrate, thawed
1 teaspoon vanilla extract

Combine all the ingredients. Put the mixture on a flat nonstick pan, spreading it evenly into a thin layer. Bake at 275 degrees for about 45 minutes, or until the mixture is dry and rather crumbly. Store in an air-tight container.

*Makes about 6 cups*

## POLENTA

1 onion, chopped
½ cup celery, diced
1 clove garlic, chopped
1 quart water
1 cup yellow cornmeal
2 to 3 tablespoons grated sapsago cheese

In a skillet, sauté the onion, celery, and garlic in a small amount of water until slightly browned. Boil the water and slowly add the corn meal, stirring constantly to avoid lumps. When mixed and smooth, put the vegetable-and-cornmeal mixture into the top of a double boiler. Cook, covered, for 30 minutes, or until thick. Pour the mixture into a nonstick 10-by-14-inch baking pan and let cool. When cool, cut the polenta into 2-inch squares and sprinkle with sapsago cheese. Bake for 20 minutes in a 400 degree oven to brown the top.

*Note:* Serve with spaghetti sauce (see Index for Our Favorite Spaghetti Sauce).

*Makes about 36 squares*


## OATMEAL WITH STEWED APPLES

2 cups "old-fashioned" rolled oats
2 cups boiling water
1 apple, thinly sliced
¼ teaspoon ground cinnamon
Skim milk

Stir the oats into boiling water in the top of a double boiler; cook and stir for several minutes. Add the apples and the cinnamon. Cook 10 minutes, mixing occasionally.

Serve hot with skim milk.

*Serves 4*

## SOUPS

### SPLIT PEA SOUP

- 2 cups dried split peas
- 2 quarts water
- 1 onion, finely diced
- 2 whole carrots, scraped
- 2 sprigs parsley, diced
- 2 celery stalks
- ¼ teaspoon pepper
- 1 bay leaf

Soak the peas in water overnight. Drain. Place them in a large soup pot with water; add the remaining ingredients. Bring to a boil, then reduce heat, and cover. Simmer for 2 hours, or until the peas have disintegrated. Rub all the soup through a food mill into another pot. Discard the bay leaf. Add extra pepper, if desired.
*Serves 8*

### LENTIL SOUP

- ½ cup garbanzo beans, dried
- 2 bay leaves
- ¾ cup chopped onion
- ¾ cup chopped celery
- ¾ cup diced carrots
- ¾ cup lentils, dried
- ¼ cup brown rice
- ½ cup blended canned tomatoes
- 2 tablespoons lemon juice
- 1 tablespoon vinegar
- 2 tablespoons unsweetened apple juice
- 1 teaspoon basil
- 1 garlic clove, minced
  Black pepper to taste
- 6 cups water or more, if necessary

Soak garbanzo beans overnight or for several hours in enough water to cover. Drain, cover again with water, add the bay leaves and cook for an hour and a half. When the beans are half-done, add the vegetables, lentils, rice, and other seasonings. Cook until tender.

*Serves 8*

## CABBAGE SOUP

   4  beef neck bones
   1  28-ounce can tomatoes
   4  cups water
  ½  small cabbage head, shredded
   1  onion, thinly sliced
   1  apple, peeled and diced
   3  tablespoons lemon juice
  ¼  teaspoon ground ginger
  ¼  teaspoon garlic powder

Place the bones, tomatoes, water, cabbage, onion, and apple in a deep soup pot. Add the lemon juice, ginger, and garlic powder. Simmer for 2 hours, covered. Skim the fat off the surface occasionally. Cut a small amount of meat from the bones into the soup.

*Note:* To remove all the fat, chill and discard the solidified top layer of fat before reheating to serve.

*Serves 6*

## LIMA BEAN SOUP

1½  cups dried lima beans
1½  cups chopped celery
1½  cups chopped carrots
1½  cups chopped onions
 ½  cup finely chopped green pepper
1½  cups green beans, cut into 2-inch lengths, or frozen or
      canned cut green beans
   2  to 3 tomatoes, chopped into small chunks, skin and
      all
      Water, as required
      Suggested seasonings: bay leaf, basil, black pepper,
      and vinegar to taste

Rinse and soak the beans overnight or for several hours

in enough water to cover. Drain. Re-cover them with water to about 3 inches above the surface of the beans. Add the bay leaf, and cook until the beans are tender. Replenish the water in the bean pot to about 3 inches above the bean surface. Add the celery, carrots, onions, green pepper, and green beans. (If frozen green beans are used, add them about 10 minutes later. Canned green beans should be added even later, when the other vegetables are almost tender.) Add more water as required to keep the soup at desired consistency and to prevent any sticking. Toward the end of the cooking period, when the vegetables are almost tender, add the seasonings and the chopped tomato. When all the vegetables are tender, remove about ⅓ of the soup and blend it in a blender. Return the blended portion to the original soup pot and mix well. Serve hot.

*Note:* You can also use 3 cups frozen lima beans instead of the dried. Simply cook the frozen beans for several minutes before adding the other ingredients.

*Serves 6 to 8*

## POTATO SOUP

    4 large peeled potatoes, diced
    1 onion, diced
    2 stalks celery, diced
    3 cups water
    2 cups skim milk
    ½ teaspoon dried dillweed
    ¼ teaspoon ground pepper
    2 tablespoons chopped chives

Place the potatoes, onion, celery, water, and milk in a saucepan. Add the dillweed and pepper. Simmer for 20 minutes or until the potatoes are soft. Ladle the soup into bowls and top with a sprinkling of chopped chives.

*Serves 6*

## EIGHT-BEAN SOUP

2 cups of dried mixed beans. Use 6–8 different kinds,
    choosing from split peas, lentils, garbanzos, kidney
    beans, pinto beans, lima beans, etc.
7 cups water, or more, if a thinner consistency is
    desired
1 cup canned or fresh tomatoes, chopped
1¼ cups chopped onion
½ cup chopped celery
½ cup chopped carrots
¼ cup chopped parsley
1 minced garlic clove
1 bay leaf
¼ teaspoon thyme
½ teaspoon each basil, thyme, and rosemary leaves
    Black pepper to taste, if desired

Rinse and soak the beans overnight or for several hours
in enough water to cover. Drain. Combine the drained
beans with the rest of the ingredients (except tomatoes)
and cook until all are tender, stirring occasionally and
adding more water, if needed. Add the tomatoes and
enough water to give the soup the desired consistency.
Heat thoroughly.
*Serves 4 to 6*

## CREAM OF CORN SOUP

2 cups cooked fresh or frozen corn niblets
2 cups skim milk
¼ teaspoon dried dillweed
⅛ teaspoon ground pepper

Put the corn in a blender or a food processor and
process it until creamy. Empty the purée into a saucepan;
add the milk, dillweed, and pepper. Stir well and heat for
several minutes.
*Note:* If you are puréeing the corn in a blender, you

may need to add some of the milk to help in the puréeing
process.
*Serves 4 to 6*


## BARLEY VEGETABLE SOUP

2 cups barley
6 cups water
2 cups chopped carrots
1 cup chopped onion
1 cup chopped rutabagas
2 cups chopped parsnips
1 16-ounce can tomatoes
2 tablespoons tomato paste
1 8-ounce can green beans, chopped, with juice
2–4 tablespoons vinegar
½ teaspoon dried marjoram
½ teaspoon celery seed
⅛ teaspoon garlic powder

In a large soup pot, cook the barley in water until done
but not mushy. Place half of the barley with a little of the
liquid in an electric blender and process until it is puréed;
return the purée to the soup pot. Add the carrots, onion,
rutabagas, and parsnips; cook until the vegetables are partially tender. Add the tomatoes, tomato paste, green
beans, vinegar, marjoram, celery seed, and garlic powder.
Add additional water, if necessary. Simmer, covered, for 1
hour.
*Serves 6 to 8*


## SOUTHERN VEGETABLE SOUP

1 medium turnip, diced
1 small rutabaga, diced
1 onion, diced
1 carrot, scraped and diced
¼ head cabbage, shredded
½ 10-ounce package frozen chopped broccoli
½ 10-ounce package frozen cauliflower

1 large tomato, chopped
1 small zucchini, diced
¼ cup fresh mustard greens, chopped (optional)
2 quarts water
¼ teaspoon oregano
¼ teaspoon marjoram
¼ teaspoon basil
1 tablespoon grated sapsago cheese

Place the turnip, rutabaga, onion, and carrot in a deep soup pot with a small amount of water to cover. Simmer, covered, until the vegetables are partially tender. Then add all the remaining ingredients, except the sapsago cheese. Simmer, covered, gently for 40 minutes. Add the cheese about 15 minutes before the soup is done.

*Serves 8 to 10*

## CHICKEN SOUP

1 soup chicken, about 4 pounds
2 quarts water
1 whole onion, peeled
2 whole carrots, scraped
4 stalks celery, including tops
1 parsnip root, cleaned
2 sprigs parsley
2 sprigs fresh dill
¼ teaspoon ground pepper

Clean the chicken and place it in a deep soup pot. Add water and the remaining ingredients. Bring to a boil, then simmer, covered, until the chicken is tender, about 2 hours. Remove the chicken, strain the soup, and chill. Skim off the fat that rises to the top of the chilled soup.

Serve with cut-up pieces of carrot and, if desired, cut-up pieces of cooked chicken. The soup may be frozen.
*Serves 8*

## MATZO BALLS

4  egg whites
½  cup matzo meal
2  teaspoons dried minced onions
½  teaspoon cinnamon
1  teaspoon dried parsley
¼  teaspoon white pepper
   Mixture of a little oil and water to lubricate hands

Beat the egg whites until stiff. Fold in the mixture of matzo meal and seasonings; let the mixture stand for 15 minutes. Mix a little oil and water to lubricate hands for forming balls. Form balls slightly larger than walnuts. Drop balls gently into boiling salted water. Cover pot. Let simmer for 30 minutes. Remove from fire and let stand for 30 minutes. Uncover and remove the balls from the water with a slotted spoon. When ready to serve, add the matzo balls to soup and heat.
*Makes about 10 medium-sized matzo balls*

## *MEAT, POULTRY, AND FISH*

### STUFFED CABBAGE

1  large leafy head cabbage
2  pounds very lean ground beef
1  onion, grated
1  apple, grated
1  cup water
2  cups cooked rice
¼  teaspoon ground pepper
1  28-ounce can tomatoes
2  tablespoons tomato paste
2  teaspoons vinegar

Juice of 1 lemon
1   onion, sliced
1   apple, diced
¼   teaspoon ground ginger

Parboil the cabbage. Cut around the core, and carefully remove the leaves one by one. Level the knife against outer side of each leaf and remove the excess of the heavy center without cutting into the leaf. Combine ground beef, grated onion, grated apple, water, rice, and pepper; mix well. Place about 2 tablespoons of the mixture in the center near the bottom of each cabbage leaf; fold the bottom up, fold over each side, and roll up. Cut up extra cabbage leaves and place them in the bottom of a deep pot. Add the tomatoes, tomato paste, vinegar, lemon juice, sliced onion, diced apple, and ginger. Add the cabbage rolls, seam-side down. Simmer, covered, for 2 hours.
*Serves 12*

## EGGPLANT PARMIGIANA

½   pound very lean ground beef
½   teaspoon onion powder
¼   teaspoon garlic powder
1   28-ounce can tomatoes
1   6-ounce can tomato paste
½   teaspoon dried oregano
1   teaspoon dried basil
1   large firm eggplant
¼   cup grated sapsago cheese

Using a nonstick skillet, cook the ground beef while breaking with a fork. Sprinkle the beef with onion powder and garlic powder; stir well. Add the tomatoes, tomato paste, oregano, and basil; cook, covered, for 15 minutes. Meanwhile, peel the eggplant and slice it into ¼-inch-thick slices. Spread a layer of the sauce to cover the bottom of an 8-by-12-inch baking pan. Top with a layer of eggplant arranged side by side. Top with the sauce and continue layering, ending with the sauce. Sprinkle with the grated

cheese. Bake in a 350 degree oven for 45 minutes, or until the eggplant is tender.
*Serves 6*


## "LITTLE BEEF" BURGERS

½  cup roasted whole buckwheat groats
6  ounces fat-trimmed flank steak, ground
2  tablespoons beet juice from cooked or canned beets
1  tablespoon dry wine
1  teaspoon soy sauce (salt-reduced variety)
1½ cups chopped onions
⅔  cup chopped mushrooms
2  tablespoons minced shallots (optional)
1  teaspoon finely minced garlic
¼  teaspoon garlic powder
¼  teaspoon ground black pepper
½  cup whole wheat pastry flour
2  egg whites

SAUCE
2  15-ounce cans tomato sauce
1  10-ounce can enchilada sauce
¼  cup prepared mustard
1  tablespoon undiluted frozen apple juice concentrate, thawed
½  teaspoon ground ginger
½  teaspoon garlic powder
½  teaspoon onion powder

Bring 1 cup water to a boil. Add the buckwheat and cook covered about 10 minutes. Turn off heat and let buckwheat steam, covered, another 10 minutes or longer. Fluff buckwheat with a fork and place 1 measured cupful into a large mixing bowl. (Freeze the extra cooked buckwheat for use the next time you make this recipe.)

In a nonstick skillet, brown the meat over moderate heat until the pinkness is gone. Pour off rendered fat, if any. Add beet juice, wine and soy sauce and heat until liquid simmers. Add onions, mushrooms, shallots, garlic and spices to the skillet. Sauté until the liquid evaporates and the vegetable-meat mixture is brown. Stir the sautéed mixture into the cooked buckwheat. Sprinkle in the flour and mix well. Beat the egg whites to soft peaks and fold them into the mixture. Shape into 6 or more patties and lay them on a nonstick baking sheet. Bake in a preheated 400 degree oven for 20 minutes, lightly covered with aluminum foil. Remove foil and bake another 10 minutes to brown tops.

*Sauce:* Combine all the ingredients in a saucepan and heat to blend the flavors. Serve hot over the patties, and freeze any extra sauce for the next batch.

*Makes 6 or more patties; 6 cups sauce.*


## FLOUNDER FLORENTINE ROLLS

4 thin slices fillet of flounder
1 10-ounce package frozen chopped spinach, thawed
¼ cup thinly sliced scallions
¼ teaspoon ground nutmeg
⅛ teaspoon ground paprika
¼ cup dry white wine or water
2 tablespoons lemon juice
1 tablespoon chopped fresh dill

Spread the flounder slices flat. Combine the thawed spinach, scallions, and nutmeg; spread the spinach mixture in a thin layer over each of the fillet slices. Roll up and fasten with toothpicks. Place the fillets in a small nonstick baking dish, just large enough to hold the fillets. Sprinkle the fish with paprika. Pour the wine and the lemon juice around the fish. Sprinkle the chopped dill over all. Bake in a 350 degree oven for 25 minutes, or until the fish flakes easily when tested with a fork.

*Serves 4*

## BAKED HADDOCK AND VEGETABLES

2   pounds haddock fillets
¼   teaspoon ground pepper
1   onion, grated
1   green pepper, diced
1   1-pound can whole tomatoes
1   bay leaf
1   carrot, scraped and thinly sliced
½   lemon, thinly sliced

Arrange the fillets in a flat nonstick baking pan. Sprinkle with pepper. Scatter the onion and the green pepper around the fillets. Break up the tomatoes with a fork and spread them in a thin layer over the fillets. Add the bay leaf and the carrot slices. Arrange thin slices of lemon over the fillets. Bake in a 350 degree oven for 25 minutes, or until the fish flakes easily when tested with a fork.
*Serves 8*

## CURRIED SALMON-RICE LOAF

1   7¾-ounce can salmon
3   cups cooked rice
⅓   cup chopped scallions
2   teaspoons curry powder
3   teaspoons lemon juice
3   tablespoons cider vinegar
1   teaspoon garlic powder
    Tomatoes, to garnish

Flake the salmon, removing any skin and bones, and add the salmon with its liquid* to the cooked rice. Add the scallions, curry, lemon juice, vinegar, and garlic powder. Pack the mixture into a small loaf pan lined with plastic wrap. Refrigerate for several hours. When ready to serve, unmold the salmon and arrange it on lettuce leaves. Garnish with sliced fresh tomatoes, if desired.
*Serves 6*

*Strain the salmon through cheesecloth to remove fat.

## CHICKEN IN THE POT

2  broiler chickens, about 3 pounds each
1  onion, thinly sliced
2  large sprigs fresh dill
1  sprig fresh parsley
2  tomatoes, peeled and diced
4  carrots, scraped, cut into chunks
4  celery stalks, cut into chunks
4  potatoes, peeled and quartered
1  cup dry white wine, or fat-free chicken broth
2  tablespoons lemon juice
1  bay leaf
¼  teaspoon ground pepper

Place the chickens in a Dutch oven. Add the onion, dill and parsley. Arrange the tomatoes, carrots, celery, and potatoes around the chickens. Add the wine, or the broth, lemon juice, bay leaf, and pepper. Cover tightly and bake in a 350 degree oven for 1½ hours, or until the chickens are tender.

*Note:* To remove the fat, chill the chicken and remove the layer of solidified fat on top. Do not eat the skin.

*Serves 12*

## OVEN-FRIED CHICKEN

6  large halved chicken breasts

BREADING
½  cup cornmeal
½  cup matzo meal
4  teaspoons whole wheat pastry flour
1  teaspoon onion powder
¾  teaspoon garlic powder
½  teaspoon paprika
½  teaspoon poultry seasoning
¼  teaspoon black pepper
2  tablespoons grated sapsago cheese

## EGG-WHITE MIXTURE DIP
 2 egg whites
 ½ cup skim milk or blend of skim and evaporated
  skim milk

## HERBED-CHICKEN MARINADE
 3 cups Tillie Lewis Italian dressing or 1 cup each of
  tomato juice, water, and wine vinegar
 ⅓ cup lemon juice
 ⅓ cup soy sauce (salt-reduced variety)
 ¾ teaspoon garlic powder
 ¾ teaspoon powdered thyme
 ¾ teaspoon Italian seasoning
 ¾ teaspoon poultry seasoning
 1½ teaspoons rosemary
 ½ teaspoon powdered oregano
 ¾ teaspoon curry powder

## TERIYAKI MARINADE
 1½ cups soy sauce (salt-reduced variety)
 1½ cups lemon juice
 2½ cups unsweetened pineapple juice
 1 tablespoon powdered ginger
 1½ teaspoon garlic powder
 1 tablespoon sherry

Remove the skin and fat from the chicken and clean thoroughly. Cut each halved breast in half again. For either marinade recipe, soak the chicken pieces in the marinade overnight in the refrigerator, or at least for several hours. For the dip recipe, you need only to dip the chicken pieces in the liquid; coat well. To bread the chicken, remove the chicken pieces from whatever liquid you have used and cover with the breading mixture; coat well. Arrange the chicken pieces on a nonstick baking sheet and place in a preheated 350 degree oven for 1¼ hours or until tender. The chicken should be covered with aluminum foil except during the first and last 10 minutes of cooking.

*Makes 6 to 12 servings*

## FRUITED TURKEY ROLL

 1 frozen turkey roll, about 4 pounds
½ cup undiluted frozen pineapple-orange-juice concentrate, thawed
½ cup water
½ teaspoon dried thyme
 2 teaspoons cornstarch

Place the turkey roll in a roasting pan. Combine the juice, water, thyme, and cornstarch in a small saucepan; bring to a boil and stir constantly until the mixture thickens and clears. Spoon half the sauce over the turkey roll. Roast the turkey in a 350 degree oven for 1½ to 2 hours, or until tender. Baste the turkey frequently with the remaining sauce.
*Serves 16*

## TURKEY POT PIE

 6 whole-wheat pita breads
 1 cup finely chopped green pepper
1½ cups finely chopped celery
 1 cup finely chopped onions
¾ cup mushrooms, thinly sliced
1½ cups cooked breast of turkey, cubed
 3 cups fat-free turkey broth
 2 cups diced cooked potatoes
 1 cup nonfat dry milk
 1 tablespoon cornstarch mixed with 2 tablespoons water
½ teaspoon curry powder
½ teaspoon celery seed
 2 small cans water chestnuts, sliced
 2 10-ounce packages frozen carrots and peas, thawed

Cut the pita breads in half, making circles. Place one half of the breads brown-side down in each of 6 small pie pans. In a skillet, sauté the green pepper, celery, onion, and mushrooms in a small amount of water. Add the turkey, turkey broth, cooked potatoes, nonfat dry milk, cornstarch paste, curry, celery seed, sliced chestnuts, and carrots and peas. Stir well. Heat and stir until the gravy thickens. Divide the mixture among the 6 prepared pie pans. Top with the other half of the pita bread, brownside up. Bake in a 350 degree oven for 15 minutes, or until hot.

*Serves 6*

## MEATLESS MAIN DISHES

### OUR FAVORITE SPAGHETTI SAUCE

8 cups blended unpeeled and fresh tomatoes
4 cups chopped onion
4 cups chopped green pepper
4 cups sliced mushrooms
8 cups tomato sauce
3 to 4 garlic cloves, minced, or equivalent garlic powder
4 tablespoons basil
2 to 4 tablespoons wine vinegar

Combine all the ingredients, except the basil, in a large saucepan or skillet. Simmer about 1 hour. Add the basil and simmer 30 minutes longer.

*Serves 6*

### SPAGHETTI

1 pound whole-wheat spaghetti
2 gallons water

Fill a 3-gallon pot ⅔ full with water. Heat the water to a rolling boil. Break the spaghetti in half and drop it little by little into the boiling water. Stir to prevent sticking. Continue to boil the spaghetti, uncovered, for 15 to 20 minutes or less, depending on the desired texture. Drain and rinse the spaghetti in a large colander. Return the spaghetti to the pot and place it over a low heat. Spoon the hot sauce over the noodles; stir and serve.

*Serves 8 to 10*

## LASAGNE

### SAUCE

2 cups canned diced tomatoes (blended in blender)
1⅔ cups tomato purée
1⅔ cups tomato sauce
2 tablespoons lemon juice
2 tablespoons dried parsley
2 teaspoons garlic powder
1 teaspoon onion powder
1 teaspoon oregano
1 teaspoon Italian seasoning
1 teaspoon basil

### FILLING

7 large lasagne-type whole-wheat noodles
2⅔ cups uncreamed cottage cheese (hoop cheese preferred)
3 egg whites, stiffly beaten
⅔ cup nonfat buttermilk
¼ cup dried parsley
½ cup grated sapsago cheese

Combine the ingredients for the sauce and cook until the flavors blend, about 20 to 30 minutes. While the sauce is cooking, begin heating enough water in a large pot to cook the noodles in. Mash the hoop cheese and buttermilk together with a fork, adding the sapsago cheese and the parsley. Fold in the egg whites. Refrigerate the egg white mixture until the noodles and sauce are ready. Put the noodles in boiling water, bring to a boil again, and pour off the water when they are almost tender but still firm. (Whole-wheat noodles, unlike their refined counterparts, break easily. Don't be dismayed if they fragment as you work with them; just put the pieces together when layering the casserole and it will taste just as good!)

To layer the casserole, place a thin layer of sauce on the bottom of a large shallow baking dish. Place a layer of drained noodles over the sauce, then a layer of the cheese. Repeat the process until all the ingredients are used up. The top-most layer should be the sauce. Bake the lasagne in a 375 degree oven for 1 hour or until thoroughly cooked and brown on top. It can also be prebaked and reheated.

*Serves 10 to 12*

## KREPLACH

3　egg whites
1　cup regular whole-wheat flour
　Chicken broth, defatted, or water
　Ground seasoned chicken or turkey for filling, cooked

Mix the egg whites into the flour. Knead for several seconds. Roll out to a thin dough and score with a knife to form 2-by-2-inch squares. Place a dab of the filling (about ½ teaspoon) in the center of each square. Make into triangles by folding each square over and pinching edges to seal. Bring enough broth (or water) to a boil. Cook the kreplach squares at a gentle boil for 20 minutes.

Serve as a vegetable, appetizer, or in a soup.

*Note:* For vegetarian kreplach, use buckwheat with onions, or any other grain-vegetable combination—all cooked—as the filling.

*Serves 4*

## GARBANZO QUICHE

1　cup dried garbanzo beans
1　cup skim milk
3　egg whites
½　cup chopped green pepper
1　cup chopped onion
1　cup chopped celery
¾　teaspoon garlic
½　cup pimiento, rinsed, drained, and chopped

Soak the garbanzo beans overnight. Do *not* cook them. The next day, drain, then grind, the beans in a blender, adding the milk to facilitate blending. (The beans should be rather coarsely ground, as opposed to being made into a thick paste). In about ½ cup water, cook the pepper and celery until tender. Do not overcook. Pour off any remaining liquid. Beat the egg whites stiff. Add the cooked vegetables, raw onion, egg whites, and garlic powder to the blended beans and stir. Add pimiento. Pour the batter into a nonstick pan and bake in a 350 degree oven for 45 minutes.

*Serves 8*

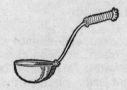

## APPLE NOODLE PUDDING

1 8-ounce package yolk-free wide noodles, cooked
3 apples, peeled and thinly sliced
2 tablespoons lemon juice
½ teaspoon ground cinnamon
1 cup hoop cheese or other uncreamed cottage cheese
2 tablespoons skim milk
1 tablespoon undiluted frozen apple juice concentrate, thawed
1 egg white

Combine the cooked noodles with the apples, which have been tossed with lemon juice and cinnamon. Mash the cheese with the skim milk and the apple juice concentrate. Beat the egg white lightly with a fork until it is frothy; add this to the cheese and whip well. Add the cheese mixture to the noodle-apple mixture; pour the noodle pudding into an 8-by-12-inch nonstick baking

dish. Bake in a 350 degree oven for 45 minutes, or until the apples are tender and the top is lightly browned.
*Serves 6*

## BROCCOLI-NOODLE CASSEROLE

1 8-ounce package yolk-free wide noodles, cooked and
    drained
2 10-ounce packages frozen chopped broccoli, cooked
2 cups hoop cheese or other uncreamed cottage cheese
¼ cup skim milk
1 egg white
1 teaspoon grated lemon rind
1 teaspoon dried dillweed

Combine the cooked and drained noodles with the chopped broccoli. Mash the hoop cheese with the milk. Beat the egg white with a fork until it is frothy; add it to the cheese. Add the lemon rind and the dillweed. Gently fold the cheese mixture through the noodle-broccoli mixture. Spoon it into an 8-by-12-inch nonstick baking pan. Bake in a 350 degree oven for 30 minutes.
*Serves 8*

## PASTA E FAGIOLI

1 cup dried kidney beans
½ cup dried lentils
1 small onion, chopped
1 stalk celery, chopped
½ clove garlic, minced
1 teaspoon dried parsley flakes
½ teaspoon dried basil
¼ teaspoon ground pepper
1 1-pound can tomatoes
2 tablespoons tomato paste
¼ cup grated sapsago cheese
1 cup yolk-free pasta bows, cooked

Combine the beans in a bowl and cover with water; soak overnight. Drain. In a skillet, sauté the onion, celery, and garlic in a small amount of water until the vegetables are tender. Add the vegetables to the beans. Add the parsley, basil, and pepper. Add the tomatoes and the tomato paste. Cook, covered, until the beans are tender, about 1 hour. Add the cooked pasta bows. Add the grated cheese. Serve hot.

*Serves 4 to 6*

## POTATO PUDDING

2½   cups grated raw potatoes
 ½   cup grated onion
 2   scraped carrots, grated
 ¼   teaspoon ground pepper
 ¼   teaspoon ground nutmeg
 1   tablespoon grated lemon rind
 ½   cup potato flour
 ¼   cup skim milk
 4   egg whites

Combine the grated potatoes, onion, and carrots. Add the pepper, nutmeg, and lemon rind. Stir in the potato flour. Stir in the skim milk. Beat the egg whites until stiff peaks form; fold the egg whites gently through the potato mixture. Pour all into an 8-by-12-inch nonstick baking pan and bake in a 350 degree oven for 45 minutes, or until lightly browned.

*Serves 6*

## CHEESE BLINTZES

CRÊPES
 1   cup whole-wheat pastry or unbleached all-purpose
     flour
1¼   cups skim milk
 4   egg whites

*FILLING*
  2 cups uncreamed cottage cheese
  ¼ cup skim milk
  1 egg white
  ½ teaspoon vanilla extract
  ¼ teaspoon cinnamon

*Crêpes:* Stir together the flour and the milk. Beat the egg whites lightly with a fork until foamy; add to the batter and mix well. Heat a small nonstick crêpe pan; pour several tablespoons of batter into the skillet and rotate the batter to distribute it evenly over the pan. Cook until the crêpe is lightly browned; turn out onto a clean surface and continue making crêpes, just browning one side, until all batter is used up.

*Filling:* Mash the cheese. Add the milk and mix well. Beat the egg white lightly with a fork until foamy; add to the cheese. Add the vanilla and the cinnamon. Fill each crêpe with about 2 tablespoons of the mixture, placing the filling on the center of the browned side of the crêpe and folding over the 2 opposite sides. Then roll up the remaining sides to enclose the filling in the crêpe. Place in a nonstick baking pan; bake in a 350 degree oven for 15 minutes, or until hot and lightly browned. Serve with Mock Sour Cream or a Fruit Topping (see Index) or applesauce, if desired.
    *Serves 8*


## CARROT PUDDING

  2 cups carrots, scraped and thinly sliced
  1 large onion, diced
  4 egg whites
  1 cup skim milk
  4 slices whole-wheat bread
  1 tablespoon grated orange rind
  ½ teaspoon ground cinnamon
  ¼ teaspoon ground allspice
  ⅛ teaspoon ground nutmeg

Steam the carrots and the onion until they are tender.
Meanwhile, beat the egg whites until stiff peaks form.
Pour the skim milk into an electric blender; add the
cooked carrots and the onions and process into a purée.
Tear up whole-wheat bread into tiny pieces; pour the
purée over the bread and mix lightly. Add the orange
rind, cinnamon, allspice, and nutmeg; mix lightly. Add
the beaten egg whites and fold through. Pour all into an
8-by-12-inch nonstick baking pan. Bake in a 350 degree
oven for 45 minutes, or until a knife inserted comes out
clean and the top is browned.
*Serves 6*

## BAKED STUFFED TOMATOES

4  large whole tomatoes
2  cups cooked rice
1  small onion, diced
½  green pepper, diced
1  tablespoon grated sapsago cheese

Scoop out the pulp of each tomato, leaving a whole
shell for stuffing. Chop the tomato pulp finely and place
in a skillet with several tablespoons of water. Add the onion and the green pepper; simmer over a low heat, stirring
occasionally until the vegetables are limp. Add the cooked
rice and mix through. Remove from the heat and spoon
the mixture into the tomato shells. Top with a sprinkling
of grated cheese. Bake the stuffed tomatoes in a 350
degree oven for 25 to 30 minutes.
*Serves 4*

## POTATO PANCAKES

2  pounds potatoes, peeled
1  onion
2  egg whites
2  tablespoons unbleached all-purpose flour
¼  teaspoon ground pepper

Grate the potatoes into a deep bowl. Grate the onions into the potatoes. Beat the egg whites lightly with a fork until they are frothy and stir them into the potatoes. Stir in the flour and the pepper, adding additional flour if necessary to firm up the batter. Drop the batter by large spoonfuls onto a nonstick griddle. When the pancakes are brown on one side, turn and brown the other side.

Serve with unsweetened applesauce and Mock Sour Cream (see Index).

*Serves 6*

# MAIN DISH VEGETABLES

## MIXED VEGETABLE STEW

      6 pearl onions, peeled
  2½ cups defatted chicken broth
      6 new potatoes
      6 small carrots, cut in half
      4 small leeks, chopped
      4 small zucchini, chopped
      4 stalks celery, chopped
      2 medium tomatoes, quartered
      1 head cauliflower, broken in florets
      2 teaspoons arrowroot
      2 tablespoons parsley flakes

Boil the onions gently in 1 cup water for 20 minutes. Add the remaining ingredients, except the arrowroot and the parsley flakes, and simmer until tender, about 1 hour. Thicken the stew with an arrowroot paste; add the parsley flakes, and serve.

*Makes 2½ quarts*

## LIMA-CORN BAKE

  1 10-ounce package frozen lima beans, thawed, or fresh
      lima beans
  1 10-ounce package frozen corn niblets, thawed, or fresh
      corn niblets

2 tomatoes, thinly sliced
1 small onion, thinly sliced
1 clove garlic, crushed
1 cup tomato juice

Place half of the lima beans in the bottom of a shallow nonstick baking dish. Top them with a layer of the corn. Then top the corn mixture with half the tomato slices and the onion and the garlic. Top with another layer of lima beans, corn, and end with the tomato slices. Pour tomato juice over all. Cover tightly and bake in a 350 degree oven for 40 minutes.
*Serves 4 to 6*

## BEAN AND TOMATO STEW

2 10-ounce packages frozen French-cut green beans, or fresh green beans
1 1-pound can tomatoes
1 small onion, sliced
¼ teaspoon dried basil
⅛ teaspoon ground pepper

Empty the green beans into a saucepan with the tomatoes, onion, basil, and pepper. Simmer, covered, for 15 minutes, or until the beans are tender, adding a small amount of water if needed.
*Serves 6 to 8*

## HAWAIIAN MIXED VEGETABLES

5 large mushrooms, sliced
½ cup green pepper, coarsely chopped
1 cup onion, diced
1 cup unsweetened pineapple chunks, with juice
4 large carrots, diagonally sliced
⅛ teaspoon basil
¼ teaspoon ground ginger
⅛ teaspoon curry powder
1 cup water chestnuts, drained and sliced

Heat a few tablespoons of water in a nonstick skillet, add the mushrooms and water-sauté until golden. Add the green pepper and sauté 3 minutes. Remove the mushrooms and green pepper and set aside. In the same skillet, add the onions and cook until golden. Drain the pineapple, reserving juice. Add the unsweetened pineapple juice, carrots, basil, ginger, and curry powder to the onions in the skillet, and simmer 35 minutes or until carrots are tender. Add the cooked mushrooms, green pepper, pineapple chunks, and water chestnuts and cook 5 minutes longer.

*Serves 4*

## CARROT FRUIT CASSEROLE

1  1-pound can whole baby carrots, drained
1  8-ounce can pineapple tidbits, water-packed, drained
1  1-pound can unsweetened applesauce
2  teaspoons lemon juice
½  teaspoon ground cinnamon
¼  teaspoon ground ginger

Combine all the ingredients together in a nonstick baking dish. Bake in a 350 degree oven for 20 minutes, or until the casserole is heated through.

*Serves 6 to 8*

## STEAMED EGGPLANT WEDGES

1  medium eggplant
¼  cup lemon juice
¼  teaspoon ground pepper

Peel the eggplant and cut it in half lengthwise. Cut each half in quarters lengthwise. Brush each piece with lemon juice and dust lightly with pepper. Place in a steamer over boiling water and cover tightly. Steam for 20 minutes, or until tender.

Serve with hot tomato sauce, if desired.

*Serves 8*

## CARROT RING

3 cups unbleached all-purpose flour
1½ teaspoons baking soda
½ teaspoon ground cinnamon
1 cup orange juice
6 egg whites
3 cups grated carrots

Sift together the flour, baking soda, and cinnamon. Stir in the orange juice. Beat the egg whites until they are just frothy; fold into the batter and mix thoroughly. Add the grated carrots. Pour the batter into a 1-quart nonstick ring mold. Bake in a 350 degree oven for 52 to 60 minutes.

*Serves 6 to 8*

## SPINACH PUFF

1 10-ounce package frozen chopped spinach, thawed
½ cup skim milk
1½ teaspoons unbleached all-purpose flour
⅛ teaspoon ground pepper
¼ cup grated sapsago cheese
4 egg whites

Stir together the spinach, milk, flour, pepper, and grated cheese. Beat the egg whites until stiff peaks form. Fold the whites through the spinach mixture, taking care not to break down the air bubbles of the whites. Pour all into an 8-inch-square nonstick pan. Bake in a 350 degree oven for 30 minutes, or until lightly browned.

*Serves 4*

## BROCCOLI WITH CURRY SAUCE

- 2 10-ounce packages frozen broccoli spears, or 1 large bunch fresh broccoli, sliced lengthwise
- 1 cup fat-free chicken broth
- 1 tablespoon cornstarch
- ¼ teaspoon curry powder
- ⅛ teaspoon dry mustard
- 2 teaspoons unsweetened apple juice

Cook the broccoli in a small amount of water until the broccoli is tender; drain. Bring the chicken broth to a boil. Dissolve the cornstarch in a small amount of water until it is smooth; add this to the chicken broth and boil, stirring constantly, until the mixture thickens and clears. Add the curry, mustard, and apple juice. Stir and cook for a moment more. Pour the sauce over the cooked broccoli and serve.

*Serves 6*

## GREEN BEANS AND ONION

- 1 cup diced onion
- 2 10-ounce packages frozen cut green beans, or 4 cups fresh trimmed and cut green beans, or canned beans
- ½ teaspoon dried dillweed

Place the onion, beans, and dillweed in a saucepan. Add a small amount of water. Cook until the beans are tender. Drain and serve.

*Serves 6*

# SWEET POTATO-SQUASH SOUFFLÉ

3 cups cooked and mashed sweet potatoes
1 cup cooked and mashed butternut squash
1 cup skim milk
1 tablespoon lemon juice
1 teaspoon grated lemon or orange rind
½ teaspoon ground cinnamon
¼ teaspoon ground nutmeg
⅛ teaspoon ground ginger
3 egg whites
⅔ cup "old-fashioned" rolled oats

Combine the sweet potatoes, squash, and skim milk, mixing to the consistency of a cake batter. Add the lemon juice, lemon rind, cinnamon, nutmeg, and ginger. Beat the egg whites until stiff peaks form; fold them into the sweet-potato batter, taking care not to break the air bubbles. Soak the oatmeal quickly in cold water to soften, then drain and lay the oatmeal in a thin layer in the bottom of a nonstick baking pan. Place the pan in a 300 degree oven for 10 to 15 minutes, or until the oatmeal layer is browned and dry. Fill the pan with the sweet-potato mixture. Raise the oven temperature to 375 degrees and bake the soufflé for 45 minutes, or until browned on top.
*Serves 6 to 8*

# ORANGE-GLAZED BEETS

2 1-pound cans sliced beets
½ cup orange juice
½ teaspoon celery seed
4 teaspoons cornstarch
2 teaspoons undiluted frozen apple juice concentrate, thawed

Drain the beet juice into a saucepan; add the orange juice, celery seed, and a paste mixture of the cornstarch and the apple juice. Mix well. Heat and stir until the mixture thickens and clears. Add the beets.
*Serves 6 to 8*

## BROWN RICE PILAF

1 cup brown rice
2 cups tomato juice
½ cup chopped onion
½ cup chopped celery
¼ cup chopped green pepper
1 teaspoon dried parsley flakes
½ teaspoon chili powder
⅛ teaspoon ground pepper

In a nonstick skillet, stir the brown rice over medium heat to toast the rice evenly. Add the tomato juice, onion, celery, green pepper, parsley, chili powder, and pepper; mix well. Simmer the rice, covered, for 35 to 40 minutes, or until all the water evaporates.

*Serves 4*

## SPICY MASHED POTATOES

3 medium potatoes
1 small onion, finely chopped
2 cloves garlic, minced
1 bay leaf
½ teaspoon rosemary
2 teaspoons dried parsley
1 cup hot skim milk
⅛ teaspoon mace

Peel the potatoes; cover with water, and bring to a boil. Add the onion, bay leaf, rosemary, and parsley. Cook 30 minutes or until done; then strain well. Add the hot milk and mace, beating with an electric mixer until a smooth texture is achieved. An alternate method for a stronger flavor is to peel the potatoes, cover with water, and bring to a boil. In a separate skillet, bring a few tablespoons of water to a boil; add onions and seasonings (except mace) and water-sauté until the onions are cooked and the water is evaporated. Strain the potatoes well and add the onion mixture. Mix. Add the hot milk and mace, beating with a mixer until a smooth texture is achieved.

*Serves 4*

## POTATO SALAD

2 pounds white or red potatoes, unpeeled
½ cup finely chopped celery
¼ cup finely chopped green pepper
1 onion, finely chopped
½ cup hoop cheese or other uncreamed cottage cheese
⅓ cup skim milk
⅛ teaspoon dry mustard
¼ teaspoon dried dillweed
¼ teaspoon celery seed
1 tablespoon vinegar
1 teaspoon lemon juice

Boil the potatoes, until they are tender, about 25 minutes. Remove the skins while the potatoes are hot; then cut them into cubes. Toss the potatoes with the celery, green pepper, and onion. Beat together the hoop cheese, milk, mustard, dillweed, celery seed, vinegar, and lemon juice. Toss the potato mixture with this dressing. Chill before serving.

*Serves 6*

## THREE-BEAN SALAD

2 cups dried garbanzo beans
2 cups dried red kidney beans
1 10-ounce package frozen cut green beans
1 stalk celery, finely chopped
1 small onion, finely chopped
1 tablespoon cider vinegar
2 teaspoons undiluted frozen apple juice concentrate, thawed
1 teaspoon lemon juice
¼ teaspoon garlic powder
¼ teaspoon dried dillweed
⅛ teaspoon ground pepper

Soak the dried beans separately for several hours, or overnight. Drain and re-cover each with water. Cook the beans separately until they are tender, about 1 to 1½ hours. Drain. Cook the green beans in a small amount of water until they are tender. Save ½ cup of the green-bean cooking water; add to it the celery, onion, vinegar, apple juice concentrate, lemon juice, garlic powder, dillweed, and pepper. Combine the cooked beans in a deep bowl and pour the dressing over all; toss well. Chill the beans for several hours before serving so that the flavors blend well. Stir occasionally.

*Serves 6 to 8*

## BAKED BEAN COMBO

    1  cup dried kidney beans
    1  cup dried great northern beans
    1  cup dried small red beans
    1  cup dried small black beans
    1  cup celery, finely chopped
    1  cup grated onion
   ⅓  cup apple-cider vinegar
   ⅓  cup unsweetened apple juice
    3  tablespoons lemon juice
    1  tablespoon grated lemon rind
    2  teaspoons dry mustard
    1  teaspoon garlic powder
    1  teaspoon celery seed
    1  teaspoon ground cloves
   ½  teaspoon ground allspice
   ¼  teaspoon ground ginger
    1  cup grated carrots
   ¼  cup grated sapsago cheese
   ½  cup potato pancake mix (check label for permissible
        ingredients)
    1  cup tomato sauce

Soak the first 3 beans together overnight. Soak the black beans separately. Drain beans and re-cover them with water, keeping the black beans separate. Cook them until they are almost tender. While the black beans are cooking, pour off and replace its blackened liquid several times, and restore it with fresh hot water. Combine all the beans after they are done. Cook the celery in a small amount of water until it is tender. Add it to the beans. Add the onion, vinegar, apple juice, lemon juice, lemon rind, and the remaining spices; mix well. Spread half the carrots and the grated cheese on the bottom of a baking pan. Cover with half the potato-pancake mix. Pour the bean mixture over this. Cover with the remaining carrots and the grated cheese. Sprinkle with the remaining potato-pancake mix. Pour the tomato sauce around the edges of the pan. Bake in a 350 degree oven for 45 minutes.

*Serves 8 to 10*

## SPICY ZUCCHINI

*This marvelous dish is quite spicy. Use it as a "relish" side dish to dress up other dishes. A little goes a long way.*

1 large zucchini, diced
1 medium onion, chopped
1 medium green pepper, chopped
1 medium tomato, chopped
1 teaspoon oregano
1 teaspoon basil
1 teaspoon chili powder
1 teaspoon garlic powder

Mix all the ingredients in pot with ¼ cup water and simmer, covered, 1 hour.

*Serves 6*

## ZUCCHINI-TOMATO COMBO

2 medium zucchini, sliced ¼-inch thick
1 1-pound can tomatoes
1 small onion, thinly sliced
1 tablespoon dried parsley flakes
¼ teaspoon ground thyme
⅛ teaspoon ground pepper

Place the zucchini, tomatoes (broken up with a fork), and onion in a saucepan. Add the parsley flakes, thyme, and pepper. Cook, covered, for 10 to 15 minutes, or until the zucchini is tender.

*Serves 6*

## *SALADS AND DRESSINGS*

### ROMAINE SALAD WITH PINEAPPLE DRESSING

1 crisp head romaine lettuce
½ cup thin Mock Sour Cream (see Index)
2 tablespoons canned crushed pineapple, water-packed
1 teaspoon undiluted frozen apple juice concentrate, thawed
¼ teaspoon dried dillweed

Tear the lettuce into pieces and arrange on salad plates. To make the dressing, combine the Mock Sour Cream, crushed pineapple, apple juice, and dillweed; mix until smooth. Serve as the dressing for the salad.

*Serves 6*

## HEARTS OF LETTUCE SALAD

4 wedges iceberg lettuce
½ cup Mock Sour Cream (see Index)
½ peeled cucumber, chopped

Arrange the lettuce wedges on salad plates. Combine the Mock Sour Cream with the chopped cucumber; pour this dressing over the wedges.
*Serves 4*

## GRAPEFRUIT BEAN SALAD

1 10-ounce package cut green beans, cooked
1 small onion, thinly sliced
1 grapefruit, peeled and sectioned
1 tablespoon grated sapsago cheese
3 tablespoons vinegar
1 tablespoon water
¼ teaspoon ground paprika
¼ teaspoon dry mustard

Combine the cooked beans, onion, grapefruit, and grated cheese in a bowl; toss well. To make the dressing, combine the vinegar, water, paprika, and dry mustard; shake the dressing well and toss with the salad. Serve at once.
*Serves 4*

## RICE SALAD

  3 cups cooked brown rice, cold
½ cup chopped green onion
  1 carrot, shredded
½ cup chopped celery

### DRESSING
¼ cup lemon juice
¼ cup cider vinegar
¼ cup unsweetened apple juice
½ teaspoon onion powder
½ teaspoon garlic powder
½ teaspoon dry mustard
  1 teaspoon Italian seasoning

Combine ingredients, pouring dressing over them to moisten well. Chill.

Serve as one of the courses in a cold meal, a buffet lunch or supper, or as a part of a brown-bag lunch.

*Serves 4*

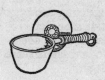

## TOMATO ASPIC

  3 cups tomato juice
  1 tablespoon grated onion
  1 teaspoon lemon juice
⅛ teaspoon ground pepper
  2 envelopes unflavored gelatin
½ cup cold water

Pour the tomato juice into a saucepan. Add the onion, lemon juice, and pepper. Bring to a boil. Meanwhile, soften the gelatin in cold water until it is dissolved; then add the gelatin to the hot tomato mixture and stir well.

Pour all into an 8-inch-square nonstick pan. Chill until the aspic is firm.

*Serves 8*

## MOCK SOUR CREAM

Skim milk or nonfat buttermilk
Hoop cheese or other uncreamed cottage cheese
Vinegar to taste (optional)

Pour about 1 cup milk or buttermilk into a blender; add a handful of the hoop cheese; blend. Stop the blender and stir. Add more liquid or more cheese, blending and occasionally stirring until the mixture resembles sour cream in smoothness and consistency and desired volume is obtained. A few teaspoons of vinegar may be added, if desired, to give a "sour-cream" tang. If a sweet topping is desired, add several teaspoons of frozen, undiluted apple juice concentrate, or substitute some fruit juice for the milk. Also, fresh bananas can be blended in for sweetness, adding cinnamon or nutmeg, if desired.

*Note:* Mock Sour Cream keeps well for several days in a tightly closed plastic container, but it has a tendency to thicken on standing. To thin, merely stir in a little more milk to bring back the desired consistency. Mock Sour Cream may also be frozen, then stirred vigorously after thawing.

## NONFAT YOGURT

1 quart skim milk
⅓ cup nonfat dry milk
1 tablespoon unflavored lowfat yogurt

Combine the milks, stirring to dissolve thoroughly. Heat to 120 degrees and place in a container (glass, crockery, or stainless steel). Allow to cool to 110 degrees. Remove about ½ cup of the warmed milk and blend into it the tablespoon of yogurt. Blend this mixture into the remaining warmed milk. Cover the container with a tea

towel. Place the container in an oven that has been preheated to 200 degrees, then turn off the heat. If you have
an electric oven, turn the light on to maintain the warmth.
(In a gas oven, the pilot light will maintain the warmth.)
Let the yogurt stand for about 12 hours or until the flavor
is tart enough for your taste. Refrigerate. The yogurt will
keep for a week or longer.

*Note:* Next time you make this recipe, use a tablespoon of the yogurt saved from this batch.

*Makes about 1 quart*


## NONFAT BUTTERMILK

*Use this recipe whenever nonfat buttermilk is required, as
commercial buttermilk is almost invariably too high in fat
even when strained.*

  1 quart skim milk
  ½ cup strained commercial buttermilk

Warm the milk to 70–80 degrees. Add the strained
buttermilk; stir well. Pour into a glass jar and cover with
a paper towel. Let it stand 5 to 8 hours or overnight at
room temperature. When the milk is clabbered and tastes
like buttermilk, cover and refrigerate. Don't let it sit out
too long after the buttermilk taste has developed or the
curd and whey will separate. Stir before using.

*Note:* Next time you make this recipe, use ½ cup of
buttermilk from this batch.

*Makes 4½ cups*


## EASY "RICOTTA" CHEESE

  ½ gallon skim milk
  ⅓ cup fresh lemon juice

Scald the milk, then remove it from the heat. Stir the
lemon juice into the milk. Let it sit for 15 minutes. Strain
to remove the liquid (whey) from the curds, pressing the
curds to remove as much liquid as possible. Chill.

*Makes about 2 cups*

# CREAMY NONFAT CHEESE

1 gallon skim milk
¼ cup nonfat buttermilk
⅛ rennet tablet, crushed and dissolved in ½ cup cold
    water

Place 1 gallon milk in a pot (don't use aluminum). Using a double-boiler arrangement, heat until milk reaches room temperature (70 to 80 degrees). Add buttermilk and rennet solution. Stir. Cover pot with cloth and let stand at room temperature 12 to 14 hours until curd breaks sharply when your finger is thrust in at an angle. (The desired consistency is like a firm custard.) Stir to break up curd into small pieces. Pour the curd and liquid (whey) into a colander lined with quadruple (4X) thickness of cheesecloth; allow it to drain. (For drier cheese, continue to drain by gathering the corners of the cheesecloth filled with cheese, tying with string or wire, and suspending it over the sink until more whey drips out.) Remove the cheese from the cloth and refrigerate it.

*Note:* For cheese with a consistency more like cream cheese, heat the milk over boiling water until the milk bubbles. Continue heating for 15 minutes. Remove the pot from heat and cool the milk until lukewarm. Continue the procedure as above, adding buttermilk, rennet, etc.

A sweeter cheese may be made by increasing the amount of rennet tablet added and reducing the time for curdling and souring. However, this produces a somewhat different cheese texture.

The cheese may also be baked, broiled, or frozen. Its flavor may be varied by mixing in any of the following after the cheese is removed from the cheesecloth: herbs, chives, dry minced onions, minced chili pepper, pimiento, or garlic powder.

*Makes about 1 quart, depending on the amount of moisture left in the cheese.*

## YOGURT-CHEESE DRESSING

1   cup nonfat yogurt
¼   cup cider vinegar
¼   cup unsweetened apple juice
2   tablespoons grated sapsago cheese
1   teaspoon dried parsley flakes
¼   teaspoon garlic powder
¼   teaspoon paprika

Combine all the ingredients and mix them until they
are smooth. Shake the dressing again just before serving.
*Makes 1⅔ cups*

## CREAMY SALSA DRESSING

2    cups hoop cheese or other uncreamed cottage cheese
¾    cup canned salsa
1½   cups canned diced tomatoes
¼    cup chopped green onion
1½   tablespoons lemon juice

Combine all the ingredients in a blender and blend.
Chill and serve.
*Makes about 3 cups*

## WINE VINEGAR DRESSING

½   cup wine vinegar
1   cup water
½   teaspoon dry mustard
½   teaspoon basil
½   teaspoon oregano
¼   teaspoon rosemary
2   teaspoons dried parsley flakes
1   clove garlic, minced

Combine all the ingredients and mix well. Shake the
dressing before each use.
*Makes about 1½ cups*

## RUSSIAN DRESSING

¾  cup cider vinegar
¾  cup water
2  tablespoons lemon juice
1  tablespoon chopped onion
1  teaspoon dry mustard
1  teaspoon garlic powder
⅛  teaspoon ground pepper
½  teaspoon ground paprika

Combine all the ingredients and mix well. Shake the dressing before each use.
*Makes about 1¾ cups*

## THOUSAND ISLAND DRESSING

1  cup Mock Sour Cream (see Index)
1  tablespoon tomato paste
2  tablespoons chopped green pepper
1  tablespoon chopped onion
¼  teaspoon garlic powder
⅛  teaspoon pepper

Combine all the ingredients and mix well. Thin the dressing with skim milk, if necessary. Refrigerate it until ready to use.
*Makes 1¼ cups*

## SAUCES

### CURRY SAUCE

*This sauce is great on Cheese Blintzes, Salmon Loaf, fish dishes, or on vegetables or rice. For variation, add dillweed.*

3¼ cups defatted chicken broth
3 tablespoons cornstarch
1 teaspoon curry powder
¼ teaspoon dry mustard
2 tablespoons undiluted frozen apple juice concentrate, thawed

Bring the chicken broth to a boil in a skillet. Dissolve the cornstarch in water in a bowl. Add this to the broth, stirring until thickened. Add the mustard and curry to the apple juice and stir in.
*Makes 3¼ cups*

### MINT SAUCE

*Use this sauce on fish or peas.*

1 cup fat-free chicken broth
1 cup skim milk
1 teaspoon lemon juice
1 tablespoon cornstarch
2 tablespoons flour
½ teaspoon mint
⅛ teaspoon lemon rind
    Dash of dried parsley, ground through a fine strainer
    Dash of dillweed

Heat the chicken broth to a boil in a skillet. Combine the cornstarch, flour, milk, and lemon juice. Pour this mixture into the skillet, stirring constantly until thickened. Add the seasonings. Stir to combine.
*Makes about 1½ cups*

## MUSHROOM CREAM SAUCE

  1 cup fat-free chicken broth
1½ cups mushrooms, thinly sliced
  ¼ cup shallots, diced
  ¾ cup onion, diced
  2 tablespoons cornstarch
  2 tablespoons nonfat dry milk
  1 tablespoon flour
1½ cups skim milk
  1 tablespoon lemon juice
  ¼ teaspoon apple-cider vinegar
  ¼ teaspoon onion powder
  ⅛ teaspoon garlic powder
    Turmeric (just enough to turn sauce a very pale yellow)

Heat the chicken broth in a skillet. Add the mushrooms, shallots, and onions. Combine cornstarch, powdered milk, and flour in a bowl. Add the milk and lemon juice. Pour all into a skillet, stirring constantly until thickened. Add vinegar and the seasonings.
*Makes about 2 cups*


## SPICY LEMON-GINGER SAUCE

*This sauce is excellent on steamed broccoli, cauliflower, carrots, or green beans.*

  ¾ cup nonfat dry milk
  1 cup water
  2 tablespoons cornstarch
  1 cup skim milk
  1 tablespoon lemon juice
  2 cups defatted chicken broth
  1 tablespoon apple-cider vinegar
  1 tablespoon curry
  1 teaspoon parsley
  ⅛ teaspoon ground ginger
  ½ teaspoon garlic powder

Blend the dry milk, water, and cornstarch until smooth. Add the lemon juice to the skim milk and combine with the cornstarch mixture. Bring the chicken broth to a boil in the skillet. Add the cornstarch mixture. Stir until thickened. Add the vinegar, ginger, garlic, curry, and parsley. Stir to combine.

*Makes about 2¾ cups*

## MUSTARD-CAPER CHEESE DIP

    1   teaspoon cornstarch blended with ¼ cup cold water
        and 1 tablespoon skim milk
 1¾   cups uncreamed cottage cheese
    ¼   cup apple-cider vinegar
    1   tablespoon lemon juice
    1   tablespoon unsweetened apple juice
    2   teaspoons capers, rinsed and drained
 1½   teaspoons prepared mustard

Blend the cornstarch with the cold water and nonfat milk to make a smooth mixture. Combine the cornstarch mixture with the other ingredients in a blender. Blend well. Chill and serve.

*Makes about 2½ cups*

## *FRUITS AND DESSERTS*

### FRUIT TOPPINGS

*Strawberry Topping.* Mix fresh or unsweetened frozen strawberries with unsweetened apple juice. Add cornstarch, mix until blended, and heat to thicken. Serve hot on hot cakes, waffles, or whole-wheat toast.

*Blueberry Topping.* Mix fresh or unsweetened frozen blueberries with unsweetened apple juice. Add cornstarch, mix until blended, and heat to thicken. Serve hot on hot cakes, waffles, or whole-wheat toast.

*Peach Topping.* Mix sliced fresh or unsweetened frozen peaches with unsweetened apple juice. Add cornstarch, mix until blended, and heat to thicken. Add a dash of nutmeg. Serve hot on hot cakes, waffles, or whole-wheat toast. (You may also use drained water-packed canned peaches instead.)

*Apple Topping.* Purée fresh apples in an electric blender with a dash of cinnamon or allspice. Serve at once. Or mix unsweetened apple juice with cornstarch; stir into puréed apples and heat until thickened, and serve hot.

*Cherry Topping.* Place fresh cherries, pitted, or unsweetened frozen cherries and unsweetened apple juice in an electric blender. Add cornstarch, mix until blended, and heat to thicken. Add ½ teaspoon vanilla extract. Serve.

*Apricot Topping.* Place fresh apricots, pitted or canned water-packed apricots, drained, into an electric blender. Add unsweetened crushed pineapple. Heat and serve as syrup or mix with cornstarch and thicken as desired.

*Strawberry-Banana Topping.* Mash fresh strawberries and bananas together; add a dash of cinnamon.

*Grape Juice-Pineapple Topping.* Combine semidiluted grape juice with unsweetened pineapple juice. Add cornstarch, mix until blended, and heat to thicken. Serve hot.

## ORANGE-PINEAPPLE SHERBET

    1  6-ounce can frozen orange juice
    1  6-ounce can frozen pineapple juice
3½  cups cold water
    2  tablespoons undiluted frozen apple juice concentrate, thawed
    1  cup nonfat dry milk

Put all the ingredients into a large mixing bowl and beat just enough to blend everything thoroughly. Pour the mixture into ice-cube trays; freeze for 1 to 2 hours until half-frozen. Remove the sherbet to a large chilled mixing bowl; with an electric mixer beat the sherbet on low speed until the mixture is softened, then beat on high speed for 3 to 5 minutes until it is creamy but not liquid. Pour the sherbet into freezer containers or ice-cube trays. Freeze the sherbet until it is ready to serve, several hours.

*Serves 12 to 14*

## PINEAPPLE WHIP

  2  envelopes unflavored gelatin
3½  cups unsweetened pineapple juice
  2  tablespoons undiluted frozen apple juice concentrate, thawed
  2  teaspoons lemon juice

In a small mixing bowl, soften the gelatin in ½ cup of the pineapple juice. Bring the remaining juice to the boil; add this to the gelatin mixture and stir until the gelatin is thoroughly dissolved. Add the apple juice and the lemon juice. Chill until the mixture begins to thicken. Beat the gelatin-juice mixture on high speed of an electric mixer until fluffy and double in volume. Chill again. Then mound the whip into 8 sherbet glasses.

*Serves 8*

## LEMON PUDDING

  ½  cup unbleached all-purpose flour
  ½  teaspoon baking powder
  ¼  cup fresh lemon juice
1½  cups skim milk
  2  tablespoons undiluted frozen apple juice concentrate, thawed
  4  egg whites

Sift the flour and the baking powder. Add the lemon juice, skim milk, and apple juice concentrate; beat well. Beat the egg whites until stiff peaks form. Fold them into the batter gently. Pour the pudding into a 1-quart nonstick baking dish. Set the baking dish in a pan of hot water. Bake in a 350 degree oven for 30 minutes. Cool. The pudding will separate into a cake layer and a sauce layer.

*Serves 6*

## ORANGE CREAM

 1 envelope unflavored gelatin
½ cup orange juice
 1 8-ounce can Mandarin oranges, water-packed
 2 cups plain nonfat yogurt (see Index)
½ teaspoon ground nutmeg

Put the gelatin into a small saucepan. Add the orange juice and mix until dissolved. Add the juice from the can of oranges. Cook this mixture until the gelatin is completely dissolved. Cool the mixture. Then stir in the orange segments (reserving a few for garnishing) and the yogurt. Mix well. Pour the cream into 4 parfait glasses. Garnish each glass with the reserved orange segments. Sprinkle with nutmeg. Chill for several hours.

*Serves 4*

## CHEESE BALLS WITH PLUMS

 1 cup hoop cheese
 1 egg white
 2 tablespoons unbleached all-purpose flour
¼ teaspoon ground cinnamon
⅛ teaspoon ground nutmeg
 1 teaspoon grated lemon rind
 1 1-pound can plums, water-packed

Mash the hoop cheese thoroughly; mix well with the egg white. Add the flour, cinnamon, nutmeg, and lemon rind; mix well. Form the mixture into small balls. Drop them gently into boiling water for 20 to 25 minutes. The balls will double in size. To test for doneness, cut 1 ball open and determine whether the center is cooked.

Serve with drained plums.

*Serves 4 to 5*


## APPLE BUNDT CAKE

  4 cups finely diced apples (5 to 6 apples)
 ½ cup undiluted frozen apple juice concentrate, thawed
 ½ cup water
 ¼ cup raisins
1¼ cups rice flour
1¼ cups whole wheat pastry flour
  2 teaspoons baking powder
  2 teaspoons baking soda
  2 teaspoons ground cinnamon
 ⅛ teaspoon ground nutmeg
 ⅛ teaspoon ground allspice
  4 egg whites
  1 teaspoon vanilla extract
  1 cup Grape Nuts cereal

Combine the diced apples, apple juice, water, and raisins in a bowl. Cover with plastic wrap and store in the refrigerator for 4 to 6 hours. Sift both flours, baking powder, baking soda, cinnamon, nutmeg, and allspice into a large bowl. Beat the egg whites until soft peaks form; fold into the flour mixture. Add the apple-raisin mixture, including the juice. Add the vanilla extract and the cereal. Stir well. Pour into a nonstick bundt pan. Bake in a 325 degree oven for 1½ hours. Turn the cake out of the pan onto a large sheet of aluminum foil. Wrap the cake completely in foil and let it sit for several hours.

*Serves 12*

## BUTTERMILK CHIFFON CHEESECAKE

3½ cups uncreamed cottage cheese (hoop cheese pre-
     ferred), loosely crumbled (approximate)
 1 cup nonfat buttermilk
 2 envelopes unflavored gelatin
 1 small can unsweetened crushed pineapple
 ½ cup undiluted frozen apple juice concentrate, thawed
 ½ cup water
 1 teaspoon vanilla extract
 3 egg whites
1½ cups Grape Nuts cereal

OPTIONAL FRUIT TOPPING
 2 bags frozen strawberries, unsweetened, or 2 boxes
     frozen blueberries, unsweetened
 ½ cup undiluted frozen apple juice concentrate, thawed
 ½ cup water
 1 teaspoon vanilla extract
   Cornstarch

Loosely crumble enough cheese into a blender to fill it
about ¾ full. Do not pack it. Add buttermilk (more than
1 cup if necessary). Blend cheese to thick but smooth
consistency. In a bowl, moisten the gelatin with the
crushed pineapple; mix well. Heat the apple juice and
water to a boil. Pour the boiling liquid over the gelatin-
pineapple mixture; stir well to dissolve. When cooled, add
the cheese mixture and vanilla. Beat the egg whites until
stiff peaks form; fold in. Pour the batter into 2 9-inch pie
pans with a bottom crust of enough Grape Nuts damp-
ened with a little additional apple juice to form a cohe-
sive layer. Refrigerate for several hours.

*Optional fruit topping:* Bring to a boil frozen strawberries or blueberries and the apple juice-water combination.
Thicken well with cornstarch which has been blended first
with a little water. Stir in vanilla. Cool, then spread over
the pies. Refrigerate until the topping is set.

*Each pie serves 6 to 8*

## APRICOT FLUFF

1 5-ounce jar strained sugar-free baby-food apricots
1 tablespoon undiluted frozen apple juice concentrate, thawed
1 teaspoon vanilla extract
1 teaspoon lemon juice
1 teaspoon unflavored gelatin
1 tablespoon cold water
2 egg whites

Mix the apricots, apple juice concentrate, vanilla, and lemon juice together. Soften the gelatin in cold water, then dissolve it over hot water in the top of a double boiler. Beat the egg whites until frothy; add the gelatin and beat until very stiff. Fold the gelatin mixture into the apricot mixture and pile it lightly into dessert dishes. Chill. Top with Mock Sour Cream (see Index), sweetened with apple juice concentrate, if desired.

*Serves 4*

## PEARS HÉLÈNE

8 pear halves, water-packed
1 cup hoop cheese or other uncreamed cottage cheese
  Several tablespoons skim milk, as needed for smooth consistency
2 tablespoons undiluted frozen apple juice concentrate, thawed
½ teaspoon vanilla extract
  Carob powder
  Nutmeg

Put a pear half in each of 8 dessert dishes. Blend together some of the skim milk with a little of the cheese; add the apple juice concentrate, vanilla, more skim milk as required, and the balance of the cheese. Blend until smooth (about 5 minutes). Spoon mixture on each of the pear halves. Refrigerate until cheese is well chilled. Just before serving, sprinkle the pears with a little carob powder and nutmeg.

*Note:* Carob has an intriguing chocolate-like flavor and may be obtained at your local health-food store.

*Serves 8*

## TAPIOCA FREEZE

### FILLING

- 1 cup dry pearl tapioca (not instant)
- 2 cups hot tap water
- 2 cups skim milk
- 1½ tablespoons potato flour
- 6 ounces undiluted frozen apple juice concentrate, thawed
- 4 teaspoons vanilla extract
- 1 15-ounce can unsweetened crushed pineapple, undrained
- ¼ cup orange juice
- 2 bananas, mashed
- 4 egg whites, stiffly beaten

### CRUST AND TOPPING

- 2 cups puffed rice cereal, unsweetened
- 2 cups Grape Nuts cereal
- ½ cup undiluted frozen apple juice concentrate, thawed
- 2 teaspoons vanilla extract
- ½ teaspoon cardamom
- ½ teaspoon cinnamon

Place the dry tapioca in the top of a double-boiler saucepan. Add the hot water and let sit for 10 minutes. Pour off the water and add the skim milk. Half-fill the bottom of the double boiler with water and cook the tapioca until the pearls are no longer opaque.

While the tapioca is cooking, prepare the crust in the following manner: Grind the puffed rice in the blender and set aside. Pour the Grape Nuts into a large serving bowl and add the apple juice concentrate, vanilla, cardamom, and cinnamon. Stir to coat the Grape Nuts and let it sit until it is no longer crunchy. Cover the bottom of a

nonstick pan with half of the Grape Nuts and rice powder.

When the tapioca is cooked, add the potato flour
blended with the apple juice concentrate, vanilla, pineapple (with its juice), orange juice, and bananas. Then fold
in the beaten egg whites until the tapioca mixture is well-
mixed and fluffy. Pour the tapioca on top of the Grape
Nuts, and sprinkle the remainder of the Grape Nuts and
rice powder on top. Freeze and eat.

*Makes 2 dozen servings*

# 29

## Recipes for the Single Cook

### DINNER IN A HURRY

Tomato Soup
Broiled Herbed Chicken
Zucchini
Grilled Potato
Banana Grape Cup

### CANDLELIGHT DINNER FOR TWO
#### (Double recipes)

Gazpacho
Veal Chop Provençal
Broccoli with Lemon-Ginger Sauce
Baked Potato with Mock Sour Cream
Romaine Salad with Wine-Vinegar Dressing
Strawberries Romanoff

### WEEKEND LUNCH

Pastina Soup
Asparagus Frittata
Spinach Salad
Pineapple-Cherry Compote

# *BREAKFASTS*

## FRENCH TOAST

1 egg white
¼ cup skim milk
½ teaspoon vanilla extract
2 slices whole wheat bread (permissible kind)
  Applesauce, unsweetened

Beat together vigorously the egg white, milk, an
vanilla. Dip the bread slices into this mixture. Cook th
bread in a nonstick skillet until browned on one side; tur
and brown the other side.

Serve hot with cold applesauce.

*Serves 1*


## EGG ON A RAFT

1 slice whole-wheat bread (permissible kind), toasted
1 egg white
  Dash of nutmeg

Cut out a circle in the center of the bread; place th
bread in a nonstick skillet. Drop the egg white into th
hole. Sprinkle with nutmeg. Cover and cook to desire
doneness.

*Serves 1*


## CHIVE-CHEESE OMELET

1 egg white
2 tablespoons Mock Sour Cream (see Index)
1 teaspoon chopped chives

Beat the egg white until soft peaks form. Stir in th
Mock Sour Cream and the chopped chives. Pour the eg
mixture into a heated small nonstick skillet and cook unt
the underside is browned; turn and cover, cooking unt
the other side is browned. Serve at once.

*Serves 1*

## EGG LORRAINE

egg white
tablespoon grated onion
teaspoon grated green pepper
teaspoon sapsago cheese, grated

Beat the egg until soft peaks form. Add the onion, een pepper, and cheese. Pour the egg mixture into a eated small nonstick skillet and cook until the underside browned; turn and cover, cooking until the other side browned. Serve at once.
*Serves 1*

## OATMEAL WITH SLICED BANANA

1 cup "old-fashioned" rolled oats
2 cups boiling water
½ banana, sliced
  Skim milk
  Dash of cinnamon

Stir the oats into boiling water; cook and stir for everal minutes. Cover and place the pot in another pot of immering water and cook, stirring occasionally, for about 0 minutes. Spoon into a bowl. Add the sliced banana, innamon and the milk.
*Serves 1 or 2*

## BAGEL SANDWICH

1 whole-wheat bagel, warmed
2 tablespoons uncreamed cottage cheese
1 tablespoon skim milk, if needed
¼ teaspoon chopped chives
1 thin slice of tomato
1 thin slice of Bermuda onion

Cut the bagel in half. Mix the cottage cheese, skim milk (to thin consistency), and chives together; spread

this on the bagel. Top with the onion and the tomato.
Top with the second half of the bagel.
*Serves 1*

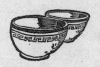

## SOUPS

### BASIC VEGETABLE CREAM SOUP FOR ONE

½  cup cooked vegetables (asparagus, broccoli, peas, etc.)
½  cup skim milk
   Dash of pepper
   Herbs (thyme, marjoram, rosemary, etc.) to taste

Put all ingredients into an electric blender and process
until smooth. Heat and serve.
*Note:* You may want to prepare extra vegetables one
night to process into a soup for the next night. Use 1 herb
at a time until you find those that suit your taste.
*Serves 1*

### GAZPACHO FOR ONE

1  tomato, quartered
½  cup tomato juice
¼  teaspoon onion powder
¼  teaspoon garlic powder
1  teaspoon vinegar
1  teaspoon lemon juice
½  cucumber, chopped
1  scallion, thinly sliced

Place the tomato, tomato juice, onion powder, garlic
powder, vinegar and lemon juice into an electric blender

d purée until smooth. Add half the cucumber and
ocess again.

Serve chilled, with the remaining chopped cucumber
d scallion floating on top.

*Serves 1*

## TOMATO SOUP

cup tomato juice
cup vegetable water
teaspoon onion powder
Dash of pepper

Heat all the ingredients together and serve. Add some
oked leftover rice, if desired.

*Note:* Vegetable water may be saved from all the vege-
bles you cook during the week by pouring small
mounts of the cooking water into a container in the re-
igerator instead of down the sink drain. At the end of
e week, cook it all together and reduce the volume by
alf by rapid boiling. Then add a small can of mixed veg-
tables and you will have a tasty vegetable soup. A pinch
f dried basil and a dash of pepper would be tasty addi-
ons.

*Serves 1*

## PASTINA SOUP

1 cup defatted chicken broth
1 tablespoon pastina
 teaspoon dried dillweed

Cook the broth, pastina, and dillweed together for at
ast 10 minutes, or until the pastina is thick.

*Note:* Keep chicken broth on hand by preparing
hicken Soup (see Index)—strained and defatted—and
eezing it into ice cubes, then storing the cubes in a plas-
c bag in the freezer compartment of your refrigerator.
Vhenever you need chicken broth, you can quickly melt
s many cubes as you need.

*Serves 1*

## MUSHROOM SOUP FOR ONE

⅛  pound fresh mushrooms
1   teaspoon grated onion
½  cup defatted chicken broth
⅛  teaspoon dried dillweed
    Dash of curry

Slice the mushrooms and place them in a small sauce
pan. Add the remaining ingredients and cover the sauce
pan. Cook the mushroom mixture over low heat for 10
minutes, or until the mushrooms are tender. Pour the
soup into an electric blender and process it until smooth.

To serve, you can save some of the mushrooms for a
garnish: slice them in thin strips and float them on the
soup.

*Serves 1*

## *MEAT, POULTRY, AND FISH*

### BROILED HERBED CHICKEN

¼  of a broiler chicken, skin removed
2   tablespoons undiluted frozen orange juice concentrate,
    thawed
⅛  teaspoon tarragon
⅛  teaspoon dried parsley flakes
⅛  teaspoon dry mustard

Arrange the chicken in a broiler pan. Combine the
concentrate orange juice, tarragon, parsley, and mustard;
mix well. Brush half the mixture over the chicken. Broil
for 6 minutes, or until the chicken is lightly browned; turn

and brush the other side with the remaining herb mixture. Broil for 6 minutes more, or until the chicken is tender.
*Serves 1*


## SHISH KEBAB

3-4 ounces lean steak, cut in 1-inch cubes
4 cherry tomatoes
½ green pepper, cut into 1-inch cubes
4 mushroom caps
1 8-ounce can boiled white onions
¼ cup tomato juice
1 teaspoon cider vinegar
¼ teaspoon dry mustard
⅛ teaspoon garlic powder
Dash of pepper

Using 1 or 2 shish-kebab skewers, thread the meat alternately with the tomatoes, green pepper, mushroom caps, and boiled onions. Place the kebabs on a broiler pan. In a saucepan, heat the tomato juice, vinegar, mustard, garlic powder, and pepper together; brush this on the skewered meat and vegetables. Broil the kebabs about 2 inches away from the heat for 6 to 8 minutes. Brush them occasionally with the remaining sauce during cooking.
*Serves 1*


## BROILED SOLE VERONIQUE

¼ cup lemon juice
1 slice fillet of sole
1 tablespoon nonfat yogurt (see Index)
⅛ teaspoon ground paprika
Dash of onion powder
8 seedless green grapes

Pour the lemon juice over the fish in a baking dish and let it stand in the refrigerator for at least 30 minutes, turning the fish occasionally. (Or this can be done in the morning and the fish can marinate all day.) Spread the fish with the yogurt and sprinkle it with the paprika and the onion powder. Arrange the grapes around the fish. Put the fish under the broiler for 10 minutes, or until the fish flakes easily when tested with a fork.

*Serves 1*

## HAMBURGER PATTY

3 ounces very lean ground beef
1 slice raw onion, diced
2 mushrooms, thinly sliced
⅛ teaspoon dry mustard
   Dash of garlic powder
1 tablespoon potato flour

Place the ground beef in a small bowl. In a skillet, simmer the onion and the mushrooms in enough water to keep the onion mixture from sticking to the pan. Cook this until the onions and the mushrooms are tender. Pour this into the beef. Add the mustard, garlic powder, and potato flour. Mix well. Form the beef mixture into a patty. Broil for 3 to 4 minutes on each side, or until done to desired degree of rareness.

*Note:* You can stretch the ground beef even more by using less beef and adding cooked rice and additional potato flour to the mixture.

*Serves 1*

## FILET MIGNON

*Your cheating ration will come into play with this recipe!*

1 4-ounce filet mignon
¼ cup red burgundy wine
¼ teaspoon onion powder
2 very large mushroom caps
¼ teaspoon dillweed
   Dash of pepper
   Dash of garlic powder

1 medium tomato
¼ teaspoon dried parsley flakes
1 teaspoon bread crumbs (permissible kind)

Soak the beef in the wine for 15 minutes, turning occasionally. Sprinkle it with the onion powder and place it on the broiler pan. Remove stems from the mushrooms and chop them finely; mix with the dillweed, pepper, and garlic powder. Stuff the mushroom caps with the chopped-stem mixture and place them on the broiler pan next to the filet. Cut the tomato in half; sprinkle each half with parsley and bread crumbs; place them next to the filet. Spoon the remaining burgundy over the meat and the mushrooms. Put the pan under the broiler for 5 minutes, then turn the filet and broil for 5 minutes more. If the tomatoes are beginning to sag, remove them to the serving platter. Then remove the filet and the mushrooms as ready.
*Serves 1*

## CHICKEN-FRUIT SKILLET

½ chicken breast, boned and skinned
1 tablespoon grated onion
¼ teaspoon tarragon
⅛ teaspoon pepper
¼ cup orange juice
1 banana, sliced into chunks
5 dark grapes, halved and seeded

Cut the boneless chicken into 1½-inch chunks and place it in a nonstick skillet. Add the onion, tarragon, pepper, and orange juice. Cook the chicken mixture over moderate heat, stirring constantly, until the chicken turns white. Add the banana and grapes. Simmer, covered, over low heat for several minutes more, adding more orange juice if necessary.

Serve on cooked rice, if desired.
*Serves 1*

## VEAL CHOP PROVENÇAL

1   veal rib chop, trimmed of excess fat
1   small tomato
½   small onion, diced
½   green pepper, diced
⅛   teaspoon rosemary
⅛   teaspoon tarragon
⅛   teaspoon basil

Place the veal chop on a broiling pan and set it under the broiler; broil about 7 minutes on each side, depending on chop size and amount of rareness desired. Meanwhile, cut the tomato into tiny pieces and place it in a nonstick skillet. Add the onion, pepper, rosemary, tarragon, and basil. Cook over low heat, stirring occasionally, and adding a small amount of water if needed. When the chop is done, remove it to a platter and top it with the sauce.

*Serves 1*

## MEATLESS MAIN DISHES

### CHEESE AND SPINACH BAKE

½   10-ounce package frozen chopped spinach
1   scallion, thinly sliced
⅛   teaspoon ground nutmeg
½   cup uncreamed cottage cheese
¼   teaspoon oregano

Cook the spinach, scallion, and nutmeg in a small amount of water; drain well. Spread the mixture on the bottom of a small baking dish. Top with the mixture of cottage cheese and oregano. Bake in a 350 degree oven for 15 minutes.

*Serves 1*

## ASPARAGUS FRITTATA

    1  8-ounce can chopped asparagus
    1  tablespoon finely sliced scallions
    1  tablespoon chopped green pepper
    4  egg whites
    2  tablespoons uncreamed cottage cheese
 1½  teaspoons skim milk
    1  teaspoon chopped parsley
  ⅛  teaspoon ground pepper

Drain the asparagus, pouring several tablespoons of its liquid into a small nonstick skillet. Chop the asparagus pieces into even smaller bits and add to the skillet; add the scallions and the green pepper. Cook over low heat until the vegetables are tender. Beat the egg whites with a fork until they are frothy; stir them into the cheese with the skim milk, parsley, and pepper. Mix until smooth. Pour the mixture over the vegetables in the skillet and stir the vegetables quickly into the mixture. Cook over low heat until the bottom is browned. Loosen the edges with a spatula and flip over to brown the other side. Place in a 300 degree oven for 15 minutes.

*Serves 2*


## GARBANZO SALAD IN PITA BREAD

    1  whole-wheat pita bread
  ½  cup cooked garbanzo beans
    1  tablespoon grated onion
  ½  cup shredded lettuce
  ½  small tomato, diced
  ¼  teaspoon garlic powder

Cut 1 side open on the pita bread to form a pocket. Combine the garbanzo beans, onion, lettuce, tomato, and garlic powder; stuff the garbanzo mixture into the pita bread.

*Note:* A small amount of water-packed tuna may be added, if desired.

*Serves 1*

## PITA PIZZA

1 whole-wheat pita bread, cut into round halves
2 ounces tomato sauce
2 ounces tomato paste
½ teaspoon oregano
4 tablespoons hoop cheese, crumbled
   Garlic and onion powder, to taste

Arrange the pita bread circles on a cookie sheet, browned side down. Stir together the tomato paste, tomato sauce, and spices. Spread some of this mixture over each bread round. Top with crumbled hoop cheese. Bake in a 350 degree oven for 15 to 20 minutes, or until the cheese is melted.

*Note:* Water-sauteed vegetables, such as chopped onions, green peppers and mushrooms, can also be added as pita toppings.

*Serves 2*

## NOODLE BOWS AND CHEESE

1 cup yolk-free noodle bows, cooked and drained
¼ cup hoop cheese, crumbled, or other uncreamed cottage cheese
2 teaspoons grated sapsago cheese
⅛ teaspoon ground nutmeg
   Dash of ground pepper
¾ cup skim milk
1 tablespoon flour
1 teaspoon parsley, chopped

Toss the cooked and drained noodle bows with the hoop cheese and the sapsago cheese. Add the parsley, nutmeg, and pepper. Combine the milk and the flour in a saucepan; cook and stir constantly until the mixture thickens. Pour the sauce over the noodles and toss well. Spoon the mixture into a small nonstick baking dish. Top with additional sapsago cheese, if desired. Bake in a 350 degree oven for 20 minutes.

*Serves 1*

## GREEN NOODLES IN SPINACH SAUCE

    4  ounces yolk-free green noodles, cooked
    3  fresh spinach leaves
    1  sprig fresh parsley
    1-2  teaspoons grated sapsago cheese
    ½  clove garlic, peeled
    2  tablespoons hot water

Place the cooked noodles on a serving plate. Place all the remaining ingredients in an electric blender and purée. Pour the sauce over the noodles and toss.

*Serves 1*

## EGG FOO YONG

    ¼  cup sliced fresh mushrooms
    ¼  cup chopped onion
    ¼  cup bean sprouts
    1  teaspoon soy sauce (salt-reduced variety)
    2  egg whites

In a skillet, sauté the mushrooms, onion, and bean sprouts in a small amount of water. Drain. Add the soy sauce and mix well. Beat the egg whites until soft peaks form; add the vegetable mixture and fold it through the egg whites. Using a nonstick skillet, drop the mixture by large spoonfuls onto the heated skillet, making several pancakes. Brown both sides.

*Serves 1*

## *MAIN DISH VEGETABLES*

### BROCCOLI WITH LEMON-GINGER SAUCE

½ 10-ounce package broccoli spears, or 1 stalk fresh
    broccoli
¼ cup skim milk
1 teaspoon cornstarch
1 teaspoon lemon juice
⅛ teaspoon ground ginger
⅛ teaspoon garlic powder

In a saucepan, cook the broccoli spears in a small
amount of water, covered, until they are tender, about 12
minutes. Drain ¼ cup of the broccoli water into another
saucepan. Stir the milk and the cornstarch together to
make a thin paste; stir it into the broccoli water. Add the
lemon juice, ginger, and garlic powder. Bring the sauce to
a boil stirring constantly, until the mixture thickens and
then clears. Pour the sauce over the broccoli and serve.
*Serves 1*

### ZUCCHINI

1 small zucchini
½ cup tomato juice
¼ teaspoon dried thyme
⅛ teaspoon ground pepper

Slice the zucchini into ¼-inch-thick rounds. Place them
in a small saucepan with the tomato juice, thyme, and
pepper. Simmer, covered, for 12 minutes, or until tender.
*Serves 1*

### MINTED PEAS

½ package (10-ounce) frozen peas, or ½ pound fresh
    peas, shelled
⅛ teaspoon dried mint
⅛ teaspoon dried grated lemon rind

Place the peas in a small saucepan with a small amount of water. Add the mint and the lemon rind. Cook, covered, for 6 minutes, or until the peas are tender. Drain and serve.
*Serves 1*


# BRUSSELS SPROUTS

½ package (10-ounce) frozen Brussels sprouts, or 1 cup fresh Brussels sprouts
½ teaspoon parsley flakes
⅛ teaspoon marjoram
  Dash of pepper

Place the Brussels sprouts in a small saucepan with a small amount of water. Add the parsley flakes, marjoram, and pepper. Cook, covered, for 8 minutes, or until the sprouts are tender but not mushy. Drain.
*Serves 1*


# CAULIFLOWER

½ package (10-ounce) frozen cauliflower
1 tablespoon lemon juice
⅛ teaspoon marjoram
⅛ teaspoon paprika

Place the cauliflower in a saucepan with a small amount of water. Add the lemon juice and the marjoram. Cover and simmer until the cauliflower is tender, about 10 minutes. Drain. Sprinkle with paprika and serve.
*Serves 1*


# SWEET POTATO WITH ORANGE

1 sweet potato
2 tablespoons orange juice
⅛ teaspoon ground nutmeg or cinnamon

Bake the sweet potato for 1 hour, or until tender. Split the top open and scoop out the potato. Mix with orange juice and nutmeg; refill the jacket and serve.
*Serves 1*

## DILLED POTATO

1 potato, peeled and quartered
1 cup water
¼ teaspoon dillweed
  Dash of pepper

Place the potato in a saucepan with the water, dillweed, and pepper. Simmer, covered, over low heat for 15 minutes, or until the potato is tender. Drain and serve.
*Serves 1*

## *SALADS AND DRESSINGS*

### SLICED TOMATO SALAD

1 medium tomato, thickly sliced
1 scallion, thinly sliced
¼ teaspoon dillweed
2 tablespoons thin Mock Sour Cream (see Index)

Arrange the sliced tomatoes on a salad plate. Sprinkle them with sliced scallion and dillweed. Drizzle Mock Sour Cream over all.
*Serves 1*

## SPINACH SALAD

6 fresh spinach leaves, trimmed
1 hard-boiled egg (yolk removed), chopped
⅛ teaspoon garlic powder
 Dash of pepper
2 tablespoons tarragon vinegar
1 tablespoon water

Arrange the spinach leaves on a plate. Sprinkle them with the cooked egg white. Stir together the garlic powder, pepper, vinegar, and water; pour the dressing over the salad and serve.
*Serves 1*

## DILLED CHILLED GREEN BEANS

½ cup cooked green beans
1 tablespoon tarragon vinegar
¼ teaspoon dillweed
 Dash of garlic powder
1 tablespoon orange juice

Place the beans in a container. Combine the tarragon vinegar, dillweed, garlic powder, and orange juice; shake the dressing well and pour it over the beans. Refrigerate the beans for several hours. Serve on a bed of lettuce.
*Note:* This is a good recipe for leftover beans, which can be served for the following night's dinner.

## LETTUCE AND EGG SALAD

1 hard-boiled egg (yolk removed), chopped
⅛ head iceberg lettuce, shredded
2 tablespoons cider vinegar
⅛ teaspoon garlic powder
⅛ teaspoon dry mustard
⅛ teaspoon ground paprika

Combine the chopped egg with the shredded lettuce. Shake the vinegar, garlic powder, mustard, and paprika together; pour the dressing over the salad and toss lightly.
*Serves 1*

## CUCUMBERS IN CREAM SAUCE

½ cucumber, sliced
¼ cup Mock Sour Cream (see Index)
1 teaspoon cider vinegar
¼ teaspoon dillweed

Combine the cucumber with the Mock Sour Cream, vinegar, and dillweed; toss well. Chill the cucumbers until they are ready to serve.
*Serves 1*

## COTTAGE CHEESE DRESSING

¼ cup uncreamed cottage cheese
1 tablespoon orange juice
1 tablespoon lemon juice
⅛ teaspoon ground cinnamon
  Dash of nutmeg
  Dash of pepper

Place all the ingredients in a blender and process until smooth. If more liquid is required to blend to a smooth consistency, add a little skim milk. Use as a dressing on crisp romaine salad or on fruit salad.
*Serves 1*

## WINE-VINEGAR DRESSING

2 ounces wine vinegar
1 ounce water
1 teaspoon undiluted frozen apple juice concentrate, thawed
  Dash of pepper

Combine all the ingredients, mix vigorously, and pour over the salad.
*Serves 1*

## *FRUITS AND DESSERTS*

### FRUIT IDEAS FOR THE SINGLE COOK

Use fresh fruit whenever possible, purchasing small amounts.

- Slice a peeled orange into circles and sprinkle it with dried mint.
- Cut Italian blue plums in half and add them to your salad.
- Cut an apple or banana into segments and serve with uncreamed cottage cheese or nonfat yogurt.
- Eat a small melon segment one day, scoop out melon balls and mix with fresh strawberries the next day.
- Mix leftover fresh strawberries with fresh sliced pear.
- Add blueberries to any fruit, but also add to a tossed green salad.
- Eat half a grapefruit for breakfast one day, broil the other half (spread with apple juice concentrate) for dessert the next day.
- Eat a banana from the peel, or slice it into any water-packed canned fruit. Broil a banana, cut in half lengthwise, along with broiled fish.

Purchase a variety of water-packed canned fruits to mix and match at whim.

- Crushed pineapple and grapefruit segments go well together.
- Mandarin oranges and pineapple tidbits are a good combination.
- Peach halves stuffed with applesauce and dusted with

cinnamon are festive. Or layer peach slices with applesauce in a parfait glass.

- Use unsweetened puréed baby-food fruits as toppings for whole canned fruits, or purée your own in an electric blender.

## STRAWBERRIES ROMANOFF

1 cup whole strawberries
¼ cup orange juice
¼ cup Mock Sour Cream (see Index)
1 teaspoon undiluted frozen apple juice concentrate, thawed

Wash and hull the strawberries; dry well. Place the berries in a dessert dish. Add the orange juice and toss the berries to coat. Top them with Mock Sour Cream mixed with the apple juice concentrate.
*Serves 1*

## BANANA GRAPE CUP

½ sliced banana
6 seedless green grapes
¼ cup orange juice
Dash of nutmeg

Combine the sliced banana and the grapes in a dessert dish. Pour the orange juice over the fruit and sprinkle with nutmeg. Chill the fruits until they are ready to serve.
*Serves 1*

## BANANA FLAMBÉ

1 banana, cut in half lengthwise
¼ cup unsweetened apple juice
½ teaspoon grated lemon rind
⅛ teaspoon ground ginger
1 tablespoon brandy

Arrange the banana slices in a large skillet. Add the apple juice, lemon rind, and ginger. Cook over low heat for 4 minutes, basting with the juice constantly. Heat the brandy and pour it over the bananas. Ignite the brandy and shake the skillet until the flames are extinguished. Serve at once.

*Serves 1*

## CREAMY FRUIT CUP

1 cup fresh cut-up fruit, such as apples, pears, bananas, melon, or berries
¼ cup Mock Sour Cream (see Index)
1 teaspoon undiluted frozen apple juice concentrate, thawed
½ teaspoon grated lemon rind

Place the fruit in a dessert dish. Stir the Mock Sour Cream and the concentrated apple juice together; swirl it on top of the fruit. Sprinkle the fruit with grated lemon rind.

*Serves 1*

## BAKED APPLE

1 apple
Dash of cinnamon
1 teaspoon undiluted frozen apple juice concentrate, thawed
1 teaspoon seedless raisins

Core the apple. Scrape off the skin from the top ½ inch of the apple. Sprinkle the cinnamon into the core cavity. Add the apple juice and the raisins. Place the apple in a small baking dish. Bake in a 350 degree oven for 30 minutes, or until the apple is fork tender.

*Note:* Using the same heat energy, it may be sensible to make 2 apples at a time and refrigerate 1 for another day.

*Serves 1*

## GINGER PEARS

⅛  teaspoon ground ginger
 2  tablespoons of the pear juice
 2  canned pear halves, water-packed

Add the ginger to the pear juice in a small saucepan and heat the mixture for several minutes. Add the pear halves and cover for 15 minutes, with the heat turned off. Serve warm.
*Serves 1*

## PINEAPPLE-CHERRY COMPOTE

 1  8-ounce can pineapple tidbits, water-packed
 1  8-ounce can Queen Anne cherries, water-packed
 1  teaspoon grated orange rind

Combine the pineapple and the cherries with their juices. Spoon a portion of the pineapple mixture into a dessert dish and top it with the grated orange rind. Refrigerate the remaining portion if you are dining alone.
*Serves 2*

# 30

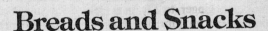

# Breads and Snacks

## *BREADS*

The Extra-Quick Yeast Bread relies on baking powder to eliminate rising time, producing a moist but fairly heavy bread. In the Quick version there is one rising prior to baking, which gives you a lighter-textured loaf. Once you've mastered these, you might want to try the Traditional Yeast Bread with two risings. It is well worth the effort!

## EXTRA-QUICK YEAST BREAD

 2 packages or 2 tablespoons dry yeast
 ¾ cup warm water
 1¼ cups soured milk (add 1½ tablespoons lemon juice to 1¼ cups nonfat milk; let stand 5 minutes), nonfat buttermilk, milk whey (leftover from making cheese, see Index), or water
 3½ to 4 cups whole wheat all-purpose flour
 1 tablespoon baking powder
    Cornmeal

In a large mixing bowl, dissolve the yeast in water. Stir in the soured milk. Mix the baking powder with 2½ cups flour. Add it to the liquid and beat well for about 2 minutes. Gradually mix in 1 cup flour. The dough should be soft and slightly sticky. Turn it onto a well-floured board and sprinkle the dough and your hands with flour. Knead the dough for about 250 strokes or 6 to 8 minutes, adding flour as required. Shape the dough for a 9-by-5-

by-3-inch loaf pan. Cover the bottom of the pan with cornmeal (instead of greasing). Place the dough in the pan and set it on the lowest rack position in a preheated oven at 375 degrees for about 45 minutes. Cool the bread for about 5 minutes on a cake rack until the bread shrinks from the sides of the pan. Remove the bread from the pan and continue to cool it on a rack.

*Variations:* Onion Bread. After the dough is kneaded, roll it out to an 8-by-10-inch rectangle and sprinkle the top liberally with dry minced onion. Roll it up from the narrow side and place it in the pan spread with cornmeal. Bake as directed above.

*Makes 1 loaf*

## QUICK YEAST BREAD

After the dough is in the loaf pan, place it in a warm spot until it has doubled in size (about 1 hour). Place the pan on the lowest rack position in a preheated oven at 400 degrees for about 35 minutes. Cool the bread following the directions above.

## TRADITIONAL YEAST BREAD

*For the more experienced baker; requires two risings.*

Follow the ingredients and directions for Extra-Quick Yeast Bread, omitting the baking powder. After kneading the dough, place it in a warm spot, such as a cool electric oven with a pot of boiling water in it to warm the area. Allow the dough to rise until it is double in bulk, about 1 hour. Remove and punch down the dough. Shape it, place it in a loaf pan spread with cornmeal, and let it rise in a warm place until it's double in bulk, about ¾ hour. Bake it on the bottom rack of a preheated 400 degree oven for about 30 minutes. Follow cooling directions as in the preceding recipe.

*Note:* Recipe may be doubled.

*Makes 1 loaf*

## IRISH SODA BREAD

*This is a delicious heavy-textured flat bread that is very simple to make with rye, graham, whole-wheat, or buckwheat flours, or any combination of these.*

2   cups flour
1   teaspoon baking powder or 1½ teaspoons low-sodium
    baking powder
½   teaspoon baking soda
½   teaspoon cream of tartar
1   tablespoon caraway or anise seeds
¾   cup (about) nonfat buttermilk

In a medium bowl stir together the dry ingredients. Make a well in the center and pour the buttermilk into it. Mix well. Knead the dough about a dozen times in the bowl; if it is too dry to form into a ball, work in a little more buttermilk. Spread the bottom of a pie pan with cornmeal. Flatten the ball into a circle 7 inches in diameter and place it in the pan. With a razor blade or sharp knife, cut an X about ¼ inch deep, dividing the dough into fourths. Bake in a preheated oven at 400 degrees until browned. about 50 minutes.
*Note:* This recipe may be doubled.
*Makes 1 loaf*


## CORN BREAD

2½   cups whole-ground cornmeal
2½   cups whole-wheat pastry flour (or brown-rice flour)
2   teaspoons baking powder
¼   teaspoon baking soda
3½   cups skim milk
¼   cup undiluted frozen apple juice concentrate, thawed
½   cup grated carrots
¾   cup egg whites (about 6), slightly beaten
½   teaspoon pumpkin-pie spice (optional)

Pour the dry ingredients into a mixing bowl; stir to mix well. Stir in the milk, apple juice, carrots, egg whites and .

pumpkin-pie spice. Pour the mixture into a nonstick baking pan. Bake at 350 degrees for 15 minutes; then turn up the heat to 375 degrees for an additional 15 minutes.

*Note:* To make corn muffins, use a nonstick muffin pan and bake the batter in a 350 degree oven for 25 to 30 minutes.

*Makes 18 pieces, 4 ounces each, or 36 muffins, 2 ounces each*

## BRAN MUFFINS

    2  cups whole-wheat pastry flour
    2  cups unprocessed Miller's bran flakes
    1  teaspoon baking soda
    ½  teaspoon baking powder
    2  egg whites
    2  cups nonfat buttermilk or skim milk
    ½  cup undiluted frozen apple juice concentrate, thawed
    ½  teaspoon cinnamon
    ⅛  teaspoon cloves
    ⅛  teaspoon nutmeg
    ½  teaspoon vanilla

Sift together the dry ingredients, except the bran, in a mixing bowl. Now mix in the bran. Beat the egg whites until stiff peaks form. Add the liquid ingredients to the dry ingredients, folding in the egg whites last. Bake 20 minutes in nonstick muffin tins in a preheated 400 degree oven.

*Serves 12*

## ESTHER'S HOT-WATER SKILLET CORN BREAD

    2  cups whole-ground cornmeal
    1  cup whole-wheat pastry flour
    ½  cup hot water
    2  egg whites
    ½  cup skim milk or nonfat buttermilk

3 teaspoons undiluted frozen apple juice concentrate, thawed
1 small zucchini, peeled and grated
1 small carrot, grated
¾ teaspoon allspice (optional)
¼ teaspoon cloves (optional)
2 teaspoons baking powder

Mix the cornmeal, flour, hot water, egg whites, milk, apple juice, zucchini, grated carrots, and seasonings, if used. Add the baking powder. Spoon the batter into a nonstick skillet. Cover with a lid or aluminum foil. Cook the corn bread over low heat for 10 minutes or until brown. Turn and brown the other side. Remove the bread from pan and wrap it in aluminum foil (to keep the bread from drying out and becoming too crusty).

*Note:* An oven-baked corn bread can be made by making the above recipe. Simply pour the batter into a nonstick square baking pan and bake the batter at 350 degrees for 30 minutes or until the bread begins to shrink away from the sides.

*Serves 6*


# SNACKS

## CRISPED TORTILLA CHIPS

1 package of 12 corn tortillas
½ teaspoon onion powder (optional)
½ teaspoon garlic powder (optional)

Arrange the tortillas in a stack. Cut all 12 in half at once, and then into quarters. Lay these wedges on a nonstick baking sheet, avoiding overlapping. Sprinkle them with onion and garlic powder, if desired. Bake in a preheated 375–400 degree oven until the chips are crisp, stirring and turning to brown evenly. Remove the wedges as they are done.

*Variation:* Barbecued Corn Tortilla Chips. Mix a little onion powder, chili powder, and paprika together to make a "barbecue" flavoring. Spread these on a flat platter and stir tortilla wedges through the mixture. Bake as above.

*Makes 4 dozen*

## OVEN-"FRIED" POTATOES

*Basic Method.* Wash and dry the potatoes, but do not peel them. Drop them into a pot of boiling water, lower the heat to a simmer, and cook until they are just barely tender. Remove from the pot and refrigerate.

When the potatoes are cold, peel them carefully and slice either lengthwise as French fries, or into round slices to make "cottage-style" fries. Spread the potatoes out on a nonstick baking sheet and season with onion powder, garlic powder, paprika, pepper, or chili powder. Brown in a 400 degree oven and then turn with a spatula to brown the other side. The potatoes should be crispy. Serve plain or with Salsa (recipe follows).

*Serves 1 person per potato*

## SALSA

1  16-ounce can whole tomatoes, undrained and chopped
1  ripe tomato, peeled and chopped
½  onion, finely chopped
½  green pepper, finely chopped
1  tablespoon diced canned green chilies
½  tablespoon cider vinegar
¼  teaspoon oregano
¼  teaspoon basil

Combine all the ingredients, stirring well. Use the Salsa as a dip, relish, salad dressing, or a baked potato topping.

*Serves 4, or more for a dip*

## BEAN DIP

Cooked and drained pinto beans
Tomato, finely chopped (optional)
Seasonings to taste: onion and garlic powder, diced green
    chilies, ground cumin

Mash cooked and drained pinto beans. Combine them
with tomatoes and desired seasonings. Serve hot or cold
with Crisped Tortilla Chips (see Index).

## EGGPLANT DIP

Whole firm eggplant
Seasonings:  Dip 1—ground cumin, nonfat yogurt
             Dip 2—chopped green onion, garlic powder,
                    lemon juice, black pepper, dillweed,
                    parsley

Bake eggplant in a 350 degree oven for 1 hour or until
it is mushy and brown on the outside. Peel and blend the
eggplant with choice of seasonings for either dip. Serve
with whole wheat pita bread cut into small wedges for
scooping dip.

## ONION DIP

Dried onion flakes
Seasonings to taste: black pepper, dillweed, garlic powder
Ground cumin and chili powder, or curry
Mock Sour Cream (see Index)

Toast dried onion flakes in the oven until lightly browned.
Mix them and seasonings into Mock Sour Cream. Serve
chilled with raw vegetables (celery, carrots, cauliflower or
broccoli, mushrooms, etc.).

## POPCORN

To make popcorn without oil, use a mesh hand-held popper that does not come in contact with the heat source, or a heavy, covered skillet. Shake the popcorn vigorously as it is popping to prevent burning. This insures perfect popcorn without the use of oil.

## FROZEN BANANA-ON-A-STICK

Peel a banana carefully, keeping it in one piece. Insert an ice-cream stick through the length of it. Wrap the banana in a plastic wrap and freeze.

To get a "nutty" texture on the outside, dip the banana in skim milk and then roll in Grape Nut "crumbs" (crushed with a rolling pin or ground in a blender) that have been flavored with a dash of cinnamon or nutmeg. Then wrap and freeze as done previously.

## TANGY DRINK

Pour sparkling mineral water or soda over ice with a twist of lime, lemon, or orange. Or mix with fruit juice for a sweeter drink.

## TOASTED CHEESE BREAD

Spread any permissible sliced bread (sourdough, wholewheat, rye) with mustard, if desired, and press crumbled hoop cheese on top, covering the surface of the bread completely. Broil the bread or place it in a 400 degree toaster oven until the cheese is soft and almost melted. Serve hot.

## ROASTED CHESTNUTS

*Chestnuts are the only nuts acceptable on the Pritikin Diet because of the sufficiently low fat content (about 6 percent of total calories).*

Make a deep slash through the shells with a sharp knife along the flat side of the chestnuts. Spread them in a single layer in a shallow pan, cut side up. Cover the pan with foil and roast in a 450 degree oven for 25 to 30 minutes. Shake the pan several times during baking. Reduce the oven temperature to 200 degrees or lower, if possible, and remove only as many chestnuts as can be peeled and eaten at a time. Keep the rest of the nuts warm until eaten.

## GARBANZO "NUTS"

Dried garbanzo beans
Onion and/or garlic powder, to taste (optional)

Rinse the dried beans in a colander, then put the beans in a covered kettle to soak for a few hours or overnight. The water level should be 3 to 4 inches above the beans, as the beans will absorb much water during the soaking process. Add more water, if necessary, during the soaking period.

When ready to cook, add additional water to bring the water level back to 3 to 4 inches above the beans. Stir well. Cook, uncovered, until the beans are almost done, then cover for the last part of the cooking. The beans should be tender.

Drain the beans well, then place them on a nonstick baking pan in a single layer. While still damp, sprinkle on onion or garlic powder, if desired. Bake in a 350 degree oven until the beans are quite dry and browned, about 45 minutes. Shake the beans occasionally while baking to brown evenly.

*Variation:* By freezing the beans after cooking, and baking later, they will be more tender.

## GARBANZO "NUT BUTTER"

4 cups cooked garbanzo beans
1½ cups liquid from cooking beans
2 tablespoons cornstarch
⅓ cup frozen apple juice concentrate, thawed
1 tablespoon vanilla extract
1 tablespoon ground cinnamon

Cook garbanzo beans until almost but not completely tender. Drain, saving 1½ cups of the cooking liquid. Place beans in a single layer on a nonstick baking pan in a 350 degree oven, stirring occasionally to toast evenly, for about 1½ hours. Grind toasted garbanzos in a food processor or blender.

Blend cornstarch, apple juice, vanilla, and cinnamon, to a smooth mixture. Mix in garbanzo bean liquid. Heat mixture in a saucepan over low heat, stirring constantly until thickened. Stir thickened mixture into the ground toasted garbanzos.

Use as stuffing for celery sticks for appetizers, or spread on bread or crackers for a snack or a sandwich.


## PITA POCKETS

Pita bread is available in whole wheat or unbleached white flour varieties. It is easy to stuff as a sandwich. Here is a list of interesting vegetarian stuffings you might consider:

Thinly sliced lettuce, any variety
Tomato wedges
Thinly sliced cucumbers
Alfalfa sprouts
Red onion slices
Grated carrot
Sliced dill pickle
Mustard
Capers
Hot peppers in wine vinegar
Mushrooms, raw or cooked

Chopped green onion
Rice, cooked
Bulgur wheat, cooked
Hoop cheese, crumbled
Sapsago or green cheese, finely grated
Leftover steamed vegetables such as chopped zucchini,
Broccoli

*To prepare:* Stuff your choice of ingredients into halved pitas that have been warmed in the oven. If desired, a dressing such as Mock Sour Cream (see Index) may be drizzled over the top.

# Appendix

## I. RATIONALE OF THE PRITIKIN DIET

Scientific literature contains much evidence supporting the thesis that excessive intake of fats, cholesterol, simple carbohydrates, and protein is deleterious to the system. The many studies cited here underlie the position that the diet of the developed nations—the Western diet—is strongly associated with degenerative diseases. The high fat and cholesterol content seems to be the primary factor; simple carbohydrates are a major secondary factor.

In the Western diet, fats generally comprise over 40 percent of total calories. Conversely, societies with a low prevalence of degenerative diseases use low-fat diets almost without exception. Usually less than 20 percent of their total calorie intake comes from fats; unrefined carbohydrates are their main calorie source.

For years, carbohydrates have been unjustly maligned. Confusion exists as to their metabolic effects because important distinctions between the rapidly absorbed simple carbohydrates—sugar, molasses, and honey—and the slowly absorbed unrefined carbohydrates—fruits, vegetables, and whole grains—are often overlooked. Carbohydrates, as grown, provide ideal body fuel and the fiber needed for a healthy intestinal tract. When starches and other polysaccharides are refined, stripped of fiber, and converted to monosaccharides and disaccharides, they create metabolic problems and potential disease. Carbohydrates, as grown, also provide ample vitamin and mineral nutrition.

# EXCESS FAT AS A FACTOR IN
# TISSUE ANOXIA

The problems of fat intake are not limited to saturated fats—all fats are implicated. Their sources include butterfat, vegetable fats, eggs, and animal tissues. Excess fats, regardless of source, are potentially damaging to the system.

The damage follows three basic modes: 1) production of tissue anoxia; 2) interference with carbohydrate metabolism; and 3) elevation of cholesterol and uric acid levels. These disturbances in body metabolism contribute to the etiology of many degenerative diseases which plague modern man.

## *Erythrocyte aggregation lowers oxygen levels in blood and tissues*

How does tissue anoxia occur? Fat is broken down in the small intestine to fatty acids and there absorbed and resynthesized into chylomicrons. The chylomicrons, almost pure triglycerides, pour into the blood from the lymph system and reach their maximum level about five hours after a meal.

An early investigator to explore the postprandial effects of fat on the blood was Swank (127), who fed hamsters heavy cream and observed the effects on their erythrocytes. In a few hours the chlomicrons caused the erythrocytes to adhere to each other and to aggregate into irregular and rouleaux formations. As the aggregation increased, the circulation slowed, stopping entirely in some capillaries. Nine to twelve hours later the clumping began to reverse; in seventy-two hours circulation was again normal. Measurements of available oxygen in brain tissues revealed a significant reduction in oxygenation—after six hours the oxygen level was 68 percent of normal. When the same test was repeated with a fat-free meal of equivalent calories and bulk, the maximum reduction in oxygen level was 5 percent.

## Precipitation of angina by ingestion of fats

Could a high-fat meal precipitate an angina attack by lowering the oxygen-carrying capacity of the blood? Kuo (84) tested this possibility with fourteen angina patients. After an overnight fast, each subject drank a glass of heavy cream, then rested while half-hour blood samples were drawn.

In five hours, the influx of chylomicrons had caused the transparent fasting blood to become six times more turbid on a plasma lactescence scale. By the time of peak lactescence, fourteen angina attacks occurred and were confirmed by electrocardiographic findings. Nearly identical lactescence curves for thirteen of the fourteen angina patients indicated a consistency in their reaction to excess fat. The same patients on another morning drank a fat-free liquid of identical calories and bulk. After five hours of monitoring, there was no increased turbidity, no angina, and no abnormality in their EKGs.

Williams (146) confirmed Kuo's experiment and showed that aggregation of erythrocytes occurred concurrently with the ischemic EKGs and angina attacks. He concluded that increased red cell agglutination following ingestion of fat was a major contributor to cardiac ischemia, coronary insufficiency, and anginal pain.

## Unsaturated fat no less harmful

In January 1961 the American Heart Association (2) published its recommendations on fats in the diet, advocating an increased ratio of polyunsaturated to saturated fats while keeping total fat intake at about the same level.

Just how beneficial are the polyunsaturates? Friedman (48) compared the effects of saturated and polyunsaturated fats on microcirculation by photographing conjunctival capillaries while monitoring blood lipids. The expected sludging and capillary blockage did indeed occur for many of the forty-four healthy subjects who ingested a cream drink following an overnight fast. On another day, the same subjects were given a safflower oil drink of equivalent fat content; the same erythrocyte aggregation and capillary blockage occurred. To complicate matters, the safflower drink elevated four-hour postprandial triglycerides and kept them high longer than did the butterfat drink.

Friedman's work demonstrated that total fat intake was more important than the degree of saturation. Although his study was completed in 1965, official enthusiasm for polyunsaturated fat diets has somehow increased in the intervening years.

## LOW-FAT DIETS

### Benefits demonstrated by population on low-fat diets

By strictly limiting total fat intake, erythrocyte aggregation can be prevented. Bantu children in South Africa, whose diet includes only 10 percent of total calories as fat, were challenged with a heavy cream drink. Walker (141), the investigator, reported that their peak triglyceride value at three hours was 78 mg./percent—about the fasting level for New York children of the same age. Bantus of all ages were found to have consistently low blood lipid levels, and were thus free from the consequences of tissue anoxia caused by erythrocyte aggregation. Kuo (84) and Williams (146) demonstrated one of these consequences: angina. Others are discussed later.

The benefits of a low-fat diet have also been shown among other populations. The diet of New Guinea natives consists of only 3 percent fat. In a study by Sinnett (118) of almost 800 adult New Guineans, there was no evidence of diabetes or hypertension. There was no measurable increase in blood pressure with age. Cardiovascular disease was essentially absent.

### How low in fat can a diet safely be?

Can a diet with less than 15 percent of total calories as fat result in deficiencies? The body can produce all the fat needed if it takes in a small quantity of linoleic acid; linoleic acid deficiency is rare. How much linoleic acid is actually required? A study by Winitz (147) gives us a good idea. His synthetic food contained only 0.7 percent fat as linoleic acid, 91 percent carbohydrate, 8.3 percent protein, and various vitamins and minerals. For six months, this diet was the sole source of food for his adult male subjects. Extensive testing was done during and after the study; there were no adverse physical or psychological effects and the subjects showed reductions in blood pressure and cholesterol levels.

When this same synthetic diet was given by McKean (93) to phenylketonuric children eight to fifteen years old, gains in height and weight occurred beyond the expected values. For two and one-half years they thrived on this diet. For example, in one year, an eight-year-old and a fourteen-year-old each grew six inches—on a diet containing less than 1 percent fat. Even the high triglyceride level normally expected to appear on a diet rich in glucose did not materialize because of the very low fat content.

In nature, a diet of adequate calories cannot be deficient in fat. Even lettuce has a fat content of over 9 percent. Fat-deficient diets simply do not exist.

## HYPOGLYCEMIA AND EXCESS INTAKE OF RAPIDLY ABSORBED CARBOHYDRATES

Although fats are the primary cause of elevated blood lipids, simple carbohydrates contribute to the effects of fat in raising lipid levels. In the process, they may also produce hypoglycemia. On a diet in which carbohydrates are consumed only as grown and mainly in the complex state, caloric fuel in the form of glucose enters the blood in a slow, steady stream. In an individual consuming 2,900 calories per day, this would provide about two calories per minute around the clock.

Ingestion of excess simple carbohydrates modifies this picture. As they are digested rapidly and quickly absorbed into the bloodstream, there is a sudden influx of glucose to the blood, perhaps 100 calories or more. Pancreatic insulin, however, adapted to handling a steady, slow glucose flow, suddenly has to increase precipitously. Although much of the glucose becomes stored in fat reserves (being in excess of immediate needs), the excess insulin continues for some time to work on blood glucose. Glucose lev-

els can thus be depressed to the hypoglycemic range
before the insulin output returns to normal. With an abnormally low glucose level, the body draws upon fat
reserves for additional fuel. Free fatty acids then enter the
bloodstream. Those in excess of immediate needs are converted into triglycerides by the liver, thereby inducing hyperlipidemia. Both hypoglycemia and hyperlipidemia can
thus be produced by excess simple carbohydrates.

The most effective way to avoid such violent metabolic
swings is to avoid simple carbohydrates and to consume a
diet high in unrefined carbohydrates. To be most effective
in providing the body with a slow, steady stream of metabolic fuel, unrefined carbohydrates should comprise 70
percent or more of the daily caloric intake.

Yet, therapy for hypoglycemia favors a high-protein
diet. Rabinowitz (110) tested eight normal women using
three different meals. A high-protein meal consisting of
27 percent protein, 31 percent fat, and 42 percent carbohydrate produced a peak insulin level twice as high as a
100-gram glucose drink. Such a meal is similar to that
recommended for hypoglycemia diets. Grasso (58) confirmed Rabinowitz's results in tests with premature infants.

## HYPERGLYCEMIA: CHEMICAL DIABETES INDUCED BY EXCESS FATS

Normal metabolism can be so disrupted by a diet high
in fat intake as to produce a chemical diabetic state. A fat
infusion can produce this effect in hours.

### Felber creates diabetics in two hours

The ability of fat to stimulate the diabetic state was
demonstrated by Felber (43), who gave five normal
young men a lipid infusion that raised free fatty acids
from an average of 500 to 700 $\mu$Eq per liter. The level of
700 is similar to that of many normals on the Western
diet. The fat infusions were started two hours before a
glucose tolerance test (GTT) and continued throughout

the test. Glucose and insulin levels were measured in advance and were identical to previous normal tests. With ingestion of the glucose, due to the elevated free fatty acids, the GTT had become diabetic and insulin peaked 50 percent higher. In these normal subjects, as fat levels increased, insulin sensitivity decreased. When blood lipids were high, even a 50 percent elevation in insulin failed to keep the glucose level in the normal range.

## Sweeney creates diabetics in two days

Sweeney (128) tested groups of young medical students on different dietary regimens. One group's diet was high in protein; another's was high in fat; a third group received no food; a fourth group was fed a high-carbohydrate diet. A GTT was made after two days. The high-protein group tested borderline diabetic; the high-fat and starvation groups were both quite diabetic (their two-hour postglucose blood values exceeded 170 mg./percent). Only the high-carbohydrate group tested normal.

## Anderson creates diabetics in two weeks

Anderson's diet (3) took two weeks to raise the lipid level high enough to stimulate diabetes. Two diets utilizing corn oil as fat and sucrose as carbohydrate were used with twenty-year-old normal men. After two weeks, the group on the 80 percent sucrose–5 percent fat diet tested normal by GTT. The other group, on a diet of 20 percent sucrose–65 percent fat, tested diabetic, with a two-hour GTT reading of 184 mg./percent. Those on the 5 percent fat diet stayed on it for seven more weeks; their GTTs at the end of the test were still normal. It is thus seen that, even with a diet high in simple carbohydrates, a low-fat content would seem to be effective in maintaining normal GTT responses. An undesirable feature of this diet was the steadily increasing triglyceride level.

# DIABETES REVERSED ON LOW-FAT DIETS

### *Rabinowitch leads the way*

Rabinowitch (109), a pioneer Canadian investigator, demonstrated the critical effect of fat intake in reversing the diabetic state. He became convinced that the then popular diabetes diet of 56 percent of total calories as fat was much too high in fat. He consequently reduced the level to 21 percent and put 1,000 diabetics on such a regimen for five years. Early in this period, he started a clinical trial with a selected group of one hundred insulin-dependent diabetics, placing fifty on the 21 percent fat diet, while the other fifty remained on the 56 percent fat diet. After five years, these were the results: on the low-fat diet, 24 percent were free of insulin, compared to 8 percent on the high-fat diet. For the low-fat group, the daily insulin dose of those still needing it had been reduced by an average of 58 percent. In the high-fat group, insulin doses remained virtually unchanged. The low-fat group also had less atherosclerosis, as well as a 20 percent lower cholesterol level.

### *Later investigations follow the lead*

Singh (117) placed eighty newly diagnosed diabetics on a sugar-free, 12 percent fat diet. In six weeks, 62 percent no longer required insulin; by eighteen weeks, 72 percent tested normal. The remainder were satisfactorily sustained on minimal insulin doses. Gulati (61) recently showed similar results on a sugar-free, 15 percent fat diet. In 50 percent of the diabetics, reductions of two to eight units of insulin per day were noted; levels of serum triglycerides and free fatty acids dropped significantly.

Kiehm (79) placed thirteen male diabetics on a 9 percent fat diet with 75 percent carbohydrates (mostly unrefined). After two weeks, nine no longer required medication and one was on reduced dosage. Medication was unchanged for the three patients who initially required forty or more units of insulin daily. The investigators concluded: "A high carbohydrate diet with generous amounts of dietary fiber may be the treatment of choice of diabetic patients requiring sulfonylureas or less than thirty units of insulin per day."

At the Pritikin Longevity Centers, patients are placed on a twenty-six day diet and exercise program. Dietary intake, as percent of total calories, is approximately 80 percent carbohydrate (mostly unrefined), 13 percent protein, and 7 percent fat. Preliminary analysis of the Center's experience with 884 patients in 1976–77 showed significant reduction in drug use over the twenty-six days. Of twenty-two maturity-onset diabetics, eleven (50 percent) were off insulin and nine of the remaining eleven were on reduced dosage. Of thirty-two diabetics on oral agents, twenty-six (81 percent) were drug-free by the end of the program.

If diabetes is readily reversible with a low-fat diet, why isn't such diet therapy widely used? West (144) relates his experience. In 1960, he doubled the carbohydrate intake, under isocaloric conditions, of a severely diabetic patient. He noted that no additional insulin was required to maintain the same blood glucose, and later wrote: "In the process of preparing a publication of this 'discovery,' I was surprised to find that very similar experiments had been done before 1935 by Himsworth, with the same results. Over and over again, this phenomenon had been rediscovered and subsequently forgotten or discarded. . . . Clinicians in India have often prescribed diets, with apparent success, that contain more than 70 percent of the calories as carbohydrates. . . . Yet most Western clinicians, dieticians and their patients believe that limiting dietary carbohydrates is the main purpose of diet therapy."

## Alleviation of symptoms of diabetics

Although it is encouraging to note the favorable chemical results with diabetics on low-fat diets, a question remains as to what effects such diets have on the symptomatology of the disease. Van Eck (138) was able to arrest and reverse retinopathy by lowering dietary fat. The correlation of retinopathy with platelet aggregation, and of platelet aggregation with dietary fat, had been demonstrated by the works of Dobbie (40) and Iacano

(70). Dobbie showed that the mean platelet aggregation index of normals is 50 percent that of diabetics with retinopathy. He further noted that the severity of retinopathy correlated significantly with the degree of platelet aggregation. Iacano placed normals on a 25 percent fat diet instead of their usual 40 percent fat intake. Not only did blood pressure and cholesterol levels drop, but there was a 50 percent reduction in platelet aggregation. When their usual diet was resumed, the platelet aggregation returned to previous levels.

Vracko (139) argues that a major threat to diabetics, basement membrane thickening in capillaries which causes microangiopathy and glomerulosclerosis, could be initiated by tissue anoxia. His hypothesis that ischemia could be the cause of basement membrane thickening appeared speculative until the work of Finney (45) was considered.

Finney introduced a dilute infusion of hydrogen peroxide into arteries of ischemic extremities. The oxygen released was equivalent to six atmospheres in a hyperbaric chamber. The resulting hyperoxygenation was found to reduce atherosclerotic plaques and lessen by 40 percent the thickness of basement membranes in diabetics in three to four weeks. In many cases this was sufficient to bring the membrane thickness into the normal range.

## EXCESS CHOLESTEROL AND ATHEROSCLEROSIS

The high cholesterol content of the Western diet is an additional problem. Western dietary intake continually produces cholesterol levels exceeding 200 mg./percent which provides the blood environment for increased risk of cardiovascular disease. In populations where cardiovascular disease is rare, cholesterol levels typically range between 100 and 150 mg./percent.

### Primate studies implicate cholesterol in the etiology of atherosclerotic plaques

Cholesterol levels of primates are similar to those in man. Dietary research with primates closely simulates results with humans. Primates, therefore, are ideal animals for atherosclerosis experiments. Wissler (148) and Armstrong (4) conducted landmark experiments with rhesus monkeys. Wissler placed one group on the Western diet, another on a reduced-fat, moderate-cholesterol diet. After two years, those on the Western diet had significantly higher cholesterol levels and significantly more arterial damage. Armstrong put one group of monkeys on a 40 percent fat, high-cholesterol diet. They untimately developed high serum cholesterol and an average 50 percent closure of the coronary arteries. To measure possible reversal of atherosclerosis, some of the group were then placed on a 42 percent unsaturated-fat diet, the balance on a 4 percent fat diet. While serum cholesterol of both subgroups returned to normal, arterial closures in the low-fat group showed more improvement than in the unsaturated-fat group. A control group which had been on a cholesterol-free low-fat diet for five years showed no significant arterial damage.

## Evidence on etiology of atherosclerosis from the past

Hints as to the role of rich diets in atherosclerosis extend back to antiquity. Moss (99) noted that mummies exhumed from Egyptian tombs were found to have plaque-filled arteries.

In the last thirty years the weight of evidence has implicated cholesterol and fats in the etiology of atherosclerotic plaques. The first clues (Hellerstein, 66) appeared during World War II in countries where food was rationed. Before 1939 they had been consuming a typical Western diet: 40 percent of total calories as fat and 600 or more mg. of cholesterol per day. During the war, even though total calories were maintained, fat was cut below 25 percent and daily cholesterol intake fell below 300 mg. Cardiovascular deaths soon declined, dropping from 20 to 50 percent. As soon as rationing was lifted, the trend reversed and cardiovascular deaths soon regained and exceeded their prewar levels.

Barnes (10) reviewed over 24,000 autopsies in Austria. He found seven times more coronary infarcts in 1958 than in 1944 and 1945. The stress of war might have been expected to cause an increase in deaths due to coronary disease. If stress was a factor, it failed to have any measurable impact on mortality.

# STUDIES CORRELATING ELEVATED CHOLESTEROL LEVELS WITH ATHEROSCLEROSIS

### The Framingham study—5,200 cases

Perhaps the largest study in this country showing an association of cholesterol levels with cardiovascular disease was started in 1948 in Framingham, Massachusetts. Over 5,000 men and women, all initially free of circulatory disease, were given physical examinations every two years. In the 30-to-49-year age group, persons with serum cholesterol levels of 260 mg./percent or higher were found in time to have four times the number of cardiovascular events as those with cholesterol levels at or below 220 mg./percent. The report by Kannel (74) also showed a similar elevation in the risk of cerebrovascular events.

### Ancel Keys's seven-country study—13,000 men

Keys (76) studied almost 13,000 men around the world for a period of years and confirmed the relationship indicated by the Framingham study. For example, he found an eight times higher rate of coronary heart disease in Finland than in Japan, while finding that Finland had seven times more men with high cholesterol levels (over 260 mg./percent) than Japan.

### Rosenman's triglyceride and cholesterol study— 3,200 men

Triglyceride level as an independent factor in etiology of atherosclerosis was demonstrated by Rosenman (111) in the early 1960s. About 3,200 men aged 39 to 59 in the San Francisco area were followed. After 4½ years, the findings were these: Those with cholesterol levels about 260 mg./percent had a four times greater incidence of coronary heart disease than those with levels below 200 mg./percent. Those with triglyceride levels of more than 176 mg./percent had almost three times the risk of coronary disease as those with levels under 100 mg./percent.

## International Atherosclerosis Project—22,000 autopsies

The International Atherosclerosis Project reported by McGill (92) was a mammoth program involving the gathering of autopsy data from fifteen cities in fourteen nations. It involved over 22,000 autopsies of persons aged 10 to 69 who died in 1960–65. To standardize the data, the same pathologists did all of the analysis. Findings were: 1) plaque damage was directly proportional to cholesterol level; 2) intimal plaque damage was proportional to coronary heart disease; and 3) surface area damaged by plaques was directly proportional to dietary intake of fats and cholesterol. The findings did not vary with race, vocation, climate, or population.

## Populations on low-fat diets have low incidence of atherosclerosis

The low incidence of atherosclerosis in populations on low-fat diets has been widely observed. The coronary heart disease rate of the Bantus (who live on a 10 percent fat diet) is almost zero. Hannah (63) reports that at one African hospital, no Bantu deaths were ascribed to coronary heart disease. In autopsies performed on forty-two Bantus and twenty-two Europeans who died suddenly for any reason, only one Bantu had atherosclerosis whereas all of the Europeans—even one youth of fifteen—had extensive damage. Of the forty-two Bantus, thirty-five lacked even a trace of a fatty streak on the intima—the earliest clinical sign of arterial damage. The cholesterol levels of the Bantus range from 90 mg./percent to 120 mg./percent.

Whyte (145) observed natives of New Guinea whose diet contained 10 percent fat and 7 percent protein. Cholesterol levels for both young and old were found to run about 100 mg./percent. Blood pressure did not rise with age; diastolic pressure was found to be somewhat lower among persons in their sixties. Autopsies performed on 600 persons revealed only one case of death attributable to coronary heart disease.

Leaf (85) studied a population in Ecuador with an unusual number of old people. Of the 800 villagers, a number were over 100 years old, as authenticated by church records. The diet was mainly unrefined carbohydrates: corn, brown rice, beans, various vegetables and fruits, with animal protein once a week. Average cholesterol level of a mature adult was 150 mg./percent; cardiovascular disease was virtually nonexistent. The pattern of the findings of this study was one becoming increasingly familiar to investigators: low-fat, low-cholesterol diet; low serum cholesterol; and a low incidence of cardiovascular disease.

Keys (75) has studied over twenty-five populations on low-fat diets; without exception, their serum cholesterol levels were low as were their heart-disease rates. However, reduction of risk in coronary heart disease would seem to last only as long as the low-fat diet was maintained. Thus, Japanese in new environments with higher-fat diets showed corresponding changes in cholesterol levels and coronary-disease death rates. In Japan, fat intake was 10 percent of total calories; in Hawaii, 30 percent of total calories; and in Los Angeles, 40 percent of total calories. The comparable coronary heart-disease death rates for Japanese and Caucasians in Los Angeles suggests that genetic factors have little association with the lower death rate exhibited by Japanese in their homeland.

## Prediction of coronary heart disease: three variables give 98 percent accuracy

Serum cholesterol has proven remarkably successful as an indicator of coronary heart disease risk as confirmed by motion-picture angiography. Welch (143) studied 723 men under forty, all of whom underwent cinecoronary angiography because of chest pain. Of the patients, 49 percent were found to have an average of two main branches of the coronary arteries significantly narrowed—that is, with more than 50 percent of the lumen closed. The percent of closure was found to be directly related to serum cholesterol levels. Serum cholesterol was thus shown to have a high order of accuracy in predicting atherosclerotic damage. Electrocardiographic results were considerably less accurate in diagnosis.

Page (102) used three risk factors: age, triglyceride level, and serum cholesterol. He found that a cholesterol level of 140 mg./percent and a triglyceride level of 60 mg./percent were associated with only 0.5 percent artery damage in men aged twenty-eight. But with a cholesterol level of 360 mg./percent and a triglyceride level of 540 mg./percent, the prevalence of artery damage at the same age rose to 73 percent.

To check the reliability of his data, Page did a predictive double-blind test on sixty new patients. Only age, cholesterol, and triglyceride levels were used in the predictions. When a comparison was made between his predictions and the angiograms which had been done independently, the predictive value proved to be 98 percent, with only one person in the group of sixty incorrectly diagnosed.

Page's conclusion based on his human angiographic studies confirmed the work of Wissler (148): "The percent of aortic surface involved with plaques was closely correlated with the serum cholesterol."

## PREVENTION OF CARDIOVASCULAR DISEASE: DIAGNOSIS OR DIET?

The high lipid levels accepted as "normal" among persons on the Western diet are probably looked upon with complacency because it is widely believed that our diagnostic procedures and medical technology make it possible to alert us to incipient cardiovascular disease before serious damage results. But even thorough physical exams may fail to warn us in time. A study by Pepine (106) illustrates this. He had observed that 30 percent of navy men dying of natural causes were under 40 years old and had no history of cardiovascular disease—yet this was the principal postmortem finding. He recruited forty-one navy and marine fliers, all under forty and certified to be in excellent health by military diagnostic tests. His plan was to

take these asymptomatic subjects and run angiograms on
them every two years to monitor any developing coronary
heart disease. His base-line findings were unexpected:
nineteen of the forty-one supposedly healthy men had advanced coronary heart disease; sixteen of them had two or
three coronary arteries that were more than 50 percent
blocked. Two years later, three of the subjects suffered
myocardial infarcts and, upon recatheterization, four others were found to have worsened.

By the time physical exams discover the presence of
heart disease, the disease may be too far advanced.

## Plaque regression in humans

Can atherosclerotic plaques be arrested and even reversed? The evidence suggests that they can be, and by
simple dietary means. Morrison (97) demonstrated this in
a twelve-year study using patients with a history of
myocardial infarction. Two closely matched groups of 50
each were put on different diets. The controls stayed on
the usual Western diet while the experimental group restricted its intake of fat to 15 percent of total calories and
of cholesterol to 100 mg.daily. Both groups started with
cholesterol levels averaging 312 mg./percent and triglycerides of 236 mg./percent. After the first year, the low-
fat group averaged 200 mg./percent for cholesterol and
120 mg./percent for triglycerides, while the controls were
unchanged. At the end of the twelve years, the entire control group had died but 38 percent of the low-fat group
was still alive.

Lyons (88) studied 280 patients with histories of
myocardial infarction. He placed 155 on a low-fat, low-
cholesterol diet and 125 continued their Western diet.
Four years later, those on the Western diet had suffered
four times the mortality and four times as many coronary
events as those on the low-fat diet.

Blankenhorn (23) used computer techniques to analyze angiographic images of twenty-five patients with
femoral atherosclerosis. Nine demonstrated regression;
their average cholesterol level was 22 percent lower than
those whose atheroma progressed.

In a case study, Basta (12) described nearly complete

regression of atherosclerotic lesions in the right renal artery of a forty-nine-year-old woman. This improvement was gained by long-term control of hyperlipidemia through diet and drug therapy.

### Lowering of cholesterol level by diet

Since serum cholesterol is so accurate a predictor of arterial damage, lowering it to safe levels is a must. How difficult is it to bring cholesterol into a safe range? Beveridge (18) noted that cholesterol levels are promptly lowered when fat and cholesterol intake is reduced. Regardless of their age, sex, or race, 95 percent of his subjects reacted rapidly to a fat- and cholesterol-free diet. When Beveridge (19) placed forty subjects on a fat- and cholesterol-free diet, their average serum cholesterol reduced from an initial level of 200 mg./percent to 150 mg./percent in just four days. Beveridge repeated the study with a group of students. Then, to demonstrate the opposite effect, he increased their dietary fat and cholesterol in a stepwise manner. Serum cholesterol levels followed accordingly, exhibiting a classical dose-response relationship.

Analysis of the Pritikin Longevity Center's experience during 1976–77 gives the following preliminary results (lipid levels expressed as milligram percent): 1) mean serum cholesterol for 884 patients—235 at admission, 175 at discharge; 2) mean serum cholesterol for 55 patients initially on Atromid-S or Questran—265 at admission, 207 at discharge (drugs discontinued at admission); 3) mean serum triglycerides for 881 patients—174 at admission, 132 at discharge; and 4) mean serum triglycerides for 54 patients initially on Atromid-S or Questran—201 at admission, 158 at discharge (drugs discontinued at admission). In general, patients with higher initial levels experienced greater decreases in their serum lipids. For example, patients arriving with cholesterol levels below 160 averaged a 9.6 percent decrease, while those arriving with levels exceeding 320 averaged a 36 percent decrease. The model class (220–240) had a 24.8 percent decrease.

## Dangers of adding polyunsaturates to the diet

The use of polyunsaturated-fat diets to lower serum cholesterol carries risks and doubtful benefits. Friedman (48) demonstrated that unsaturated fats interfere with circulation as effectively as saturated fats. Grundy (60) has shown that the reduction in serum cholesterol levels associated with polyunsaturates is due in part to a transference of cholesterol from the plasma into body tissues. Bischoff (22) had warned of the inherent danger of this situation by showing that cholesterol crystals can act as a solid-state carcinogen in animals and humans. Dayton's (39) eight-year controlled clinical dietary trial of saturated vs. polyunsaturated fats resulted in a higher cancer mortality and a 2.5 times increase of gallstone disease for those on polyunsaturates. These figures, although interesting, were not statistically significant because of the small numbers involved.

The American Heart Association recommends increasing the dietary ratio (P/S ratio) of polyunsaturates to saturated fats. An ongoing mass test of these recommendations is actually taking place in Israel, where much of the diet is a model of the AHA recommendations. A test of these recommendations was funded by the U.S. Department of Agriculture to evaluate the benefits of the Israeli diet as compared to the diet of West Germany. The latter diet is low in polyunsaturates but high in saturated fats. It was assumed that a higher cardiovascular mortality would be associated with the West German diet. Such, however, was not the case. The data, gathered abroad, analyzed at the Rockefeller Institute, and reported by Blondheim (24), indicated that Israel had a higher cardiovascular death rate than West Germany. Blondheim noted that the expected benefits of the Israeli diet and the harmful effects of the West German diet failed to materialize; the data appeared to contradict accepted hypotheses.

Israeli research includes investigation of disease among Bedouin tribesmen (82). The Bedouins, gradually acculturating to the life-style of their fellow Israelis, are also acquiring their diseases—especially coronary heart disease. This is particularly noticeable among Bedouins living in close contact with Jewish communities, much less so among those living a traditional life-style in relative isolation. The former have adopted a high-fat (mostly polyunsaturated) Western diet; the latter retain their low-fat (mostly saturated) traditional diet. This evidence tends to support the hypothesis that total fat is more important than P/S ratio in the etiology of coronary disease.

## Recommended diet for lowering blood lipids to safe levels

What specific dietary recommendations should be followed to prevent, to arrest, and possibly to reverse atherosclerosis? Based on the overwhelming evidence, these should be as follows: reduce fat intake to less than 15 percent of total calories; limit cholesterol to 100 mg. daily; minimize simple carbohydrates. These rules would make it possible to bring serum lipids into a truly safe range—below 160 mg./percent for cholesterol and below 80 mg./percent for triglycerides. This range is lower than that considered normal today in the United States. The so-called "normal" range has been a passport to disability and death for too many persons.

## Carbohydrates and dietary fiber

These dietary recommendations automatically deliver an important bonus: the large amount of fiber present in unprocessed carbohydrates.

The important role of dietary fiber, or "roughage," has not been appreciated. Insufficient dietary fiber, the indigestible fraction of unprocessed carbohydrates, has been implicated as a substantial factor in the degenerative diseases by Hill, Burkitt, Trowell (68), and others. Its role in diverticular disease and colitis has been so convincing that wheat bran is the treatment of choice for diverticulitis in England. Burkitt has written that "the most likely cause of bowel tumors seems to be carcinogens produced by bacterial action of the normal intestinal flora on bile salts."

This is a special problem for those on the Western diet since the high fat content requires a greater secretion of bile. Fecal concentrations of bile and steroids on a

Western diet were shown to be eleven times higher than on a low-fat, high-unrefined-carbohydrate diet. The high fiber content of unprocessed carbohydrates results in a much faster transit time (from ingestion to evacuation). The typical eighty- to ninety-hour transit time of a Western diet is reduced to thirty-five hours. Thus, if bile-derived carcinogens are formed, their contact with bowel tissues would be relatively brief.

### Exercise as an adjunct to diet in reversing athero-sclerosis

Cardiovascular conditions associated with atheromatous plaques are subject to dramatic improvement with the appropriate dietary changes. Improvement is especially facilitated when physical activity is added to the regimen. A systematic, carefully supervised walking or jogging program helps to develop collateral circulation and hasten cardiovascular improvement. Restoring circulation in the coronary arteries can relieve angina; restoring circulation in the renal arteries can reduce hypertension. Hunt's study with one hundred hypertensives (69) demonstrated how this could be done surgically; a low-fat diet plus exercise may achieve similar results nonsurgically.

Boyer (25) placed twenty-three hypertensive men from forty-two to sixty years old on an exercise program (one hour twice weekly for six months with no dietary changes) and achieved significant blood pressure reductions. Kidera (78) applied a walking-and-running exercise regimen to airline pilots who were experiencing ischemic ST-wave depressions on their EKGs. The EKGs were brought back to normal and remained there three years later. Hellerstein (66) has had good results since 1958 with his physical activity program for coronary patients.

# OTHER DEGENERATIVE DISEASES AND THE WESTERN DIET

### Gallstone formation and diet

Many studies have demonstrated the association between a high-fat diet and fatty infiltration of the liver. Linscheer (86) showed how a lithogenic bile is associated with a fatty liver. Sunzel (126) observed that the liver triglycerides of twenty-five patients undergoing cholecystectomy were eight times higher than normal and that all had the fatty livers closely associated with gallstones. Bischoff (22), in turn, implicated gallstones in the etiology of gallbladder cancer.

### Elevated uric acid levels in gouty arthritis

Elevated uric acid is another condition which is responsive to dietary change. Feldman (44) and Berkowitz (17) have each reported on the rise of uric acid in relation to the high intake of fats in the Western diet; the mechanism has been clarified by Alderman (1). The significance of raised uric acid levels appears in Hall's (62) population study. He found that with uric acid levels of 6–7 mg./percent, 2 percent had gouty arthritis; at 7 to 8 mg./percent, 12 percent had gouty arthritis; and above 8 mg./percent, 36 percent were arthritic.

## TISSUE ANOXIA: A BASIC FEATURE IN MANY DEGENERATIVE DISEASES

The tissue anoxia produced by elevated lipid levels is fundamentally involved in a wide range of degenerative diseases.

*In atherosclerosis:* Tissue anoxia in atherosclerosis is associated with increased permeability of arterial walls that develop in oxygen-deficient environments. This permits lipids and cholesterol readily to penetrate the walls, thereby increasing anoxia. The feedback mechanism then accelerates the development of atheromatous plaques. Astrup (6) reported that lowering blood-oxygen levels only

15 to 20 percent produced increased permeability and subintimal edema, which deposited two and one-half to five times more cholesterol on the arterial wall than in controls whose oxygen levels were unchanged. Astrup also reported that other anoxic agents, such as carbon monoxide from cigarettes, may also contribute to increased arterial permeability.

*In angina:* The magnitude of the anoxic effect of smoking on ten angina patients was measured by Aronow (5). Non-nicotine cigarettes were smoked until carboxyhemoglobin levels reached 8 percent; oxygen available to the myocardium decreased proportionately. On a standardized exercise protocol, the patients experienced angina pains 25 percent sooner than they did on nonsmoking days.

*In fibrillation:* Bellet (16) found that a moderate lowering of blood oxygen induced ventricular fibrillation in dogs 40 percent sooner than when blood oxygen was not lowered.

*In senility:* General symptoms of senility, including memory loss, can be improved by oxygen inhalation, as in Jacobs's (71) study. However, the reversal of symptoms disappears a few days after withdrawal of treatment. Could anoxia be a factor in schizophrenia? Gordon (57) tested cerebral oxygen uptake in schizophrenics and found that twenty-one of twenty-four had a subnormal uptake.

*In visual field loss:* Reduction of the visual field is often considered an inevitable consequence of aging. Wolf (149) demonstrated that this loss had an anoxic base. He had twenty-year-old subjects breathe air of reduced oxygen content. In ten minutes their visual fields narrowed to the size characteristic of sixty-year-olds. Reversing this process, Johnson (72) persuaded habitual smokers to quit for two weeks. As their circulation was now free of the deoxygenation effects of carbon monoxide, they had a 36 percent enlargement of the visual field. Loss of visual field with age may now be explainable in terms of increased blood lipids, which reduce the oxygen-carrying capacity of the blood.

*In hearing loss:* Depressed blood oxygen levels may also be associated with hearing loss. Zelman (152) carefully matched 126 smokers and 126 nonsmokers and found that the smokers had more hearing loss at each frequency, especially the higher ones. He suspected that the reduced oxygen-carrying capacity of the blood from carboxyhemoglobin made the difference; this was confirmed by Miyake (94), who restored hearing loss by increasing oxygen tension in the blood.

*In malignancy development:* Tissue anoxia is known to interfere with normal cell metabolism. Goldblatt (55) was able to produce malignant cells from normal cells *in vitro* by lowering the oxygen content of their environment. Warburg (142) demonstrated that a 35 percent reduction of oxygen was capable of producing malignant cells. Malignant cells propagate poorly in an oxygen-rich environment. Exner (42) has used this principle successfully in treating skin cancer with hydrogen peroxide, whereby a highly oxygenated environment selectively destroys only the cancerous tissue.

Chapman (35) demonstrated that beta-lipoprotein can inhibit the phagocytotic activity of macrophages with respect to tumor cells. He was able to replicate his results by pretreating macrophages with cholesterol alone.

A high-fat diet with resulting tissue anoxia may contribute to the risk of lung cancer. Stamler's (124) study of 876 cigarette smokers indicated that persons with cholesterol levels over 275 mg./percent had a seven fold greater risk of lung cancer than those with levels below 225 mg./percent.

*In rheumatoid arthritis:* Synovial anoxia is a necessary condition for the development or rheumatoid arthritis. Lund-Oleson (87) measured more than 120 synovial fluid samples from the knees of patients and found that those with rheumatoid arthritis had average oxygen levels of 30 percent of normal, some with no measurable oxygen. Those with oxygen levels of 25 percent or less could not bear weight on their joints. Gilly (51) treated severe arthritis with oxygen at two or three atmospheres and was able to reverse inflammation and joint immobility until the effects of the oxygen wore off and the arthritis symptoms returned.

*In hypertension:* Provisional analysis of the Pritikin Longevity Center's 1976–77 experience indicates the following: 1) mean systolic blood pressure for 535 normotensive patients—117.1 at admission, 110.6 at discharge; 2) mean diastolic for the normotensives—69.4 at admission, 64.4 at discharge; 3) mean systolic blood pressure for 315 diagnosed hypertensive patients—137.6 at admission, 132.4 at discharge; 4) mean diastolic blood pressure for the hypertensives—78.1 at admission, 73.5 at discharge. At admission, there were a total of 218 persons on hypotensive medication; at discharge, 186 (85 percent) were no longer on medication, and were normotensive.

# CONCLUSIONS AND RECOMMENDATIONS

## Concept of lipotoxemia*

As people on the Western diet age, their blood lipid levels rise. As they rise, blood oxygen levels are depressed. The resulting anoxia is associated with a variety of degenerative diseases from the least catastrophic, such as impaired hearing, to life-threatening myocardial infarctions and ventricular fibrillation.

This one etiology—excess serum lipids associated with the fat and cholesterol intake of the Western diet—appears to be responsible, at least in part, for many of the conditions generally regarded as distinct disease. Atherosclerosis, hypertension, diabetes, gout, arthritis, gallstones and other degenerative states should not be viewed as separate disease entities, but as the symptoms of a single disease. This disease can be thought of as a poisoning of the blood by elevated fat and cholesterol. Thus, "lipotoxemia" is the disease, and the degenerative diseases are the principle symptoms. That is why one diet can reverse the many symptoms, since it reverses "lipotoxemia," the plague of the developed nations.

## Dietary implications of the studies

The foregoing analysis provides a rationale for the nutritional recommendations of the Pritikin Longevity Cen-

* A one-hour tape cassette is available from Pritikin Research Foundation, P.O. Box 5335, Santa Barbara, CA 93108, for $5.95.

ter's diet, which are translated into practical suggestions for patients' daily diets. These suggestions stem from the following general formula:

Fats—10 percent of total calories (maximum)
Cholesterol—100 mg. per day (maximum)
Omit—simple carbohydrates such as sugar, honey, molasses, and syrup
Omit—salt (except as already present in prepared foods, e.g., canned or frozen)
Omit—highly processed foods
Emphasize—fresh fruits, vegetables, whole grains, legumes, and tubers

## Blood tests: criteria for normality

The foregoing also provides the basis for revised criteria or normality for blood tests, as follows:

| Test | Pritikin Longevity Center Standard (per 100 ml) | General Population Standard* (per 100 ml) |
|---|---|---|
| Total lipids | <525 mg | 450–1,000 mg |
| Serum cholesterol | <160 mg | <315 mg† |
| Serum triglycerides | <100 mg | <135 mg |
| Glucose | <100 mg | 70–110 mg |
| Hemoglobin | | |
| Men | 10.5–15 gm | 13–18 gm |
| Women | 10.0–14 gm | 11–16 gm |
| Uric acid | | |
| Men | <7.0 mg | 4.0–8.5 mg |
| Women | <6.0 mg | 2.8–7.5 mg |

* Per Bioscience Labs., Van Nuys, Calif.
† At age 40.

## II. DISEASES THAT MAY REGRESS ON THE PRITIKIN PROGRAM

### by Hugh Trowell, OBE, MD, FRCP†

  1.   Addison's disease, primary hypocorticalism
\*2.   Angina pectoris
\*3.   Atherosclerosis, all manifestations: hypercholesterolemia and hypertriglyceridemia
  4.   Autoimmune diseases
  5.   Cerebrovascular disease, if due to atherosclerosis\* and hypertension\*
  6.   Crohn's disease
  7.   Deep-vein thrombosis (DVT) and pulmonary embolism
\*8.   Diabetes mellitus, maturity-onset
  9.   Diverticular disease
 10.  Endocrine disease, excluding endemic goiter and neoplasms
 11.  Gallstones, cholesterol, and mixed varieties
 12.  Gout, hyperuricemia
 13.  Hemorrhoids
 14.  Hiatus hernia
\*15.  Hypertension, primary essential hypertension
\*16.  Ischemic heart disease, all manifestations
 17.  Irritable colon syndrome
 18.  Multiple sclerosis (MS)
 19.  Myxedemia
\*20.  Obesity
 21.  Osteitis deformans, Paget's disease
 22.  Osteoarthritis (OA), at certain sites
 23.  Osteoporosis, senile
\*24.  Peripheral vascular disease, atheromatous

---

† Physician at Makere University Medical School, Uganda, 1935–58; Primary witness in Dietary Fiber Hearings, U. S. Senate Select Committee on Nutrition and Human Needs, 1977. Publications: *Kwashiorkor*, 1952, republished by Nutrition Foundation, 1978. *Non-Infective Disease in Africa*, 1960. *Refined Carbohydrate Foods and Disease*, co-edited with D. P. Burkitt, 1975.

\* These diseases have been reported to show significant regression on the program.

25.  Pernicious anemia (PA) and subacute combined
     degeneration
*26.  Rheumatoid arthritis (RA), Still's disease, anky-
     losing spondylitis
*27.  Senile dementia, arteriosclerotic variety
28.  Thyrotoxicosis
29.  Ulcerative colitis (UC)
30.  Varicose veins (VV) and ulcer

If structural changes have occurred in any disease and
are marked, such as the stretched incompetent valves
present in varicose veins, then no regression is likely to
occur. Again, there is no evidence that the diverticula in
diverticular disease decrease in size if bran or high-
cereal-fiber diets are taken, but symptoms improve considerably. In other diseases, like maturity-onset diabetes
mellitus, the structural changes in the organs may not be
marked and then much remission can occur.

A detailed explanation follows.

1.  *Addison's disease,* primary hypocorticalism (8, 32,
    49, 129). See Autoimmune diseases.

4.  *Autoimmune diseases.* Includes Addison's disease,
    Crohn's disease, many endocrine diseases, multiple
    sclerosis, myxedema, pernicious anemia, rheumatoid
    arthritis, primary thyrotoxicosis, Hashimoto's thy-
    roiditis, and probably ulcerative colitis. Epidemiolo-
    gical evidence of rarity in African blacks (8, 32, 49,
    59, 129) and the rise of serum globulins, 1gG and
    1gM (115, 152).

6.  *Crohn's disease.* Epidemiological evidence of rarity
    in African blacks (32, 38, 52, 98, 101), Iran (32),
    India—rural areas (32), and Brazil (32). No ex-
    perimental data or dietary trials have been traced.

7.  *Deep-vein thrombosis and pulmonary embolism.*
    Epidemiological evidence of decreased frequency in
    African blacks (9, 32, 47, 50, 64, 81), also Thai
    women (36) and Andes Plateau inhabitants (34).
    Decreased incidence in Norway during wartime ra-
    tions of low-fat, high-fiber rye bread (125, 137). A
    small amount of experimental data (137), but no
    prospective experiments. In many of the countries
    having low DVT incidence, fibrinolysis is more

rapid than in Western populations (32, 114) but
becomes less rapid if persons from these countries
consume Western diets (11).

9. *Diverticular disease.* Epidemiological evidence from
several continents (32, 104, 134), dietary trials in
man (26), and a recent book on diverticular disease
(103), which summarizes experimental data on man
and animals, relate this disease to a lifelong consumption of low-fiber diets, especially a lack of fiber
derived from cereals.

10. *Endocrine diseases.* Excluding endemic goiter and
neoplasms. Epidemiological evidence of the rarity of
all endocrine diseases is strong (20, 32, 41, 49, 105,
112, 133). See also Addison's disease, myxedema,
and thyrotoxicosis.

11. *Gallstones, cholesterol and mixed-varieties.* Heaton
(32, 65, 107, 136) has discussed the epidemiological and experimental evidence relating cholesterol
gallstones to the consumption of refined low-fiber
carbohydrate foods. Epidemiological evidence from
tropical regions reports decreased incidence but sel-
dom reports separately the common pigment stones.
Some experiments in animals (136) and in man
(107) support the role of fiber-depleted carbohydrate foods.

12. *Gout, hyperuricemia.* Epidemiological evidence from
different ethnic groups in Polynesia (108), also urban and rural South African blacks (13, 14), and
the rarity of the disease in rural African blacks
(77) and its association with diabetes (89, 108) is
well documented. Serum uric acid concentrations
have fallen in patients eating Pritikin diets. No other
experiments or therapeutic trials in man or in animals have been traced.

13. *Hemorrhoids.* Epidemiological evidence of the rarity
of hemorrhoids in African blacks and in certain developing Indian communities is well documented
(31, 32). Anatomical studies suggest that hemorrhoids are produced by hard, small stools pressing
on the venous plexus of the anal cushions (132).
No experimental studies or therapeutic trials have
been traced.

14.  *Hiatus hernia.* Epidemiological data (28, 32) of the great rarity of hiatus hernia in rural African blacks suggests that raised intra-abdominal pressures, associated with straining to defecate small, hard fecal masses, causes hiatus hernia and other "pressure diseases" such as diverticular disease and varicose veins (29). No experimental or therapeutic trials have been traced.

15.  *Hypertension.* The rapid, marked fall of essential hypertension in many patients, even those not losing weight, treated with Pritikin high-unrefined, high-fiber diets, to which no salt is added, has been reported (73) and endorsed in all 1976 monthly Pritikin reports. Epidemiological studies in the world's populations suggest a linear relationship between salt intake and blood pressure (54). Other unidentified dietary factors, also cultural change and industrialization, introduce essential hypertension as a new disease at an early stage of the Westernization of developing countries. Hypertension was rare in rural African blacks in Kenya in the 1920s (133). Currently in Kenya there is much hypertension, and even more in South African and West African blacks and U.S. blacks. In these blacks the disease is more severe and more common than in whites. No experimental or therapeutic trials, except those of the Pritikin diets, have been traced.

17.  *Irritable bowel syndrome.* Epidemiological studies in rural Africans (133) stress the rarity of this disorder, even in urban South African Bantu, examined in Johannesburg's largest gastroenterological clinic (113). A recent controlled trial concluded that high-cereal-fiber diets are the treatment of choice in this disorder. These diets decrease intracolonic pressures and symptoms and accelerate transit (90).

18.  *Multiple sclerosis.* An infective agent, probably viral, appears clearly implicated in the etiology of MS. The presence of MS, albeit of low incidence, in South African whites, but the absence of any recorded case in South African blacks (21) and rarity in other developing communities (27), suggests that, like other autoimmune diseases (*q.v.*), protective

factors exist (27). Whether these factors are high-carbohydrate, high-fiber diets remains speculative. No experimental studies or therapeutic trials have been traced.

19. *Myxedema, also Hashimoto's thyroiditis.* These diseases have not yet been recorded in African blacks, but incidence in U.S. blacks and whites is equal (53, 83, 130). No experimental studies or therapeutic trials have been traced.

20. *Obesity.* Many obese patients eating *ad libitum* Pritikin diets lose weight. It has been postulated that man preserves a slim and healthy body weight if he feeds on his ancient traditional diet, composed largely of high-unrefined, high-fiber plant foods. Food-gatherers/hunters could not have survived if they became obese. The ancient diet of man had a low energy:fiber (E/F) ratio (32). Modern fattening foods, such as sugar and fat, also refined white flour and white rice, have a high E/F ratio. The inhabitants of all developing countries are slim, even when foods, largely unrefined and of low E/F ratio, are consumed freely. There is a close link between diabetes and obesity (135). More observations are required concerning body weight in persons consuming Pritikin diets *ad libitum*. It is considered that these diets may prove those of choice to cure obesity and maintain nonobese body weight.

21. *Osteitis deformans, Paget's disease.* Many radiologists have never seen Paget's disease in an African black; the first case in a Southern African black has been recorded recently (90). Little epidemiological data has been traced and no experimental studies are known.

22. *Osteoarthritis.* Many factors, including such known factors as obesity and occupational trauma, influence OA prevalence, severity, and sites. The hip joint, commonly affected in aging Western populations, is far less commonly attacked in South African blacks (121). Little other epidemiological data has been traced. No experimental data has been found.

23. *Osteoporosis, senile.* Although the average intakes

of calcium in African black adults are 200-500 mg./day and blood calcium levels are a little lower than in Western adults (140), an orthopedic surgeon has estimated that aging blacks experience about one-tenth the fractures of the femoral neck and less collapse of vertebral bodies (120). Little other epidemiological studies and no experimental data have been traced.

24.  *Pernicious anemia, subacute combined degeneration.* PA is a very rare disease in African blacks (46, 67, 95) and subacute combined degeneration even more so (151). No experimental data or therapeutic trials have been traced.

26.  *Rheumatoid arthritis, Still's disease, and ankylosing spondylitis.* Sophisticated prevalence surveys in West Africa and in South Africa have confirmed the rarity and mildness of RA in all African black adults (14, 121). Rural South African blacks eating high-carbohydrate, high-fiber diets had about a quarter of the RA incidence of a comparable urban group of blacks, members of the same tribe, who ate a lower-fiber, partially Westernized diet (15, 121). Concerning RA, no experimental or therapeutic studies have been traced. Rarity of ankylosing spondylitis in African blacks has been confirmed (121).

28.  *Thyrotoxicosis.* Epidemiological evidence, clinical and pathological, emphasizes the rarity of thyrotoxicosis in African blacks of many countries (37, 53, 83, 100, 115, 131). Incidence is increasing in urban groups (53, 115, 150). Incidence in U.S. blacks equals that of U.S. whites. Thyroid autoantibodies are less common in African blacks than in whites (59). No experimental or therapeutic studies have been traced.

29.  *Ulcerative colitis.* Epidemiological evidence of rarity of UC in African blacks (7, 32, 119, 123), also Iranians (56) and Indonesians (154). Many consider that autoimmune factors occur in UC. Experimental studies in baboons have reported that a low-fiber diet caused chronic inflammation of the cecum and sometimes of the colon (80). No controlled trials of high-unrefined carbohydrate foods

rich in fiber in treatment of UC have been reported.

30. *Varicose veins, varicose ulcer.* Epidemiological evidence of the rarity of VV in African blacks (32), in India (30), Pakistan, New Guinea (32), also Thailand (33) and the South Pacific Islands (33), is unchallenged. Raised intra-abdominal pressures, during years of straining to defecate hard stools, have been suggested as a cause (29). No experimental or therapeutic studies have been traced.

# REFERENCES

1. Alderman, M.H., *et al.* 1965. Hyperuricemia in starvation. *Proc. Soc. Exp. Biol. Med.* 118:790.

2. American Heart Association. 1961. Dietary fat and its relation to heart attack and strokes. *Circ.* 23:133–36.

3. Anderson, J. W., *et al.* 1973. Effect of high glucose and high sucrose diets on glucose tolerance of normal men. *Amer. J. Clin. Nutr.* 26:600–607.

4. Armstrong, M. L., *et al.* 1970. Regression of coronary artheromatosis in rhesus monkeys. *Circ. Research* 27:59.

5. Aronow, W. S., *et al.* 1971. Carboxyhemoglobin caused by smoking non-nicotine cigarettes. *Circ.* 44:782–88.

6. Astrup, P. 1973. Carbon monoxide, smoking and cardiovascular disease. *Circ.* 48:1167–68.

7. Awori, N. W., *et al.* 1972. Causes of chronic diarrhea in Kenya and their relationship to ulcerative colitis. *E. Afr. Med. J.* 49:604–13.

8. Bagshawe, A. F., and Forrester, A. T. T. 1966. Addison's disease in Kenya. *E. Afr. Med. J.* 43:525–29.

9. Baker, L. W., and Houlder, A. 1973. Deep vein thrombosis in Bantu and Indian patients. *S. Afr. Med. J.* 47:1689–92.

10. Barnes, B.O., *et al.* 1960. Arteriosclerosis in 10,-000 autopsies and the possible role of dietary protein. *Fed. Proc.* 19:19.

11. Barr, R. D., *et al.* 1973. The blood coagulation

and fibrinolytic enzyme systems in healthy Africans and Europeans. *Scott. Med. J.* 18:93–97.

12. Basta, L. L., *et al.* 1976. Regression of atherosclerotic stenosing lesions of the renal arteries and spontaneous cure of systemic hypertension through control of hyperlipidemia. *Amer. J. Med.* 61:420–23.

13. Beighton, P., *et al.* 1973. Serum uric acid concentrations in a rural Tawana community in Southern Africa. *Ann. Rheum. Dis.* 32:346–50.

14. ———, *et al.* 1974. Serum uric acid concentrations in an urbanized South African Negro population. *Ibid.* 33:442–45.

15. ———, *et al.* 1975. Rheumatoid arthritis in a rural South African Negro population. *Ibid.* 34:136–41.

16. Bellet, S., *et al.* 1970. The effect of cigarette smoke inhalation on the ventricular fibrillation threshold. *Circ.* 42 Sup. 3:135.

17. Berkowitz, D. 1964. Blood lipid and uric acid interrelationships. *JAMA* 190:856–58.

18. Beveridge, J. M. R., *et al.* 1956. Dietary factors affecting the level of plasma cholesterol in humans: The role of fat. *Canad. J. Bio. & Phys.* 34:441.

19. ———, *et al.* 1960. The response of man to dietary cholesterol. *J. Nutr.* 71:61.

20. Billinghurst, T. R. 1966. Intracranial space-occupying lesions in African patients at Mulago Hospital, Kampala. *E. Afr. Med. J.* 43:385–93.

21. Bird, A. V., and Kerrick, J. E. 1969. Multiple sclerosis in South Africa. *S. Afr. Med. J.* 43:1031–33.

22. Bischoff, F., and Bryson, G. 1964. Carcinogenesis through solid state surfaces. *Exp. Tumor Res.* 5:85–133.

23. Blankenhorn, D. H., *et al.* 1978. The rate of atherosclerosis change during treatment of hyperlipoproteinemia. *Circ.* 57:355–61.

24. Blondheim, S. H. 1973. High P/S fat ratio fails to cut Israeli heart ills. *Med. Trib.* Feb. 7.

25. Boyer, J. L., and Hasch, F. W. 1970. Exercise

therapy in hypertensive men. *JAMA* 211:1668–71.

26. Brodribb, A. J. M., and Humphreys, D. M. 1976. Diverticular disease; three studies. *Brit. Med. J.* 1:424–30.

27. Brody, J. 1972. Epidemiology of multiple sclerosis and a possible virus etiology. *Lancet* II: 173–76.

28. Burkitt, D. P., and James, P. A. 1973. Low-residue diets and hiatus hernia. *Ibid.* II:128–30.

29. ———. 1975. Dietary fibre and "pressure diseases." *J. Roy. Coll. Phys.* (London). 9:138–46.

30. ———, *et al.* Varicose veins in India. 1975. *Lancet* II:765.

31. ———, and Graham-Stewart, C. W. 1975. Hemorrhoids—postulated pathogenesis and proposed prevention. *Postgrad. Med. J.* 51:631–36.

32. ———, and Trowell, H. C., eds. 1975. *Refined carbohydrate foods and disease: some implications of dietary fibre.* London: Academic Press.

33. ———, *et al.* 1976. Varicose veins in developing countries. *Lancet* II:202–3.

34. Caen, J. P., *et al.* 1973–74. Thrombosis, platelet behavior, fibrinolytic activity, and diet in the Andes plateau. *Haemostasis* 2:12–20.

35. Chapman, H. A., and Hobbs, J. B. 1977. Modulation of macrophage tumoricidal capability of components of normal serum: a central role for lipid. *Science* 197:282–85.

36. Chumnijarakij, T., and Poshyachinda, V. 1975. Postoperative thrombosis in Thai women. *Lancet* I: 1357–58.

37. Dancaster, C. P. 1970. Thyrotoxicosis in the Bantu, with special reference to myopathy. *S. Afr. Med. J.* 44:695–97.

38. Davis, R., *et al.* 1974. Crohn's disease in Transvaal blacks. *Ibid.* 48:480–586.

39. Dayton, S., *et al.* 1969. A controlled clinical trial of a diet high in unsaturated fat. *Circ.* 62 Supp. 2:1–63.

40. Dobbie, J. G., *et al.* 1973. The role of platelets in pathogenesis of diabetic retinopathy. *Trans. Amer. Acad. Ophthal. Otolaryn.* 77:43–47.

41. Edozien, J. F. 1960. Biochemical normals in Nigerians: urinary steroids. *Lancet* I:258–59.

42. Exner, F. B. 1972. Immunoresistance and radiation therapy. *Med. Tribune,* November 18.

43. Felber, J. P., and Vannotti, A. 1964. Effects of fat infusion on glucose tolerance and insulin plasma levels. *Med. Exp.* 10:1536.

44. Feldman, E. B., *et al.* 1964. Hyperglyceridemia in gout. *Circ.* 29:508.

45. Finney, J. W. 1969. Localized $O_2$ aids ischemic limbs. *JAMA* 207:2363.

46. Forbes, J., and Gordon, J. A. 1969. *Centr. Afr. J. Med.* 18:92.

47. Franz, R. C., *et al.* 1975. The histochemical localization and assay of plasmogen activator in the venous wall. *S. Afr. Med. J.* 49:1423–24.

48. Friedman, M., *et al.* 1965. Effect of unsaturated fats upon lipemia and conjunctival circulation. *JAMA* 193:882–86.

49. Gelfand, M. 1975. The pattern of disease in African and the western way of life. *Centr. Afr. J. Med.* 21:145–52.

50. ———. 1975. Venous thromboembolism in the blacks of Rhodesia. *S. Afr. Med. J.* 49:1432–33.

51. Gilly, R. 1971. Hybaroxia held useful in easing rheumatic joints. *Med. Tribune,* January.

52. Giraud, R. M., *et al.* 1969. Crohn's disease in the Transvaal Bantu. *S. Afr. Med. J.* 43:610–13.

53. Gitau, W. 1975. An analysis of thyroid diseases seen at Kenyatta National Hospital. *E. Afr. Med. J.* 52:564–70.

54. Gleibermann, L. 1973. Blood pressure and dietary salt in human populations. *Ecol. Food & Nutr.* 2:143–56.

55. Goldblatt, H., *et al.* 1953. Induced malignancy in cells from rat myocardium subjected to intermittent anaerobiosis during long propagation *in vitro.* *J. Exp. Med.* 97:525–52.

56. Goligher, J. C., *et al.* 1968. *Ulcerative colitis,* pp. 1–4, 47–61, 265. London: Bailliere, Tindall & Cassell.

57. Gordon, G. S., *et al.* 1955. Cerebral oxygen uptake

in chronic schizophrenic reaction. *Arch. Neurol. Psychiat.* 73:544–55.

58. Grasso, S., *et al.* 1973. Insulin secretion in the premature infant. *Diabetes* 22:349–53.

59. Greenwood, B. M. 1968. Autoimmune disease and parasitic infections in Nigerians. *Lancet* II:380–82.

60. Grundy, S. M., and Ahrens, E. H. 1970. The effects of unsaturated fats on absorption, excretion, synthesis and distribution of cholesterol in man. *J. Clin. Invest.* 49:1135–53.

61. Gulati, P. D., *et al.* 1974. Diet for diabetics. *Lancet* II:297–98.

62. Hall, A. P., *et al.* 1967. Epidemiology of gout and hyperuremia: a long time population study. *Amer. J. Med.* 42:27.

63. Hannah, J. B. 1958. Civilization, race and coronary atheroma with particular reference to its incidence and severity in copperbelt Africans. *Centr. Afr. J. Med.* 4:1–5.

64. Hassan, M. A., *et al.* 1973. Postoperative deep vein thrombosis in Sudanese patients. *Brit. Med. J.* 1:515–17.

65. Heaton, K. W. 1972. *Bile salts in health and disease,* p. 184. Edinburgh: Churchill Livingstone.

66. Hellerstein, H. K. 1967. *Atherosclerotic vascular disease,* p. 115. Salt Lake City: Meredith.

67. Hift, W., and Moshal, M. C. 1973. Pernicious anemialike syndromes in the nonwhite population of Natal. *S. Afr. Med. J.* 47:915–18.

68. Hill, M. J., *et al.* 1971. Bacteria and etiology of cancer of large bowel. *Lancet* I:95–100.

69. Hunt, J. C., *et al.* 1967. Factors determining diagnosis and choice of treatment of renovascular hypertension. *Circ. Res.* 20, Supp. 2:211.

70. Iacono, J. M. 1975. Lipid Research Laboratory, U.S. Department of Agriculture. Beltsville, Md. Private communication.

71. Jacobs, E. 1972. Retaining memory in older people. *Sci. News,* 101:188–89.

72. Johnson, D. M. 1965. Preliminary report of the effect of smoking on size of visual fields. *Life Sci.* 4:2215–21.

73. Joint FAO/WHO *Ad Hoc* Expert Committee. 1973. *Energy and protein requirements.* World Health Org. Techn. Rep. Series No. 522, p. 20.

74. Kannel. W. B., *et al.* 1965. Vascular disease of the brain—epidemiologic aspects: the Framingham study. *Amer. J. Pub. Health* 55:1355-66.

75. Keys, A., *et al.* 1958. Lessons from serum cholesterol studies in Japan, Hawaii, and Los Angeles. *Ann. Int. Med.* 48:83-94.

76. ———. 1970. Coronary heart disease in seven countries. *Circ.* 41, Supp. 1.

77. Kibukamusoke, J. W. 1968. Gout in Africans. *E. Afr. Med. J.* 45:378-82.

78. Kidera, G. J., and Smith, J. W. 1968. Exercise aids in converting ECG to normal. *JAMA* 204:31.

79. Kiehm, T. G., *et al.* 1976. Beneficial effects of a high carbohydrate, high fiber diet on hyperglycemic diabetic men. *Amer. J. Clin. Nutr.* 29:895-99.

80. Klerk, W. A., and Du Bruyn, D. B. 1975. Chronic typhlitis in baboons fed a semisynthetic low-fibre diet. *S. Afr. Med. J.* 49:2233-34.

81. Kloppers, P. J. 1975. Intercultural aspects of venous thromboembolic disease. *S. Afr. Med. J.* 49:1430-31.

82. Kretzmer, M. 1978. Bedouin diet mystifies MDs. *Hadassah,* Feb., pp. 10ff.

83. Kungu, A. 1974. The pattern of thyroid disease in Kenya. *E. Afr. Med. J.* 49:449-67.

84. Kuo, P. T., and Joyner, C. R., Jr. 1955. Angina pectoris induced by fat ingestion in patients with coronary artery disease. *JAMA* 158:1008-13.

85. Leaf, A. 1971. Hard labor, low cholesterol linked to unusual longevity. *Med. Tribune,* June.

86. Linscheer, W. G. 1972. Malabsorption in cirrhosis, *Amer. J. Clin. Nutr.* 23:488-92.

87. Lund-Oleson, K. 1970. Oxygen tensions in synovial fluids. *Arthritis Rheum.* 13:769.

88. Lyons, T. P., *et al.* 1956. Lipoproteins and diet in coronary heart disease. *Calif. Med.* 84:325.

89. Malins, J. 1968. *Clinical diabetes mellitus,* p. 347. London: Eyre & Spottiswode.

90.    Manning, A. P., *et al.* 1976. Communication to
       British Society of Gastroenterology, Annual Meet-
       ing, October.

91.    Matheson, A. T., and Kossack, P. 1967. Osteitis
       deformans in the Bantu. *S. Afr. Med. J.*
       41:931–33.

92.    McGill, H. C., Jr., ed. 1968. The geographic pa-
       thology of atherosclerosis. *Lab. Invest.* 18:463.

93.    McKean, C. M. 1970. Growth of phenylketonuric
       children on chemically defined diets. *Lancet* I:148.

94.    Miyake, H. 1973. Oxygen for deafness. *Med.
       Tribune,* January 10.

95.    Mngola, E. N. 1968. Two cases of pernicious ane-
       mia among Africans. *E. Afr. Med. J.* 45:669–72.

96.    Morrison, L. M. 1952. Diet and atherosclerosis.
       *Ann. Int. Med.* 37:1172.

97.    ————. 1960. Diet in coronary atherosclerosis.
       *JAMA* 173:104.

98.    Moshal, M. G., *et al.* 1973. Malabsorption and its
       causes in Natal. *S. Afr. Med. J.* 47:1093–1103.

99.    Moss, O. J. 1961. Ballistocardiographic evaluation
       of the cardiovascular aging process. *Circ.* 36:434.

100.   Nevill, G., and Kungu, A. 1969. Goiter in Kenya.
       *E. Afr. Med. J.* 46:598–603.

101.   Novis, B. H., *et al.* 1975. Incidence of Crohn's dis-
       ease at Groote Schuur Hospital during 1970–1974.
       *S. Afr. Med. J.* 49:693–97.

102.   Page, I. H., *et al.* 1970. Prediction of coronary
       heart disease based on clinical suspicion, age, total
       cholesterol and triglyceride. *Circ.* 42:625–45.

103.   Painter, N. S. 1975. *Diverticular disease of the
       colon.* London: Heinemann.

104.   ————, and Burkitt, D. P. 1975. Diverticular dis-
       ease of the colon, a 20th century problem. *Clin.
       Gastroent.* 4:3–21.

105.   Parkinson, L., *et al.* 1960. Adrenocortical response
       of Bantus and Europeans to surgical stress. *Trans.
       Roy. Soc. Trop. Med. Hyg.* 54:366–72.

106.   Pepine, C. J. 1972. Coronary heart disease discov-
       ered in asymptomatic men. *JAMA* 221:241.

107.   Pomare, E. W., *et al.* 1976. The effect of wheat

bran upon bile salt metabolism and upon the lipid composition of bile in gallstone patients. *Amer. J. Diges. Dis.* 21:521–26.

108. Prior, I. A., *et al.* 1966. Hyperuricemia, gout, and diabetic abnormality in Polynesian people. *Lancet* I:333–38.

109. Rabinowitch, I. M. 1935. Effects of the high carbohydrate low calorie diet upon carbohydrate tolerance in diabetes mellitus. *Canad. Med. Assoc. J.* 33:136–44.

110. Rabinowitz, D., *et al.* 1966. Patterns of hormonal release after glucose, protein and glucose plus proten. *Lancet* II:454–57.

111. Rosenman, R. H., *et al.* 1967. Comparative predicted value of three serum lipid entries in a prospective study of IHD. *Circ.* 35, Supp. 2.

112. Saffer, D., *et al.* 1974. Acromegaly presenting with hemiplegia. *S. Afr. Med. J.* 48:684–86.

113. Segal, I., and Hunt, J. A. 1975. The irritable bowel syndrome in the urban South African Negro. *S. Afr. Med. J.* 49:1645.

114. Shaper, A. G. 1972. Cardiovascular disease in the tropics. IV. Coronary heart disease. *Brit. Med. J.* 2:32.

115. Shee, C. J., and Houston, W. 1963. Thyrotoxicosis in Southern Rhodesia. *Centr. Afr. J. Med.* 9:267–70.

116. Shulman, G., *et al.* 1975. Serum immunoglobulins G, A and M in white and black adults in the Witwatersrand. *S. Afr. Med. J.* 49:1160–64.

117. Singh, I. 1955. Low-fat diet and therapeutic doses of insulin in diabetes mellitus. *Lancet* I:422–25.

118. Sinnett, P. F. 1969. Primitive life keeps tribesmen's hearts strong. *JAMA* 210:1687–88.

119. Sobel, J. D., and Schamroth, L. 1970. Ulcerative colitis in the South African Bantu. *Gut* 11:760–63.

120. Solomon, L. 1968. Osteoporosis and fracture of the femoral neck in the South African Bantu. *J. Bone Joint Surg.* 50:2–13.

121. ———, *et al.* 1975. Rheumatic disorders in the South African Negro. I: Rheumatoid arthritis and

ankylosing spondylitis. *S. Afr. Med. J.* 49:1292–96.

122. ———, *et al.* 1975. Rheumatic disorders in the South African Negro. II: Osteoarthrosis. *S. Afr. Med. J.* 49:1737–40.

123. Spencer, S. S., and Nhonoli, A. M. 1972. Ulcerative colitis in East Africans. A report of three cases. *E. Afr. Med. J.* 49:163–69.

124. Stamler, J. 1969. Elevated cholesterol may increase lung cancer risk in smokers. *Heart Res. Letter* 14:2.

125. Stormoken, H. 1973–74. Epidemiological studies: relation between dietary fat and arterial and venous thrombosis. *Haemostasis* 2:1–12.

126. Sunzel, H., *et al.* 1964. The lipid content of human liver. *Metabolism* 13:1469–74.

127. Swank, R. L. 1961. *A biochemical basis of multiple sclerosis*. Springfield, Ill.: Charles C. Thomas Publishers.

128. Sweeney, J. S. 1927. Dietary factors that influence the dextrose tolerance test. *Arch. Int. Med.* 40:818–30.

129. Taube, E., and Buchanan, W. M. 1970. Two African cases with Addison's disease. *Centr. Afr. J. Med.* 16:101–4.

130. Taylor, J. R. 1968. The thyroid in Western Nigeria. I: Anatomy. *E. Afr. Med. J.* 45:383–89.

131. ———. 1968. The thyroid in Western Nigeria. II: Pathology. *Ibid.*, 45:390–98.

132. Thomson, W. H. 1975. The nature of hemorrhoids. *Brit. J. Surg.* 62:542.

133. Trowell, H. C. 1960. *Non-infective disease in Africa,* p. 465. London: Edward Arnold.

134. ———, *et al.* 1974. Aspects of the epidemiology of diverticular disease and ischemic heart disease. *Amer. J. Diges. Dis.* 19:864–73.

135. ———. 1975. Dietary fibre hypothesis of the etiology of diabetes mellitus. *Diabetes* 24:762–65.

136. ———. 1976. Definition of dietary fibre and hypotheses that it is a protective factor in certain diseases. *Amer. J. Clin. Nutr.* 29:417–21.

137. ———. 1976. Fibre inadequate replaced by cellulose or other forms of roughage in animal experimental diets. *Thromb. Haemost.*, Nov.

138. Van Eck, W. F. 1959. The effect of a low-fat diet on the serum lipids in diabetes and its significance in diabetic retinopathy. *Amer. J. Med.* 27:196.

139. Vracko, R. 1974. Basal lamina layering in diabetes mellitus. *Diabetes* 23:94–104.

140. Walker, A. R. P. 1972. The human requirement of calcium: should low intakes be supplemented? *Amer. J. Clin. Nutr.* 25:518–30.

141. ———. 1970. Glucose and fat tolerance in Bantu children. *Lancet* II:51.

142. Warburg, O. The prime cause and prevention of cancer. English ed. by Dean Burk. National Cancer Institute, Bethesda, Md.

143. Welch, C. C., *et al.* 1970. Cinecoronary arteriography in young men. *Circ.* 62:625.

144. West, K. M. 1973. Therapy of diabetes: an analysis of failure. *Ann. Int. Med.* 79:425–34.

145. Whyte, H. M. 1958. Body fat and blood pressure of natives in New Guinea. *Austr. Ann. Med.* 7:36–54.

146. Williams, A. V., *et al.* 1957. Increased cell agglutination following ingestion of fat, a factor contributing to cardiac ischemia, coronary insufficiency and anginal pain. *Angiology* 8:29.

147. Winitz, M., *et al.* 1970. Studies in metabolic nutrition employing chemically defined diets. *Amer. J. Clin. Nutr.* 23:525–45.

148. Wissler, R. W., *et al.* Aortic lesions and blood lipids in rhesus monkeys fed "table-prepared" human diets. *Circ.* 32: (Supp. II) 220, 1965.

149. Wolf, E. and Nadroski, A. S. 1971. Extent of the visual fields. *Arch. Ophthal.* 86:637–42.

150. Wong, R. A., and Outim, L. 1974. Thyrotoxicosis in Eastern Cape blacks. *S. Afr. Med. J.* 48:1993.

151. Woods, J. D., and Rymer, J. J. H. 1955. Pernicious anemia in the South African Bantu. *Lancet* II: 1274–75.

152. Zelman, S. 1973. Correlation of smoking history with hearing loss. *JAMA* 223:920.

153. Zoutendyk, A. 1970. Auto-antibodies in South African whites, colored, and Bantu. *S. Afr. Med. J.* 44:469–70.
154. Zuidema P. J. 1959. Ulcerative colitis in an Indonesian. *Trop. Geogr. Med.* 11:246–52.

# Glossary

**Achilles tendon** The large tendon attaching the two major calf muscles to the heel bone.

**Additive** Any chemical substance added to foods to improve nutritional quality or palatability, or to suppress deterioration. Additives may be vitamin or mineral supplements, flavoring agents, preservatives, emulsifiers, stabilizers, thickeners, acids, alkalies, or buffers.

**Adhesion** Tissues abnormally joined by a fibrous tissue, often formed during wound healing.

**Adrenal glucocorticoid** A hormone produced by the adrenal gland, which raises the concentration of liver glycogen and blood glucose. Cortisol and corticosterone are two such hormones.

**Adrenalin** A trade name for synthetic epinephrine, q.v.*, an adrenal hormone which stimulates the sympathetic nervous system.

**Aldomet** A trade name for an oral antihypertensive drug.

**Amino acid** Any one of a class of acids of which proteins are built. Of twenty-odd amino acids found in protein, eight are called essential and must be consumed in food, since they cannot be synthesized in the body.

**Amphetamine** A stimulant to the central nervous system, producing increased blood pressure, elation and euphoria, and reduced appetite. Its abuse may result in mental depression and sleeplessness.

**Anerobic bacteria** Microorganisms which grow in the absence of oxygen.

**Angina pectoris** A sudden onset of chest pain, sometimes accompanied by a feeling of suffocation and impending death.

**Angiogram** An X ray of blood vessels treated to show their shape.

**Animal fat** Fat obtained from tissues of animals.

**Antidepressant** A drug that prevents or alleviates depression.

* q.v. = see cross-reference

**Anxiety neurosis** A state in which apprehension or fear is out of proportion to any apparent cause.

**Apgar Score** A number evaluating a newborn infant's heart rate, respiratory effort, muscle tone, and other values.

**Arlidin** Trade name of a vasodilating drug which increases cardiac output.

**Arterial plaque** A plaque formed in the wall of an artery.

**Arthritis** Inflammation of the joints.

**Atherogenic** Producing atherosclerosis.

**Atheroma** A plaque or lesion which thickens the lining of an artery.

**Atherosclerosis** An extreme form of arteriosclerosis in which plaques, containing cholesterol crystals and fat particles, are formed in the linings of large- and medium-sized arteries.

**Atromid** Usually called Atromid-S, a trade name for a drug that reduces serum cholesterol and blood lipids.

**Behavioral modification** A method to make changes in a life-style, which may include food selection and physical activity.

**Beta-lipoprotein** A compound of lipid and protein, found in blood plasma, which carries more cholesterol than a related compound, alpha-lipoprotein.

**Biofeedback** A technique of using visual or auditory signals to enable one to perceive the status of one or more body functions, such as heartbeat, blood pressure, temperature, etc., so as to enable one to control these functions.

**Blind testing** A method of testing one drug or procedure against another, in which the monitor does not know the identity of the samples or the expected results. Usually, a presumably effective agent is tested against a placebo, q.v.

**Blocked coronary bypass** A closure in a graft which replaced a previously closed portion of a coronary artery.

**Blood cholesterol level** The amount of cholesterol, in blood plasma or serum, measured in mg./percent, or milligrams per 100 milliliters.

**Blood plasma** The fluid portion of blood in which blood cells and other components circulate. Serum is the fluid obtained after clotting has removed the cells and fibrinogen.

**Blood profile** The results of laboratory analysis of blood. It may include values for as many as thirty-three constituents.

**Bypass surgery** An operation to remove a section of a blood vessel and rejoin the two remaining parts by means of a transplanted vessel or synthetic material. Bypass surgery may also refer to removal of a portion of intestine and rejoining the remaining parts.

**Caffeine** A bitter stimulant to the central nervous system, found mainly in coffee, tea, and cola drinks.

**Caffeinism** A diseased condition due to ingestion of excessive amounts of caffeine.

**Calcified aorta** A hardened condition of the large artery leaving the heart, due to the deposit of calcium salts in the walls.

**Calorie** A measure of the energy released when a nutrient or food is oxidized or digested in the body.

**Capillary** A tiny blood vessel that connects the smallest arteries and veins. Their walls are semipermeable, allowing exchange of substances between the blood and tissue fluids.

**Carbohydrate** A chemical composed of carbon, plus hydrogen and oxygen in the same proportions as water. Starches, sugars, cellulose, and gums are carbohydrates.

**Carbon monoxide** A colorless poisonous gas, formed by burning fuels with a scanty supply of oxygen.

**Carboxyhemoglobin** A compound formed when carbon monoxide combines with hemoglobin in the blood, thus decreasing the amount of oxygen carried in the blood.

**Carcinogenicity** The capacity to cause cancer

**Cardiac ischemia** The lack of blood supply to the heart tissues.

**Cardiogram** A graphic record of heart movements.

**Cardiologist** A physician specializing in the diagnosis and treatment of heart conditions.

**Cardiovascular disease** A disease affecting the heart and/or blood vessels.

**Cardiovascularity** Relating to the circulatory system, i.e. the heart and blood vessels.

**Carotid artery** One of the large arteries on each side of the neck, which supply the external and internal tissues of the head and neck with blood.

**Cartilage** A tough, fibrous tissue found in the joints of adults, and in structures that keep passages rigid, such as in the nose, larynx, trachea, and ears. In the fetus, it is the model for the skeleton, later replaced by bone.

**Catapres** A trade name for an oral antihypertensive drug.

**Cerebral cortex** The outer gray-matter layer of the largest lobes of the brain, responsible for movement, visceral functions, perception, and highest mental functions.

**Cholesterol** A fatlike substance found in animal fats, bile, blood, brain tissue, milk, egg yolk, nerve fiber sheaths, liver, kidneys, and adrenal glands.

**Chromosomal** Pertaining to chromosomes, the structures in the nucleus of cells which carry and transmit genetic characteristics.

**Cocarcinogen** An agent that increases the effect of a cancer-causing substance.

**Collagen** A protein in skin, tendon, bone, cartilage, and connective tissue. It is converted into gelatin by boiling.

**Collateral circulation** One or more side branches of a blood vessel developed to go around a blockage in the vessel.

**Common duct** The common opening for the pancreas and gall bladder that exits into the duodenum.

**Complex carbohydrate(s)** A carbohydrate, q.v., whose molecules are composed of a large number of monosaccharides (sugars) joined together. Starches are complex carbohydrates. The term as used in the book is meant to describe unrefined grains, vegetables, and fruit.

**Congestive heart failure** Failure of the heart to pump enough blood.

**Coronary artery closure** Blockage of one of the vessels that supplies blood to the heart itself.

**Coronary artery disease** Any abnormality in the vessels that supply blood to the heart.

**Coronary bypass** Replacement of a diseased portion of a coronary artery by grafting a portion of a healthy vessel taken from another part of the body.

**Coronary heart failure** Failure of the heart to pump blood adequately due to obstructed coronary arteries; also called ischemic heart disease.

**Coronary insufficiency** Insufficient blood flow to the heart owing to blockage or narrowing of coronary arteries.

**Decaffeinated** Beverages from which most of the caffeine has been removed.

**Degenerative disease** Disease caused by breakdown of function due to dietary or other life-style abuse.

**Demerol** A narcotic sedative for relief of severe pain.

**Deoxycholic acid** A breakdown product of bile.

**Diabetes** A general term for disorders characterized by excessive urine secretion.

**Digital image processing** A computer-assisted method of determining degree of narrowing of arteries.

**Digoxin** A drug obtained from the leaves of *Digitalis lanata*, used for congestive heart failure.

**Diuretic** An agent that increases the secretion of urine.

**Diverticulosis** An abnormal pouch or sac formed in a weakened muscular wall of the intestine.

**Dyazide** Trade name for a diuretic and antihypertensive drug.

**Edema** Abnormally large amounts of fluid between the cells of a body tissue.

**EKG** Abbreviation for electrocardiogram.

**Electrocardiogram** A graphic tracing of the electric current produced by heartbeats.

**Electrolyte imbalance** Abnormal amounts of metallic salts relative to water in the body fluids.

**Elevated blood sugar** A higher than normal amount of sugar in the blood, due to inability to metabolize ingested carbohydrate.

**Emphysema** A pathological accumulation of air in tissues or organs. Pulmonary emphysema is enlargement of the air spaces at the end of the bronchial branches, causing breathing difficulty.

**Endocrine** Pertaining to ductless glands or their secretions which go directly into blood or lymph.

**Enzyme** A protein which initiates or speeds up a metabolic process, such as digestion, coagulation, etc.

**Epinephrine** An adrenal hormone which stimulates contraction of arteries, accelerates heart rate, increases blood pressure, heart output, and sugar release.

**Esidrix** Trade name for an antihypertensive drug.
**Esophageal** Pertaining to the esophagus, the tube that leads from the pharynx to the stomach.
**Estrogen** Female sex hormone.

**Fatty acid** One of a class of compounds which are the building blocks of fats (phospholipids and glycolipids).
**Femur** The thigh bone.
**Fetal gonad** The immature sex gland in an unborn infant.
**Fibrillate** To contract or twitch involuntarily, usually at a rapid rate.
**Flatulence** Air or gas in the stomach or intestine.
**Food fiber** The indigestible parts of plant cells.

**Gallstone** A solid mass, usually of cholesterol formed in the gall bladder or bile duct.
**Gastric acid** Hydrochloric acid secreted by the stomach for digestion.
**Gerontologist** A specialist in the study of the process of aging.
**GI tract** Gastrointestinal tract.
**Glucose** The simplest form of sugar
**Glucose tolerance test** A blood test which measures the efficiency of glucose absorption.
**Glycogen** The chief form of carbohydrate storage in animals. It is released as glucose when needed.
**Gout** A disease condition resulting from excess uric acid in the blood, usually manifesting as attacks of arthritis.

**HDL** Abbreviation for high-density lipoprotein, q.v.
**Heart attack** The death of a portion of the heart tissue due to blockage of a coronary vessel.
**Heel bone spur** A growth of bone on the lower surface of the heel bone, frequently causing pain when walking.
**Hemoglobin** The oxygen-carrying pigment of red blood cells.
**Hemorrhoid** A dilated vein in the anal or rectal region, caused by excessive venous pressure.
**Hiatus hernia** Protrusion of any structure through the esophageal hiatus of the diaphragm.
**High-density lipoprotein** A combination of a lipid and a protein with relatively more protein and less cholesterol

and triglycerides. A low-density lipoprotein has relatively more cholesterol and triglycerides and less protein.

**Hormone** A chemical substance secreted by a ductless gland, which regulates certain functions.

**Hyperglycemia** Abnormally increased sugar in the blood.

**Hypertension** Persistently high arterial blood pressure.

**Hypoglycemia** Abnormally low sugar in the blood.

**Inderal** Trade name for an antihypertensive drug, which also is used to lessen angina pain.

**Insulin** A protein hormone, produced in the pancreas, which regulates carbohydrate, lipid, and amino acid metabolism.

**Intermittent claudication** Pain in the legs when walking due to poor circulation.

**Intestinal bypass surgery** Called ileal bypass, the disconnection of a portion of the small intestine and rejoining of the remaining portions in order to decrease absorption of nutrients.

**Intestinal flora** Bacteria which live in the intestines.

**Intravenous** Within a vein or veins.

**Ischemia** Lack of blood in a tissue, due to blockage of a blood vessel.

**Isometrics** Muscle contraction without a change in length of the muscle, the force developed being dissipated as heat.

**Isordil** Trade name for a drug to reduce pain of angina pectoris.

**Isotonic exercise** Exercise involving muscles contraction, movement, and work.

**Ketoacidosis** Accumulation of acid and ketone bodies in body tissues and fluids. Sometimes occurs in diabetes.

**Ketone** Chemical containing a carbonyl group, CO. Acetone, acetoacetic acid, and beta-hydroxybutyric acid are ketone bodies, and are products of fat digestion.

**Ketosis** Abnormally high concentration of ketone bodies in tissues and fluids, occasionally producing loss of valuable minerals through kidney excretion.

**Kidney toxicity** Poisonous to the kidneys.

**K-Lyte** Trade name for a potassium supplement.

**Lasix** Trade name for a diuretic drug.

**Laxative** An agent that promotes evacuation of the bowel.

**LDL** Abbreviation for low-density lipoprotein, q.v.

**Lecithin** A group of phospholipids (fats containing phosphoric acid) present in nerves, liver, egg yolk, and other tissues.

**Linoleic acid** The most important of the three essential fatty acids. The other two, linolenic acid and arachidonic acid, can be made from linoleic acid.

**Lipids** Fats, a group of organic substances, insoluble in water, but soluble in ether, alcohol, or chloroform.

**Lipoprotein** A combination of a lipid (fat) and a protein.

**Low blood sugar** An abnormally low concentration of glucose in the blood.

**Low-density lipoprotein** A lipoprotein which contains relatively more cholesterol and triglycerides and less protein.

**Lowfat** Usually refers to diet or foods having a low concentration of fats with no butter, fats, or oils added.

**Lymphocyte** One type of white blood cell.


**Master Two Step** Master "2-step" exercise test; an electrocardiographic test, the tracings made while the patient exercises on two steps, each nine inches high.

**Menopause** Cessation of menstruation in the human female.

**Metabolism** The sum of all physical and chemical life processes involved in nutrition.

**Metabolize** To utilize or process a substance for the maintenance of life function.

**Mineral Balance** A state of the body in which the mineral intake equals the mineral excretion.

**Molecular cross-linkage** The joining together of simple molecular structures to form long chains or more complex structures.

**Mutagenic** Causing genetic change.

**Myocardial infarction** Death of a portion of the myocardium (the main muscular tissue of the heart), due to blockage of the blood supply to the area.

**Myocardium** The middle and thickest layer of the heart wall.

**Neuropathy** Any disease of the nervous system.

**Nicotinic acid** Another name for niacin, a member of the vitamin B complex.

**Nitrobid paste** Trade name for 2 percent nitroglycerin ointment, used in treatment of angina pectoris.

**Nitrogen balance** A condition in which net protein intake is equal to protein utilization.

**Nitroglycerin** A chemical used in treatment of pain of angina pectoris.

**Nonfat** Usually refers to milk or food products in which all fat has been removed.


**Obesity** Excessive body weight due to accumulation of fat.

**Osteoporosis** Abnormal loss of bone or skeletal atrophy.


**Pancreas** A gland behind the stomach and between the spleen and small intestine. It secretes a number of digestive juices, as well as the hormone insulin which controls carbohydrate metabolism.

**Pathology** A branch of medical science concerned with the essential nature of disease, the structural and functional changes in the body which cause, or are caused by, disease.

**Peptic ulcer** A lesion of the lining of the stomach or duodenum (small intestine) caused by the acid gastric juice.

**Percodan** Trade name for a pain-relieving drug containing a narcotic.

**Peroxidation** An oxidation reaction in the presence of a peroxide.

**pH** A symbol relating hydrogen ion activity to a standard, used to indicate acidity (pH 1–6) or alkalinity (pH 8–14). pH 7.0 is neutral.

**Placebo** An inactive substance, resembling a drug in appearance, given in controlled studies to determine the comparative effectiveness of medicinal substances, or given to satisfy a patient's psychological need for a drug.

**Placenta** An organ during pregnancy joining mother and fetus, providing exchange of certain soluble substances through their respective circulatory systems.

**Plaque** A flat patch or area. In blood vessels, plaques are formed from deposits of cholesterol, fats, and calcium.

**Platelet** A small disk-shaped structure in blood which is active in blood coagulation.

**Polysaccharide** A carbohydrate made up of complex sugars.

**Polyunsaturate** A fat or oil having unfilled carbon bonds and tending to be liquid at room temperature.

**Posterior wall myocardium** The middle muscular layer of the back side of the heart.

**Precancerous** Pertaining to a pathological process that tends to become malignant.

**Preservative** A substance added to a product to destroy or inhibit the growth of microorganisms.

**Preventricular contraction** Premature beat of the heart's ventricle, often resulting from oxygen deficiency.

**Progesterone** A hormone whose function is to prepare the uterus for the reception of the fertilized ovum.

**Prostate** A gland in the male, located around the neck of the bladder and urethra. Its secretions go into the seminal fluid.

**Protein** A large group of compounds, containing nitrogen, which are the main constituents of animal cells, but are also found in plant cells. Proteins are large compounds made up of various combinations of amino-acid linkages.

**Protein metabolite** A product of protein digestion.

**Pulse rate** Rhythmic expansion of an artery which reflects the beat of the heart.

**Red blood cell** Blood cell containing hemoglobin for transport of oxygen. Also called erythrocyte.

**Refined carbohydrates** Carbohydrates, usually cereal grains, from which the coarse parts, such as bran and germ, have been removed. Sugar is a refined carbohydrate.

**Roughage** Indigestible fibers of foods.

**Runner's knee** A condition among runners associated with excessive irritation of the kneecap at the joining of the thigh bone. The malady is thought by some doctors to be due to faulty weight-bearing function of the foot.

**Safrole** The principle ingredient of sassafras oil.

**Saturated fatty acid** A fatty acid in which all available carbon bonds of the hydrocarbon chain are filled with hydrogen.

**Serum cholesterol** Amount of cholesterol measured in blood serum (the liquid that separates from blood on clotting), usually expressed in mg./percent (milligrams per 100 milliliters serum).

**Serum triglyceride level** Amount of triglycerides measured in blood serum, usually expressed in mg./percent.

**Shin splints** Strain of lower leg muscle, accompanied by pain along the shin bone.

**Simple carbohydrate** A class of carbohydrates composed of sugars.

**Sludging** Sticking together of blood cells.

**Steroid** A group of compounds which includes progesterone, some hormones, bile acids, and sterols (such as cholesterol).

**Sterol** A steroid, such as cholesterol or ergosterol.

**Stress** Reaction to adverse external influences, including trauma and infection.

**Stress treadmill test** An electrocardiographic record of a patient's performance on a treadmill, operated at increasing velocity and slope, to elucidate the patient's heart function under stress.

**Stroke** Brain impairment due to hemorrhage in the brain or lesion in a blood vessel supplying the brain.

**Tachycardia** Excessively rapid heart beat, above 100 per minute.

**Tannin** Tannic acid, found in ordinary tea, which may cause liver damage.

**Teratogenic** Tending to produce malformed embryos.

**Theobromine** An alkaloid with properties similar to caffeine, found in cocoa.

**Theophylline** An aklaloid found in tea.

**Thyroid function** The regulation of metabolism by the secretions of the thyroid gland.

**Toxic** Poisonous.

**Toxin** A poisonous substance.

**Tranquilizer** An agent which quiets or calms the emotional state of a patient without changing clarity of consciousness.

**Triglyceride.** A compound containing three fatty acids. It is formed from carbohydrates and is stored in fat cells. When broken down, it releases free fatty acids into the blood.

**Triple coronary bypass** Surgical bypass of three coronary arteries (see Bypass surgery).

**Unsaturated fatty acid** Fatty acids in which the available carbon bonds of the hydrocarbon chain are not all filled.

**Urea** A compound containing nitrogen, found in urine, blood, and lymph. It is a product of protein metabolism.

**Urethra** The tube from the bladder to the exterior of the body for discharge of urine.

**Uric acid** A product of protein metabolism, insoluble in water, but soluble in alkaline solutions. Excessive amounts in the blood are associated with gout.

**Valium** Trade name for a tranquilizer.

**Varicose veins** Abnormally distended veins.

**Vasodilator** An agent that causes dilation of the blood vessels.

**Ventricular fibrillation** Rapid, repetitive involuntary contraction of the myocardial fibers without coordinated contraction of the ventricle.

**Vitamin** A group of unrelated organic compounds, occurring in foods, that are necessary for normal metabolic functions of the body.

**Xanthine** A compound found in most body tissues and fluids, a stimulant, especially to heart muscle.

**Zyloprim** Trade name for a drug used in treatment of gout and uric acid stone formation.

# Recipe
# Index

# Recipe Index

## Index for Maximum Weight Loss Recipes

## Index for the Gourmet Cook

## Index for the Family Cook

## Index for the Single Cook

## Index for Breads and Snacks

# General Index

# General Index

## ABOUT THE AUTHORS

NATHAN PRITIKIN is the founder and director of the Longevity Center and the Pritikin Research Foundation. During the last twenty years he has done research in worldwide literature in the fields of nutrition, exercise and degenerative diseases, followed by clinical studies that corroborated the concepts he had developed. Mr. Pritikin, who has more than two dozen patents (U.S. and foreign) in chemistry, physics and electronics, is an Honorary Fellow of the International Academy of Preventive Medicine and coauthor of the bestselling *Live Longer Now*. Mr. Pritikin and his wife, Ilene, who helps direct diet research and is in charge of food preparation demonstrations and lectures at the Longevity Center, live in Santa Barbara, California.

PATRICK M. MCGRADY, JR. is a writer specializing in medical and scientific subjects. He was Moscow bureau chief for *Newsweek* and is past president of the American Society of Journalists and Authors and a member of the board of directors of the American Aging Association. Mr. McGrady is the author of *The Youth Doctors* and *The Love Doctors*.

# Bantam Book Catalog

Here's your up-to-the-minute listing of over 1,400 titles by your favorite authors.

This illustrated, large format catalog gives a description of each title. For your convenience, it is divided into categories in fiction and non-fiction—gothics, science fiction, westerns, mysteries, cookbooks, mysticism and occult, biographies, history, family living, health, psychology, art.

So don't delay—take advantage of this special opportunity to increase your reading pleasure.

Just send us your name and address and 50¢ (to help defray postage and handling costs).